ADVANCED PRAISE FOR MEDICINAL PLANTS OF THE SOUTHERN APPALACHIANS

This is a priceless guide that makes Southern plant alchemy accessible to everyone. Howell's book is healing and exhilarating because it contains vital knowledge we all need as we face significant earth changes and political unrest. Though the sheer beauty of this book will captivate you, it overflows with wisdom that may one day save your life.

— Janisse Ray, author of *Ecology of a Cracker Childhood*

Nearly 20 years ago, Patricia Kyritsi Howell published Medicinal Plants of the Southern Appalachians, an essential resource for herbalists and foragers. Blending scientific and folk knowledge, it has been celebrated for its comprehensive coverage of native medicinal plants. Howell's new edition includes vibrant color photographs and updated information, making it an invaluable reference for those interested in Southern Appalachian medicinal plants.

— T. J. Smith, editor of *The Foxfire Book of Appalachian Cookery* and *Foxfire Story: Oral Tradition in Southern Appalachia*

I often refer to my copy of the first edition of this book, as its dog-eared corners and sticky yellow notes clearly show. Therefore, I was excited to learn that a second edition is on the way. If you live in the Southern Appalachians, use herbs from the region, or want to learn how to identify, find, harvest, and utilize native botanicals, this accessible guide is for you. Patricia is a highly experienced and respected herbalist who shares her extensive knowledge in this easy-to-read, full-color second edition, tailored to meet your specific needs and interests.

— Jeanine Davis, PhD, author of *Growing and Marketing Ginseng, Goldenseal, and Other Woodland Medicinals*

Patricia Kyritsi Howell's book is a vital guide to the medicinal plants of the Southern forests and fields. In this revised and updated second edition with stunning photographs, she highlights herbs like American Ginseng and Black Cohosh and lesser-known plants like Turtlehead and Rabbit Tobacco, sharing their traditional uses, preparation methods, and sustainable harvesting practices.

— David Winston, RH(AHG), primary author of *Adaptogens, Herbs for Strength, Stamina and Stress Relief*

Drawing on decades of clinical experience, Patricia Kyritsi Howell has crafted an indispensable resource for beginner and advanced herbalists, native plant enthusiasts and historians. This book features a stunning layout and captivating photos in a clear, concise, and accessible style. It also provides practical guidance on medicinal uses, preparation methods, harvesting techniques, identification tips, and easy-to-follow recipes for 44 native plants.

— Christa Sinadinos, author of *The Essential Guide to Western Botanical Medicine* and Director, Northwest School for Botanical Studies

This pharmacopeia of relatively common medicinal plants in the Southern Appalachians answers everything you ever wondered about them. Combining the legacies of Cherokee healers with herbals from Europe and Asia, Howell details the historical and current importance of 44 species. Each account is beautifully photographed and rich in ethnobotanical content from many cultures. After reading *Medicinal Plants of the Southern Appalachians*, I'm reminded why the stories of leaves, roots and seeds reveal some of the most consequential results of natural biochemical selection.

— Paul Manos, PhD, Professor of Biology, Duke University

Patricia has accomplished something truly remarkable with this book. She has crafted a beautiful text that speaks to all plant lovers. Clinicians, wildcrafters, botanists, and wildflower enthusiasts will repeatedly be drawn back to this gem. The book's true value lies in the decades of stories, experiences, and deep connections with plants that Patricia has cultivated over her lifetime. With its visually stunning presentation, this book will become a timeless, cherished reference.

— Kat Maier, RH(AHG), author of *Energetic Herbalism: A Guide to Sacred Plant Traditions Integrating Elements of Vitalism, Ayurveda, and Chinese Medicine*

In a world where thousands of plants are used as medicine, this book's value lies in its focused scope and deep regional expertise. Patricia has chosen to write deeply about what she knows best: the rich medicinal flora of the Southern Appalachians. This dedication to place and personal experience creates an increasingly rare authenticity in herbal literature.

The intimate understanding of each plant's habitat, growth patterns, and medicinal applications reflects years of careful observation and practical experience: a documentation of a living relationship with the land and its healing plants. The second edition offers refined insights, updated information and stunning photography while maintaining the accessible, experience-based approach that made the first edition valuable.

This book is an indispensable resource for anyone interested in the medicinal plants of the Southern Appalachians, whether as a beginner or an experienced herbalist. It's the kind of work that grows with you — revealing new layers of insight with each reading and season of practical application.

— Thomas Easley, Eclectic School of Herbal Medicine

Nothing replaces the knowledge gained from a lifetime among the plants of Southern Appalachia, except perhaps the joy of quickly accessing this treasure in Patricia's book. This revised edition provides practical and inspiring information for students, academics, and anyone wanting to learn about the plants around them. It's a book everyone who enjoys learning about herbal medicine should have!

— Bevin Clare, Professor and Program Director MS in Clinical Herbal Medicine, Maryland University of Integrative Health

Medicinal Plants of the Southern Appalachians is already a beloved classic, but this new edition brings the plants to life with vibrant, full-color photographs that leap off the pages. Patricia skillfully integrates her skills as a clinical herbalist into the rich fabric of our cherished Appalachian traditions with her deep understanding of the region's native flora. As I peruse these pages, I feel a deep connection to the winding medicinal plant trail, a part of our Appalachian heritage!

— Mimi Prunella Hernandez, author of *National Geographic Herbal*

Second Edition

MEDICINAL PLANTS
OF THE
Southern Appalachians

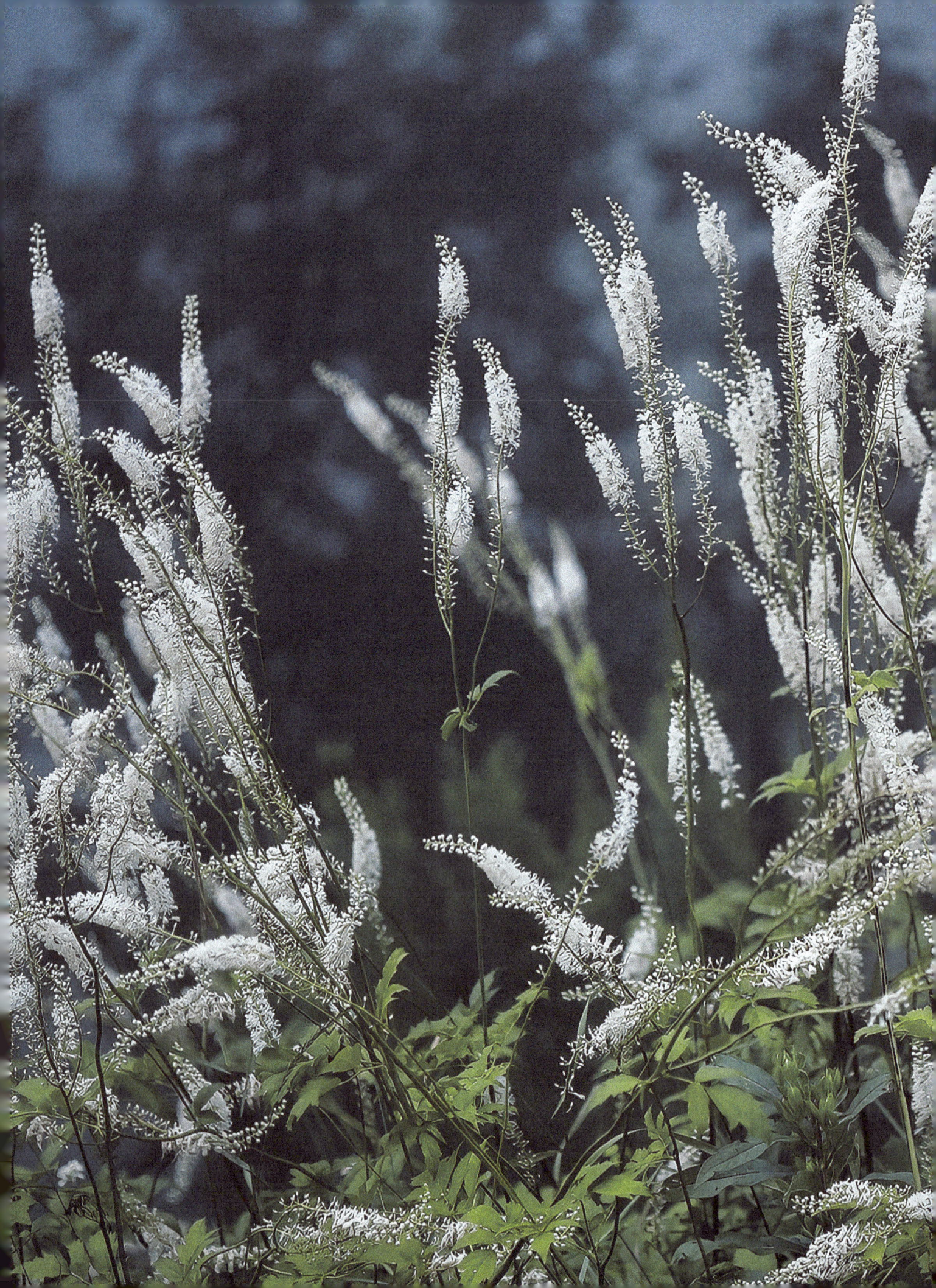

Second Edition

MEDICINAL PLANTS
OF THE
Southern Appalachians

Patricia Kyritsi Howell

BotanoLogos Books
Tiger, Georgia

Note to the Reader

The information provided in this book is not a substitute for professional medical advice or treatment. It is intended to help you make informed choices. The remedies, approaches, and techniques described here are meant to supplement, not replace, professional care. They should not be used to treat serious medical conditions without prior consultation with a qualified healthcare professional. Such consultation is not just recommended; it is essential for your health and safety.

Dosage information is provided as a general guideline. The opinions expressed in this resource do not guarantee specific results. While care has been taken to ensure the accuracy of the information and to describe generally accepted practices, the author and publisher are not responsible for any errors or omissions or any consequences arising from the application of this information. They make no warranties, expressed or implied, regarding the contents of this publication.

Copyright First Edition 2006
Copyright Second Edition 2025

ISBN 979-8-218-59875-4
LCCN 2025902575

All rights reserved. No portion of this book, except for a brief review, may be reproduced, stored in a retrieval system, or transmitted by any form or by any means, electronic or mechanical, including photocopying, recording, or by any information storage or retrieval system without written permission of the publisher.

For permission, contact the publisher at:
BotanoLogos Books
info@wildhealingherbs.com

Cover and Book Design by Barbara Lande
Cover Photo by Steven Foster
Edited by Leslie Williams

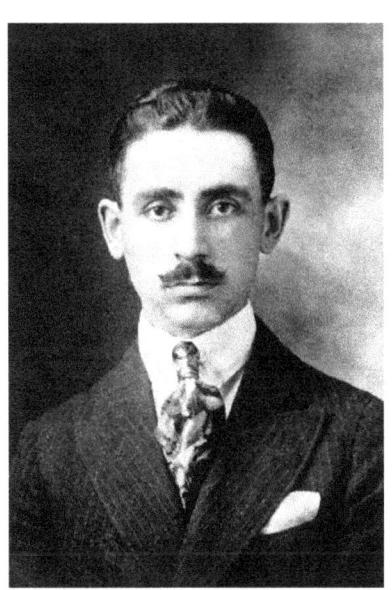

In memory of my grandfather,
Ioannis E. Kyritsis,
whose love for learning continues to inspire me.

"There is no doubt that much of what we know of medicine comes from very ancient times, and from the birds and animals we have watched. Myself, I do not know enough to say how or why one certain weed will calm a fever…All I can do is wonder, and everything that I have remembered and recorded here has made me do that.

—*A Cordiall Water: A Garland of Odd and Old Receipts to Assuage the Ills of Man and Beast* by M. F. K. Fisher

Preface to Second Edition

I am delighted to introduce the second edition of *Medicinal Plants of the Southern Appalachians!* First published in 2006, this updated version has been expanded to include more valuable information and features over 200 breathtaking color photos that vividly depict 44 native plants.

Unlike conventional field guides that only feature plants in full bloom, this book is uniquely designed for herbalists, foragers, and native plant enthusiasts. It caters to the need to identify medicinal plants at every stage of their life cycle, from gnarled roots to tender spring shoots, autumn-kissed leaves, and fruit-laden branches. This seasonal approach provides an intimate introduction to herbs used in traditional healing for thousands of years.

As a clinical herbalist with over 30 years of experience, I've shared what I've learned about these herbs in the field, in the classroom, and working with clients. You'll find practical guidance on their safe and effective use peppered with insights from my years of using them to address everyday health issues. Plus, instructions for making herbal remedies, dosage recommendations, and cautions, all designed to equip you with the knowledge you need.

For those interested in foraging, I've provided sustainable harvesting tips and bloom and harvest calendars to guide you through the seasons.

While this book focuses on plants native to the Southern Appalachians, nearly all of them grow in wild places throughout North America, making it an indispensable resource for everyone.

Whether you're an herbalist, forager, gardener, or simply a plant lover, this book is for you. I hope it inspires you and gives you the confidence to appreciate and use these remarkable remedies.

—*Patricia Kyritsi Howell*

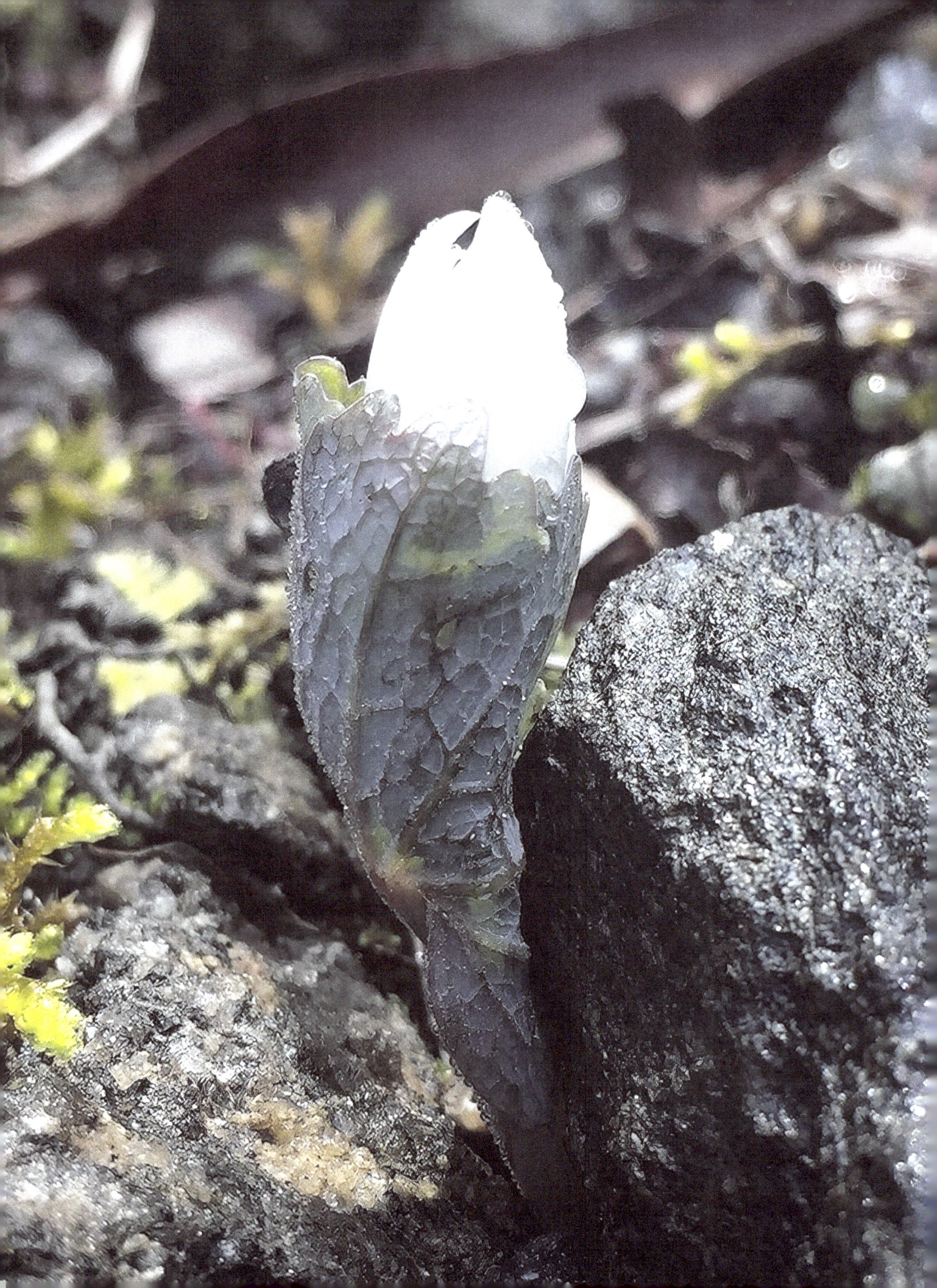

Table of Contents

1	INTRODUCTION
7	HOW TO USE THIS BOOK
15	THE SIMPLE ART OF MEDICINE MAKING
29	THE MEDICINAL PLANTS
31	Bee Balm – *Monarda spp.*
35	Black Cohosh – *Actaea racemosa*
39	Black Haw – *Viburnum prunifolium*
43	Black Walnut – *Juglans nigra*
47	Bloodroot – *Sanguinaria canadensis*
51	Blue Cohosh – *Caulophyllum thalictroides*
55	Boneset – *Eupatorium perfoliatum*
61	Devil's Walking Stick – *Aralia spinosa*
65	Elder – *Sambucus canadensis*
71	Evening Primrose – *Oenothera biennis*
75	Fringetree – *Chionanthus virginica*
79	Gentian – *Gentiana spp.*
83	Ginseng, American – *Panax quinquefolius*
89	Goldenrod – *Solidago spp.*
93	Jewelweed – *Impatiens capensis*
97	Joe Pye Weed – *Eutrochium spp.*

101	Lobelia – *Lobelia inflata*
107	Mountain Mint – *Pycnanthemum incanum*
111	Partridgeberry – *Mitchella repens*
115	Passionflower – *Passiflora incarnata*
119	Pipsissewa – *Chimaphila maculatum*
123	Pleurisy Root – *Asclepias tuberosa*
127	Poke Root – *Phytolacca americana*
133	Rabbit Tobacco – *Gnaphalium obtusifolium*
137	Ragweed – *Ambrosia artemisiifolia*
141	Red Root – *Ceanothus americanus*
145	Sarsaparilla – *Aralia nudicaulis*
149	Sassafras – *Sassafras albidum*
155	Skullcap – *Scutellaria spp.*
159	Solomon's Seal – *Polygonatum biflorum*
163	Spicebush – *Lindera benzoin*
167	Stoneroot – *Collinsonia canadensis*
171	Sumac – *Rhus spp.*
175	Sweetfern – *Comptonia peregrina*
179	Sweetgum – *Liquidambar styraciflua*
185	Turtlehead – *Chelone spp.*
189	Wild Cherry – *Prunus serotina*
195	Wild Geranium – *Geranium maculatum*
199	Wild Ginger – *Asarum arifolium/Hexastylis spp.*

203	Wild Hydrangea – *Hydrangea arborescens*
207	Wild Yam – *Dioscorea spp.*
211	Witch Hazel – *Hamamelis virginiana*
215	Wood Betony – *Pedicularis canadensis*
219	Yellowroot – *Xanthorhiza simplicissima*
223	GLOSSARY AND INDEXES
224	BLOOM CALENDAR
226	HARVEST CALENDAR
229	GLOSSARY
237	THERAPEUTIC INDEX
243	BIBLIOGRAPHY
247	INDEX
265	ACKNOWLEDGMENTS
267	PHOTO CREDITS
269	ABOUT THE AUTHOR

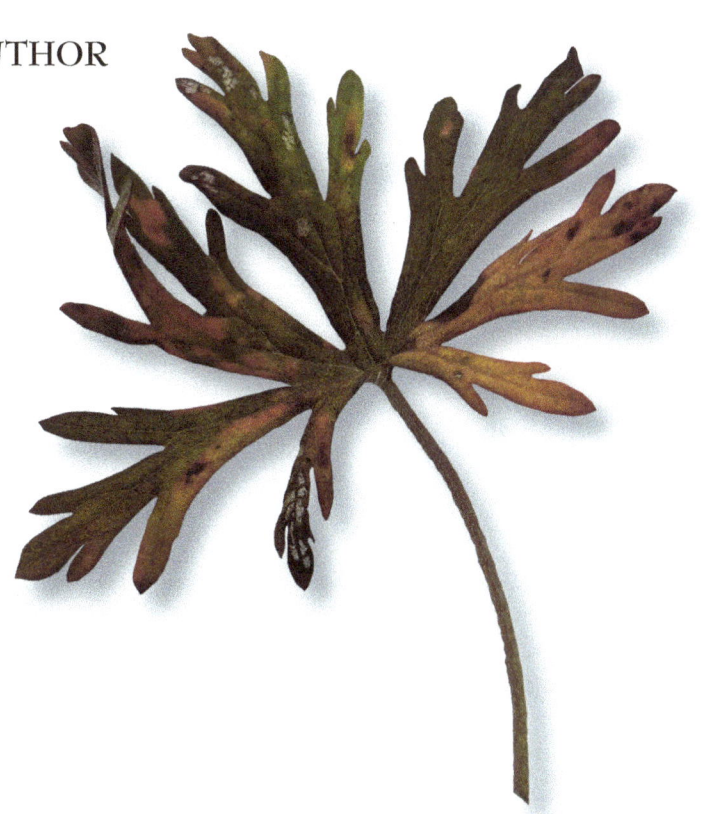

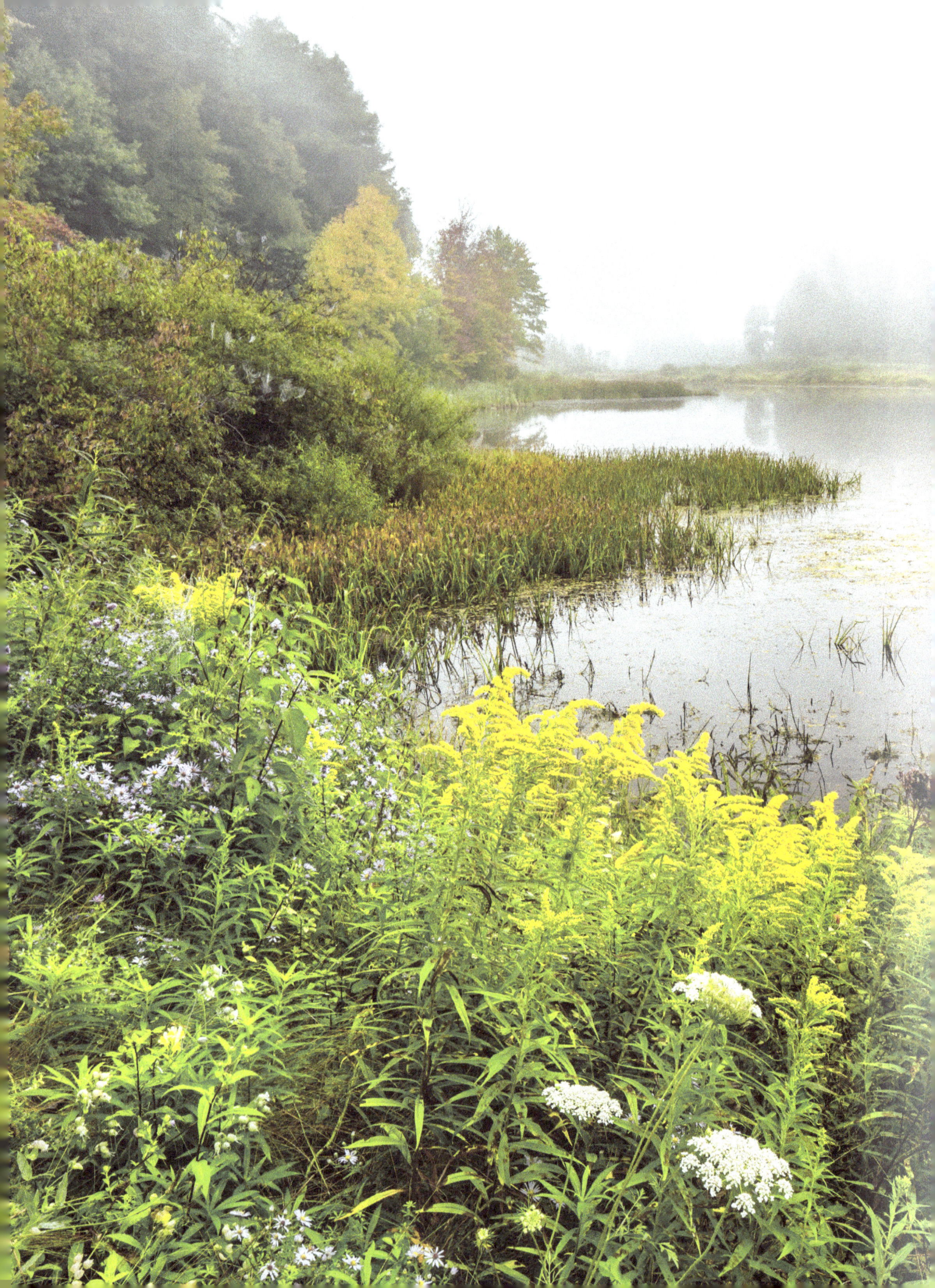

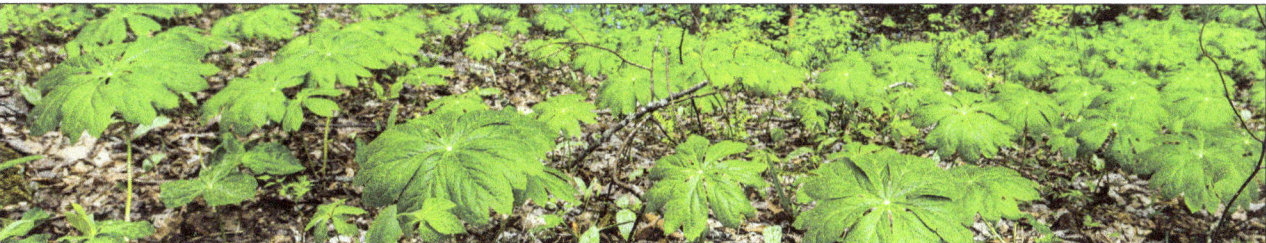

Introduction

I grew up on the tall grass prairies of northern Illinois and was well into my thirties the first time I experienced a deciduous cove forest in the southern Appalachian Mountains. I remember the exact moment I realized I was walking along a path lined with many medicinal plants I often used in clinical practice. The hillside above me was crowded with black and blue cohosh, partridgeberry, Solomon's seal, and maidenhair fern. Plants that had just been names in books or dried green things in jars were suddenly gloriously alive. I felt I was among friends.

A few years later, I moved to the southern Appalachians. The seasonal rhythm of the wild herbs growing around my forest home are now markers of the passing seasons. When my sister calls to tell me she is coming south for a visit, I think: When the lady's slipper blooms, she will be here; when the first goldenrod blooms in late summer, I know I must start preparations for winter. This seasonal cadence is ancient.

The Appalachians are some of the oldest mountains on Earth, having formed from 1.2 billion to 250 million years ago by geological uplift from shifting tectonic plates. Since then, this ancient formation has eroded from its former stature into undulating ridges interspersed with many deeply forested coves. The cove forest ecosystem is a unique sanctuary, blessed with rich soils and abundant rain. It shelters one of the world's most botanically diverse temperate rainforests and many species of plants and animals found nowhere else.

Botanists refer to the southern part of the Appalachian region as Southern Appalachia. This area of the Southeast ecoregion spans ten states, starting in the New River Valley in southwestern Virginia and extending through parts of West Virginia, Kentucky, North Carolina, South Carolina, Georgia, Tennessee, and northeast Alabama. These iconic highlands traverse the lower Piedmont, Blue Ridge, Ridge and Valley, and Appalachian Plateau, incorporating sections of the Allegheny Plateau and Mountains, then progressing into the Shenandoah Valley, the Cumberland Plateau and Mountains, and most of the Piedmont Uplands as well as the entire southern range of the Blue Ridge Mountains. The Southern Blue Ridge comprises multiple sub-ranges, including the famous Great Smoky Mountains.

More than 3,000 trees, shrubs, and herbaceous plants thrive here. Of these, 100 genera are endemic. Sassafras, blue cohosh, ginseng, witch hazel, and many other genera native to the eastern deciduous woodlands are species that grow here and in two other places: the Ozark mountains of Arkansas and east Asia. This phenomenon, known as floristic disjunction, is the only remaining evidence of a vast ancient forest that covered the Northern Hemisphere millions of years ago. The unique mountain geography of the Ozarks, eastern Asia and the southern Appalachians appears to have harbored plants in relative isolation, allowing them to survive millennia of environmental changes, evolve into unique species and, over geologic time, spread out into the surrounding lands.

This book focuses on medicinal plants native to the southern Appalachians, although their range extends throughout North America, as far north as Nova Scotia, west to the Pacific Ocean, and throughout the Southeast. These mountains are also home to a diverse population of endemic plants, such as yellow root, which are rarely found in other regions.

Plants with Deep Roots

The historical use of southern Appalachian medicinal plants is rooted in the sophisticated healing practices of the Cherokee people who lived here until many were forcibly removed from their ancestral homes along with the Creek, Chickasaw, Choctaw, and Seminole people. Cherokee knowledge of the region's flora is legendary. Historical accounts of their plant use indicate most Cherokee knew how to recognize and use several hundred medicinal and edible plants, and tribal healers may have been skilled in using many more. Enslaved Africans who survived the Middle Passage across the Atlantic brought their healing traditions and religious practices with them. And out of necessity, they learned to use local herbs to survive the horrors of slavery. Much of today's knowledge about healing with native and naturalized plants owes an outstanding debt to the practical wisdom of Native American and African American traditions, wisdom that still informs our understanding of herbalism today.

European colonists integrated native plants into their healing traditions and exploited the botanical wealth of the eastern woodlands. European botanists, including William Bartram, Andre Michaux, and others, traveled through the southern Appalachians, documenting plants they saw and collecting seeds, roots and cuttings for export to European botanists, doctors and gardeners.

The bark and roots of the sassafras tree *(Sassafras albidum)* were among the first North American exports to Europe. As early as 1603, British merchants from Bristol organized expeditions to collect the roots. They were brewed into a tea called saloop, a beverage considered a panacea capable of restoring health and vitality that was popular in European cafes.

For the next 400 years, Europeans plundered North American forests, harvesting and exporting vast amounts of Appalachian medicinal plants. The roots of ginseng, goldenseal, bloodroot, lady's slipper, and other native plants were exported by the ton to Europe. The roots of most of these plants are quite small, making it almost impossible to imagine how many were destroyed.

Overharvesting of woodland herbs continues today. In 2001, an estimated 420,000 pounds of wild black cohosh root were harvested from the forests of western North Carolina. Those numbers continue to increase with the growing demand for herbs. As a result, many woodland herbs, once abundant, are now classified as endangered or threatened.

Healing Practices in the Southern Appalachians

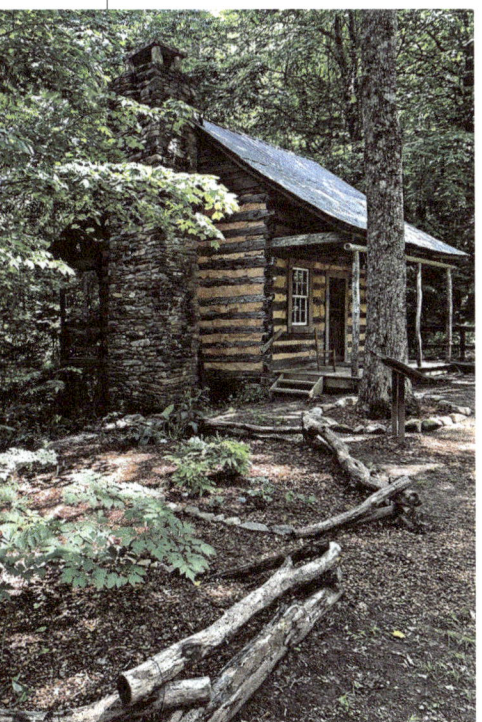

Until recently, the mountain terrain and rough roads made travel difficult in the southern Appalachians. Native plant medicines were essential for health care as isolated communities had little access to other forms of health care. The Southern folk medicine tradition relied on native plants and cultivated garden herbs used in European folk medicine, such as peppermint, horehound, and comfrey. The books written about Tommie Bass give us a detailed picture of the many plants he used from both sources.

Anthony Cavender's study of folk medicine in southern Appalachia found that many people living in rural communities relied on herbal folk remedies as recently as the years following World War II. He notes that many folk healers throughout the region had thriving practices using herbal remedies. Stories recorded in the famous Foxfire books also document the importance of herbal medicines in north Georgia and western North Carolina.

My 94-year-old neighbor, Maude, and her family have lived in northeast Georgia for seven generations. Maude still lives in the house where she was born, keeps chickens, and grows and cans most of her family's food. When she has a cold, Maude brews a strong pot of boneset tea *(Eupatorium perforatum)* and tells me the bitter tea, mixed with a liberal amount of honey from her husband's bees, has never let her down. Her grown children still ask her to brew it for them when they are sick. Maude doesn't remember the names of all the plants she used to collect with her mother and grandmother, but she says that they worked better than anything she'd been given by a doctor. However, Maude also reports that no one in her family is interested in learning about the plants, and she feels certain that the little she remembers will die with her. Within her lifetime, herbal remedies have become a quaint reminder of times gone by, like churning butter or dipping candles by hand.

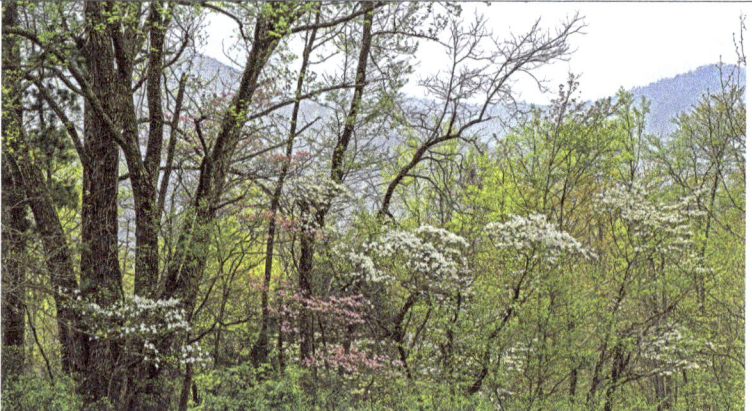

The Illusion of Abundance

Herbalism and the herbal products industry depend on a continuous supply of wild and cultivated herbs. This is nothing new; medicinal herbs and spices have been traded throughout human history. As early as 2,000 BCE, the Minoan people on the Greek island of Crete exported vast amounts of wild sage, thyme and others to all parts of the Mediterranean.

European botanists battled through rhododendrons and dog hobble thickets three hundred years ago to "discover" new plants and ship them across the sea. Today, we can purchase herbs from anywhere with a click of a button. Sophisticated marketing has convinced consumers that rare, expensive plants from exotic places are more effective than the plants growing all around them. As a result, the latest trending herbs from other parts of the world are being overharvested in ways that destroy their native habitats to meet consumer demand.

Our sacred obligation as herbalists is to reject the idea that we need the latest new miracle herb from far away and instead focus on the native and naturalized plants growing in abundance all around us.

As I learned more about these serious issues, I questioned my herb choices. This led me to wonder what I would do if I could only use the plants around me. How different would my herbal apothecary be if I resisted the convenience of herb shops and the vast array of online shopping options?

With these questions in mind, I became a dedicated student of the medicinal plants that thrive in the southern Appalachians, leading me to write this book. The plants I've included are those I used in my thirty years of clinical practice and introduced to thousands of students. As I learned about them, I discussed their uses with my colleagues, collected anecdotes from numerous local sources, and, most importantly, became a patient daily observer of the plants around me.

The plants that intrigue me most are those with roots deep in the folk medicine culture of southern Appalachia and those that are an essential part of the local ecosystem. Of course, that also included studying and using many medicinal plants introduced from other parts of the world—such as dandelion, plantain, chickweed, and mullein. They are now so prevalent in the landscape that it is hard to believe that they, like me, are relative newcomers to these mountains.

Does it really matter whether a plant is native or naturalized? To an herbalist, both include essential remedies. And because herb books that describe the many naturalized plants from Western or European herbalism are easy to find, this book's unique contribution to herbalism is that it celebrates plants native to the southern Appalachians.

Reclaiming an Old Path

In recent years, the Centers for Disease Control have cautioned doctors and other medical professionals against the overuse of antibiotics as this practice leads to virulent, untreatable bacterial infections. While antibiotics have saved many lives and definitely have a place in modern healthcare, the overuse of pharmaceuticals is rampant in conventional medicine. I don't need to point out the reality that iatrogenic causes, that is, the result of mistakes made by licensed doctors, cause a significant number of deaths each year. The Food and Drug Administration recalls widely used pharmaceutical drugs yearly due to dangerous or life-threatening side effects. Polypharmacy, the regular use of five or more medications, is now standard practice, especially for older patients. This is uncharted territory rife with side effects and other dangerous outcomes. Drug companies now market prescription drugs directly to consumers to create more demand. If you watch any commercial television, you have been subjected to a glut of drug commercials flooding the airwaves.

The questionable marketing practices and rampant overuse of drugs make it appear that legitimate medical care is limited to drugs and surgery. As a result, we've lost touch with the powerful simplicity of herbal remedies.

While at first glance, this book may appear to be a guide to using the native medicinal plants of the southern Appalachians, that is only one of the reasons I wrote it. Ultimately, it is a practical, no-nonsense book designed to cure amnesia and restore your innate ability to use plants for healing. I challenge you to expand your capacity for intuitive, instinctive ways of knowing as you learn about herbs until they become a part of your everyday life. My hope is that this book will restore and nourish your relationship with plants and their magic.

When possible, I invite you to consider reducing your reliance on pharmaceutical drugs—and other health-destroying practices—and rely on teas, salves, tinctures, and other simple home remedies to heal yourself, your family and your community.

The path that leads to an understanding and appreciation of medicinal plants is old, and many have traveled it before you. But it is still easy to find your way if you slow down enough to appreciate the healing powers of plants growing around you.

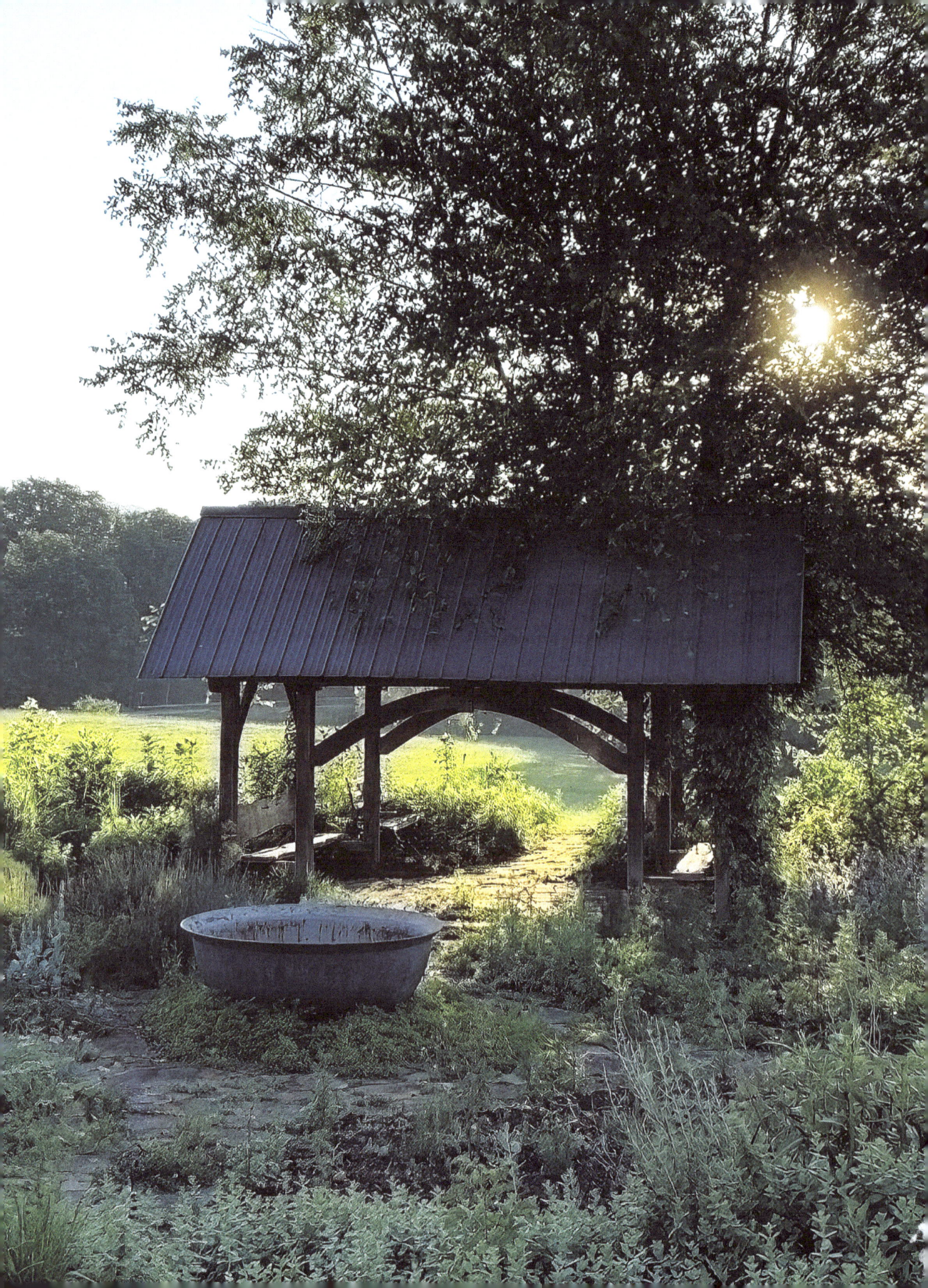

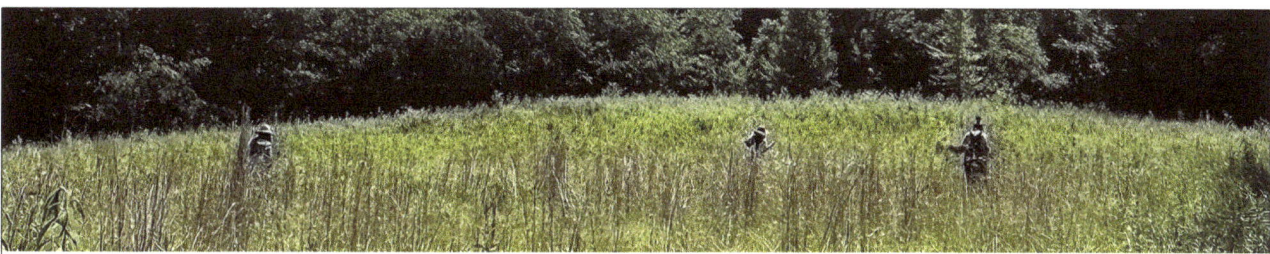

How To Use This Book

This book explains how to use 44 medicinal plants native to the southern Appalachians. Anyone who has spent time in the area may be familiar with some of them, including many of the region's most famous wildflowers. I have deliberately omitted several plants considered threatened or endangered, such as goldenseal *(Sanguinaria canadensis)*, false unicorn root *(Chamaelirium luteum)* and lady's slipper *(Cypripedium spp.)*; these fragile native plants must be allowed to regenerate themselves in peace.

Information about each plant is presented in monograph form for easy reference and includes the common name, botanical or scientific name and description, plant family, medicinal actions, energetics and the part of the plant used. You'll also find information about each plant's traditional and current uses, instructions for making medicinal preparations, sustainable harvesting tips, therapeutic guidelines and any cautions or contraindications for their use.

The information about harvesting is intended for you if you collect them for personal use. If you use native plants for commercial purposes, please don't rely on wild plants, instead find reputable sources of cultivated and sustainably harvested herbs. To learn more about the sustainability issues related to medicinal herb sourcing, I invite you to explore the work being done by United Plant Savers and the American Botanical Council's Sustainable Herbs Program.

Plant Names

The plants in this book are organized by the common names most frequently used in the southern Appalachians. Though common names are often colorful and descriptive, they are unreliable for accurately identifying specific plants. To positively identify and use plants you must know the scientific name (genus and species).

Often, only one genus and species of a plant is used medicinally. In other cases, several or all species of a particular genus may be used, as in the case of the genus *Solidago* or, as you probably know it, goldenrod. With 90 species of *Solidago* in North America and about 60 species in the southeast, the good news is that all have similar properties, with a long history of medicinal use, and they provide an important source of nourishment for pollinators. When referring to goldenrod, it is common to see its scientific name written as *spp.;* the abbreviation *spp.* indicates that more than one species is being referenced.

Related Species lists other medicinal plants in the same genera (the word used to indicate more than one genus) that are used similarly. Some related species are also native to the Southern Appalachians; others are naturalized or introduced; some are not found in the wild, though they may be cultivated in gardens.

Even if scientific names are new to you, I hope you will take the time to note the genus and species given for each plant (in italics) to be sure that you are collecting or buying the correct plant. To learn more about scientific names, plant families, etc., an excellent introduction can be found in *Botany in a Day* by Thomas Elpel. (See the Bibliography.)

Botanical Descriptions

Scientific methods for learning plant identification ask us to override our intuitive awareness of nature's sensual dimensions in favor of an objective approach that describes plants in precise botanical terms. This compartmentalizing is neither easy nor pleasurable for most of us, but this skill is needed to positively identify plants.

In contrast, hanging out with wild plants can be a feast for the senses, resulting in a different kind of knowing. Henry David Thoreau, a great observer of the natural world, described the value of allowing nature to soften his sensual awareness like this:

> *I must walk more with free senses…I must let my senses wander as my thoughts, my eyes see without looking…the more you look the less you will observe…Be not preoccupied with looking. Go not to the object; let it come to you…What I need is not to look at all, but a true sauntering of the eye.*

Actively enlisting all your senses as you learn to recognize plants reconnects you with an ancient, time-honored way of knowing. When you engage your senses, you experience texture, color, taste, and aroma, creating a visceral experience of the plant that expands your ability to know it. When you allow your senses to lead the way, you begin to see the natural patterns around you.

After you have identified a plant using botanical descriptions or a botanical key in a field guide, enlist your senses. Close your eyes and lightly touch the surface of a leaf or dig your fingers into the damp earth to touch the shape of the root or pick a leaf from a plant (one you have identified as safe, of course) and taste or smell it. I like to stretch out flat on my back on the ground beside plants to see the world from their point of view. Or get up close and personal by observing it from just inches away and try a jeweler's loop or magnifying glass for a butterfly perspective.

My botanical descriptions are designed to nudge you towards both ways of knowing plants; they include botanical and sensual descriptions. I invite you to refer to the Glossary for definitions of botanical terms as needed.

Photos of each plant are included to help with identification. The wise herbalist also consults regional field guides, asks someone familiar with local plants, or uses a reliable app to help with identification. If you take a photo of a plant, be sure it is easy to see the type of flower (if there is one), number of flower parts, leaf arrangement and shape, and habitat; this will make it easier for someone to help you ID it later.

Key Actions

European herbal traditions, also called Western herbalism, are rooted in classic Greek texts on botanical medicine that classified plants according to their actions. Actions are code words that describe a plant's physiological effect and help you understand its medicinal properties. Knowing how to match the right herbal action to a specific symptom and combining herbs with various actions may take years to master. But as you become more familiar with the herbal actions of each plant, it gets easier. Actions included here are listed in descending order of importance, with primary actions first. Keep in mind that some herbs have more than one primary action. Refer to the Glossary for definitions. To learn about herbal actions and how to apply them, refer to one of the general herb primers in the Bibliography.

Energetics

A more sensual way to understand how herbs work is by noticing their energetic qualities. Energetic terms categorize herbs based on their sensations, flavors, and how they manage or enhance fluids. The most used energetic terms describe the temperature they generate in the body, hot, warm, neutral, cool, or cold, and whether they restore or astringe moisture and fluids. The quality of flavor is also a consideration. When you taste an herb, receptors on the tongue are stimulated, generating a physiological response in parts of the body. For example, when you taste a bitter herb, like turtlehead *(Chelone glabra),* your body responds with increased secretions in your digestive system to better absorb nutrients. The bitter flavor also stimulates immune function and helps regulate blood sugar. And this happens whether you swallow the herb or not!

The terms used to describe the taste of herbs include bitter, sweet, salty, acrid, and pungent, each eliciting a unique physiological response. The tricky thing is that while many herbal traditions have codified their descriptions of herbal energetics based on generations of practical experience, there may be differences of opinion about many herbs, especially those used in the indigenous and folk traditions of the southern

Appalachians. I've provided energetic qualities based on common practice and my clinical experience; you are welcome to take this as a jumping-off point for your own experience of the individual plants.

Part Used

Different parts of the same plant may have very different actions. For example, a leaf may be used to soothe skin irritation, while the root of that same plant may induce vomiting, as is the case with elder *(Sambucus canadensis)*.

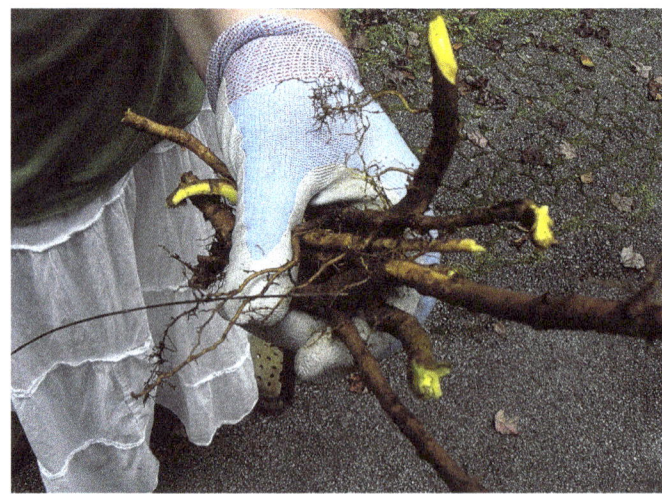

One or more parts of each plant are categorized as the official part used in herbal practice. How this is determined is based on tradition and research about plant constituents. Most commercial herb products contain the official parts, though folk tradition may have relied on entirely different parts of the plant. In these monographs, I've included the official part and details about other plant parts that may have been used in regional folk traditions.

But the most important point is this: you need to know exactly which part of the plant provides the action you need before harvesting or buying herbs. Plant parts generally used are the root and/or rhizome, leaf, flower, leaf with flower, flowering tops, bark, and seeds or fruits.

Traditional and Current Uses

A plant's historical use often reveals how it was used in the past when people were using herbs to treat the health challenges they were facing. For example, a hundred years ago, when immediate access to health care was uncommon, especially in rural areas, knowing how to use herbs to manage the symptoms of common conditions like influenza and colds was essential for everyday home health care. Many acute conditions can now be addressed with a visit to an urgent care center, emergency room or 24-hour drug store. The focus in herbalism today has shifted to emphasize tonic herbs to address issues caused by the long-term effects of stress and exposure to environmental toxins. In short, the herbs we rely on change as our world changes.

Historical uses described here are drawn from ethnobotanical and anecdotal accounts of how indigenous and enslaved peoples used regional plants and from clinical records documented by Europeans as they incorporated them into medical practice. While skewed by prejudice and cultural bias, we can still discern familiar patterns that help us understand the essential nature of these herbs.

The contemporary use of Appalachian herbs is indebted to the late A. L. Tommie Bass, Alabama herbalist, who used over 300 herbs in his practice. His knowledge was extensively documented in several excellent books; see the Bibliography.

As we study the historical uses and expand our understanding of plant medicines in response to current health challenges, we contribute to the dynamic, ever-evolving art of herbal healing. The traditional and current plant uses are offered here as a starting point to hopefully point you in the right direction as you embark on your own herbal adventures.

Harvesting

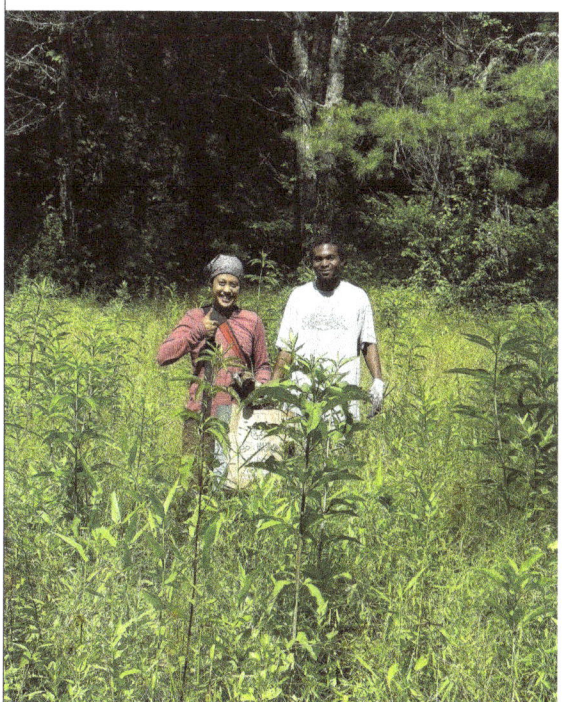

To harvest medicinal plants, whether they are in your garden or the wild, takes some planning and observation to determine when and how to harvest them. And if you are gathering wild plants, you first need to know their conservation status. Wild herbs are endangered and protected in many places due to centuries of overharvesting and extreme habitat loss. Fortunately, we have resources to help us embrace sustainable practices. United Plant Savers, a non-profit based in Ohio, monitors wild medicinal plant populations and shares critical guidelines about the status of medicinal plants.

Plants are generally harvested when the part used is most potent. The ideal plant harvest time varies depending on its growth habits and the parts used. Our ancestors based their harvesting practices on observation and sometimes moon cycles. Science has now verified that these traditional practices accurately identified the ebb and flow of chemical compounds during various stages of growth. For example, an emerging leaf in early spring contains more active compounds than it does later in the growing season after the plant has flowered and gone to seed. Careful observation is always needed to track a plant's growth cycle through the seasons, which takes patience to learn. Generally, plants harvested at the right time and carefully processed produce strong medicines, while plants harvested before or after their peak potency may result in weak or ineffective medicines

The charts on pages 224 and 226 provide an easy-to-use reference for each plant's bloom and harvest times.

However, the best time to harvest herbs may vary from year to year according to regional weather and as we continue to see the impact of climate change on our environment. Examples of harvesting instructions include "dig the entire root after the first frost" or "collect the leaves before the flowers appear." Other traditional ways to determine when to harvest include the moon's phases and other astrological, astronomical, and environmental signs. You may need to devote a season or two to observing a plant before you get in sync with the rhythms of its growth cycle.

If you are new to identifying plants in the wild, I strongly suggest you find an experienced herbalist or native plant enthusiast to assist you. Basic botany books and field guides with identification keys are helpful, but it is best to learn the subtleties of plant identification from someone who knows them well. Please see the basic botany and field guide suggestions in the Bibliography.

Detailed instructions are given about when and how to harvest each plant for peak medicinal potency. Before collecting any plants, be certain you know exactly what part of the plant is medicinal. This book contains information about how to harvest each plant sustainably. Even when harvesting roots, replanting a section of the root or rhizome or a ripe seed is sometimes possible so that the plant regenerates itself.

When preparing for a harvesting expedition, you'll need tools like knives, clippers, and shovels, but don't forget that you'll also need a way to keep plants in a cool place, protected from heat and sunlight until you can process them. I store my harvested plants in individual baskets or paper bags; avoid using plastic bags to store fresh plants as they will wilt and lose much of their potency. As you harvest each plant, place it in a labeled bag or basket; wilted plants look remarkably similar. As you harvest, garble or sort your plants, discard yellowed or dead leaves and shake or wipe off any dirt—especially important when gathering roots. The wise herbalist always wears gloves when harvesting, as contact with fresh plants can cause skin irritation and other unpleasant symptoms.

Sustainable Harvesting

For hundreds of years, large quantities of medicinal plants have been removed from fields and forests of the southern Appalachians for sale on the commercial market. Today's plant populations in the region are a mere shadow of the abundance that once existed. Threats to their survival have only increased over the last 30 years due to renewed interest in herbal medicine and the large-scale manufacture of herbal products.

The destruction of fragile mountain ecosystems has also contributed to the decline of many wild plant populations.

Because many of the plants included here are only found in the wild—they will not grow outside their native habitat or are not widely cultivated—it is critical that you only harvest from places you have carefully observed for a long period of time. In fact, Tim Blakely, one of my first herb teachers, advised us to observe wild plants in a particular place for at least one year before harvesting them. Tim taught us that we shouldn't harvest plants we have just "discovered" until we observe whether a plant is part of an established, abundant community of plants or one that has just managed to establish itself.

Guidelines for Harvesting Wild Plants:

Before harvesting wild plants, verify their conservation status by checking their botanical names against lists published by various state and federal agencies or local conservation groups, like United Plant Savers.

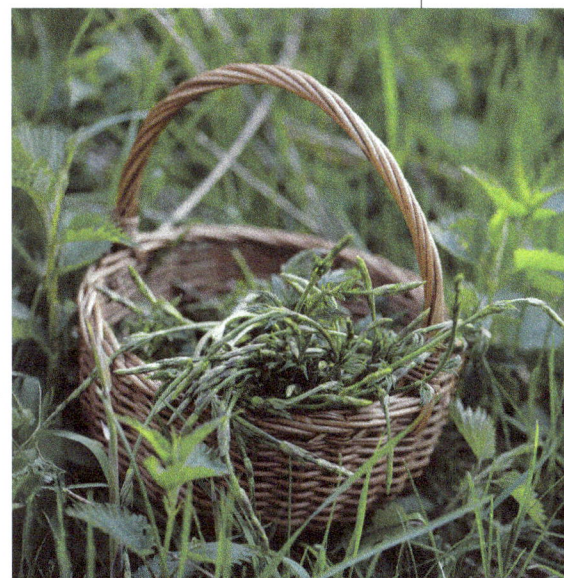

Avoid harvesting along roadways, railway lines, beneath electrical lines, or other areas regularly sprayed with or exposed to toxic chemicals.

It is illegal to collect plants from National Forests, state parks, recreation areas, wildlife management areas, nature preserves, etc. These lands are held in the public trust, and removing plants is strictly prohibited and punishable by fines. However, you can obtain permits to collect specific medicinal plants from National Forests in some areas. Inquire at your local U.S. Forest Service office for details.

If there is a native plant society or wildflower group in your area, they may be a reliable source of native plant information. In addition, botanical gardens often sponsor symposia and lectures about regional and native plants. Many gardens feature well-labeled collections of native plants. Local conservation groups sometimes sponsor plant rescues to remove native plants from land scheduled for development. Plant rescues can be heartbreaking, but relocating native plants can safeguard their survival and add to your garden.

Do not harvest on private property without permission from the landowner. You could be prosecuted for theft or trespassing. Introducing yourself and explaining what you want to gather and why is better. Although they probably think you are crazy to be interested in their weeds, reassure them that you will collect them without damaging their property, and most will let you help yourself. I've even had people offer to pay me to remove them!

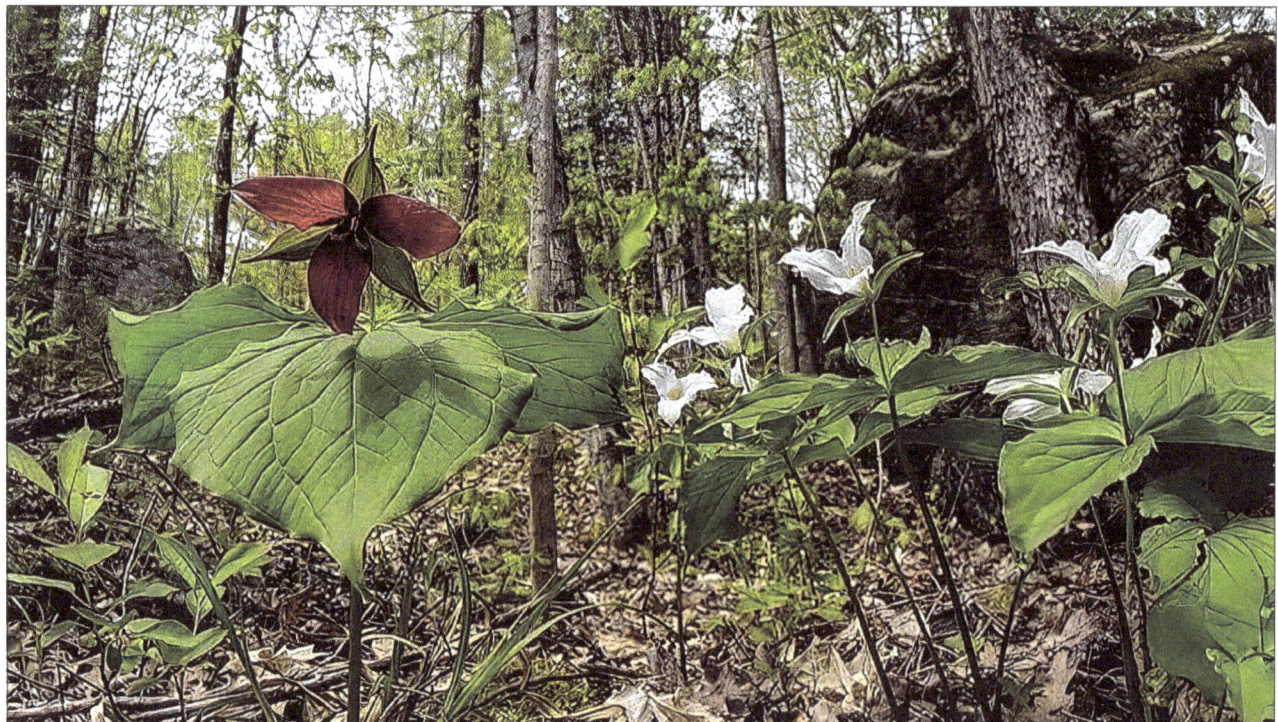

Herbal Preparations

It is so satisfying to make your herbal medicines! It is true 'homeland security' to know you can care for yourself and your family and friends with your cupboard full of dried herbs for teas, bottles of honey-rich cough syrup, potent tinctures, and skin salves. For each plant included here, I've included information about making herbal preparations based on historical and current use. Medicine-making at home requires a small investment in tools and supplies and yields a handsome return, not to mention saving you lots of money! See The Simple Art of Medicine Making for detailed instructions.

Herbal Basics and Dosages

This book's information assumes that you have a basic understanding of herbalism. If you are new to working with herbal medicine, before using any of the plants described here, I invite you to peruse one of the basic herbals in the Bibliography to learn more.

For suggestions about using herbs in this book for specific health conditions, please see the Therapeutic Index.

The dosages given throughout are approximations based on my clinical experience and information I've gathered from other practitioners and herbal reference books. Use these recommendations as a starting point for creating herbal therapies. The herbal information in this book is not intended to replace healthcare from a skilled healthcare practitioner.

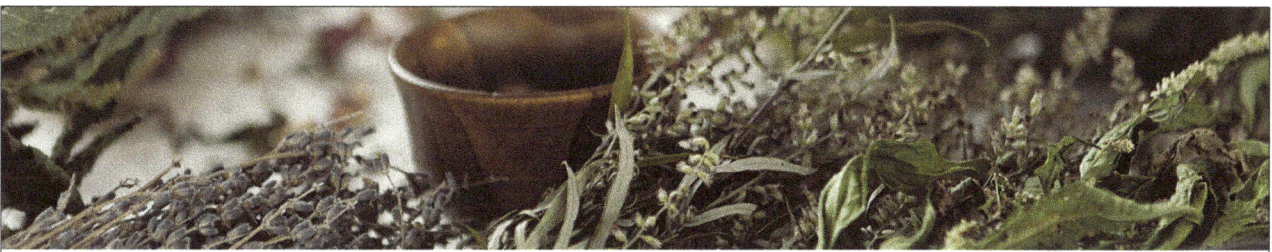

The Simple Art of Medicine Making

Making herbal preparations for home use is no more complicated than cooking a meal. All you need are the right tools, quality ingredients, a clearly written, easy-to-follow recipe, and the willingness to learn from mistakes! The information given here will help you get started.

There are many ways to transform herbs into medicinal preparations; this section provides instructions for making some of the most common ones. Start with one or two preparations, and as you learn about more plants and their uses, keep creating more medicines to build your apothecary. I've included a few excellent books with more detailed herbal medicine-making methods in the Bibliography. And I want to give you my biggest tip for successful medicine-making: Label everything. Few things are more frustrating than an unlabeled jar or bottle you must discard because you can't remember what is in it. But for now, please roll up your sleeves and give herbal medicine-making a try. Making your own remedies is incredibly satisfying!

Water-Based Medicines (Infusions and Decoctions)

Herbal teas are one of the most common ways to use herbs. What we refer to as tea is further divided into infusions and decoctions, the two methods used to extract herbal properties into water. An infusion is an herbal tea prepared by steeping fresh or dry herbs in hot or cold water for a specific period. A tea is a decoction if fresh or dry herbs are prepared by boiling or simmering them. The infusion method is best when working with delicate or aromatic parts of plants, such as flowers and leaves. Fibrous parts like roots, seeds, and barks are best when decocted. When plant parts of both types are used to make a tea, each may be prepared separately and combined using the appropriate method.

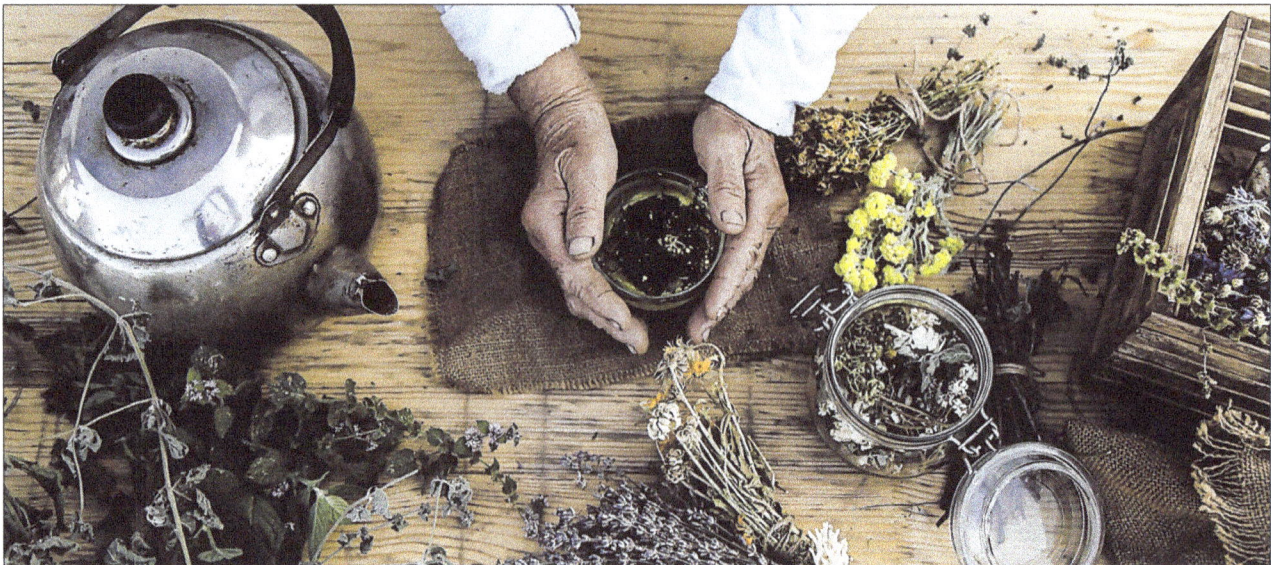

Drink infusions or decoctions at room temperature, warmed slightly or as recommended for each herb.

Remember that the weight-to-volume measurements used in the examples given are general guidelines. Use the specific recommendations I've provided for each herb for the best results.

Infusions and decoctions may be the starting point for various preparations such as gargling for throat and mouth, cleaning wounds, soothing itchy skin, as a vaginal douche or enema and as the first step in preparing syrup.

The amount of herb used to make an infusion or decoction for a therapeutic tea is much greater than what is used to make a beverage tea; as a result, these therapeutic teas have a stronger, more distinctive flavor and are potent remedies. If you find the flavors too strong, feel free to sweeten them with a small amount of honey or dilute them with water or fruit juice. Avoid the use of refined sugar or artificial sweeteners.

The weight-to-volume method is best for preparing infusions or decoctions. The herbs are weighed using a kitchen scale; the water is measured with a measuring cup. The weight of the herbs determines how much water is needed. You can use either fresh or dry herbs to make infusions and decoctions.

Once you have weighed your herbs, use the formula outlined below to determine the volume of water you need. The amount of water needed depends on whether the herbs are fresh or dry. You need a larger quantity of fresh herbs, as they contain water. When using dry herbs, the quantity of herbs needed is less, as they contain no water.

When making infusions, decoctions, and some other herbal preparations, the ratio of herb to water is described in parts. The total weight of your herbs is a part, and the total volume of water is also calculated in parts.

When making an infusion or decoction with fresh herbs, combine 2 parts herbs to 16 parts water; with dry herbs, combine 1 part herb to 16 parts water. This is easier to understand by example.

You have some fresh black cohosh root that weighs two ounces. This is considered one part. You need to combine it with 16 times as much water by volume. So, if making an infusion or decoction with two ounces of fresh black cohosh root, you will need 32 ounces of water. The mathematical equation is 2 parts fresh herb (two ounces by weight) x 16 = 32 ounces of water (by volume). This is written as 1:8.

When using dry herbs, the ratio of herb to water changes. You have some dry black cohosh root that weighs one ounce. This is considered one part. You need to combine it with 16 times as much water by volume. So, you will need 16 ounces of water for one ounce of dry black cohosh root. The mathematical equation is 1 part dry herb (one ounce by weight) x 16 = 16 ounces of water by volume. This is written as 1:16.

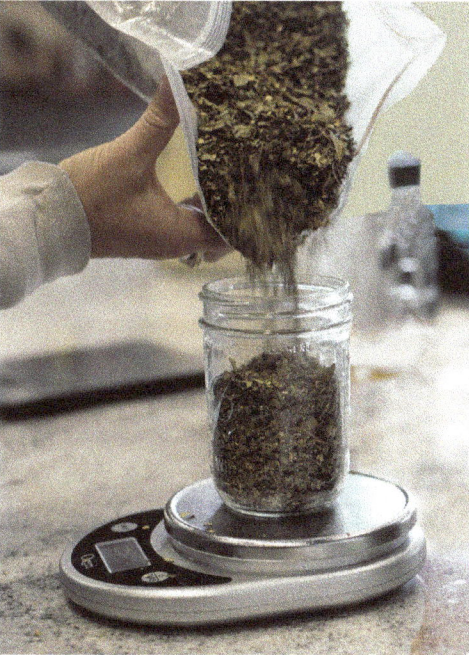

Remember, a part can be any amount of herb or water, but the ratio of herb to water remains constant: 1 part dry herb to 16 parts water or 2 parts fresh herb to 16 parts of water.

To be honest, working with Imperial weights (ounces and pounds) is a challenge. As you continue to make herbal preparations, you will find it easier to use the Metric system as it allows much more accurate measurements. Refer to any of the medicine-making books in the Bibliography for guidance on working with the Metric system. But if you are learning to make herbal medicines for the first time, go ahead and start using the methods for measurements described here.

Water-based preparations have a short shelf life and should be prepared daily if possible. In hot weather, store them in the refrigerator. You can also freeze them for future use or if you make more than you need.

Making an Infusion

Chop fresh or grind dry herbs. Weigh the herbs and place them in a container (a teapot or one-quart canning jar). Add the correct volume of water needed to make a therapeutic infusion. Cover and steep for the time indicated for each herb (see herbal monographs). When ready, strain out the spent herb and discard. Store infusions in the refrigerator and use within 24 hours. Infusions may be made using hot, boiling water (a standard infusion) or cold water. Cold water infusions should be steeped for one or more hours.

Making a Decoction

Chop fresh or grind dry herbs. Weigh them and place them in a saucepan with a tight-fitting lid. Do not use aluminum pans or any with non-stick coatings. Add the volume of cold water needed to make a therapeutic decoction. Bring to a boil and immediately reduce to a simmer; cover and decoct for 20 minutes or as indicated for each herb. Cool the decoction; strain out the spent herb and discard. Store decoctions in the refrigerator and use within 24 hours.

Always use cold water to make decoctions. Immersing herbs in hot water causes the cell walls to contract, resulting in a weaker preparation.

Tinctures (Alcohol Extracts)

Tinctures are easy to make! Learning this simple technique will save you lots of money. To make a tincture, you only need your herbs and a solvent, or menstruum, to extract the active compounds from the herbs. Here's an overview of the steps needed to make a tincture.

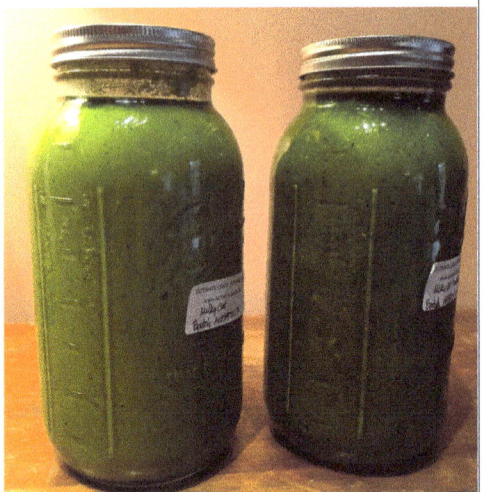

Chop fresh or grind dry herbs. Weigh the herbs to determine the ratio of alcohol and water needed for the menstruum. Combine the herbs and the menstruum in a glass container; a canning jar works well here. The mixture needs to steep or macerate for at least two weeks. Then, the spent herbs, known as the marc, are strained out of the menstruum and discarded. The menstruum has extracted the active compounds from the herbs, resulting in an alcohol tincture. Tinctures should be stored in a cool, dark place in a glass container. Tinctures remain potent for eight to ten years or more when properly stored.

About Menstruums

A menstruum is usually made with a combination of alcohol and water. Other liquids like vegetable glycerin and apple cider vinegar are also used to make alcohol-free tinctures but result in a weaker preparation with a shorter shelf life. See the Bibliography for medicine-making resources. The ratio of alcohol to water used varies according to the chemical compounds contained in the individual plants. For example, to make a tincture from herbs with a high resin content, such as sweet gum, the menstruum is almost all alcohol with very little water. Conversely, skullcap, an herb traditionally prepared as an infusion, is almost completely soluble in water, so the amount of alcohol needed is very low. But to make a tincture shelf-stable, a menstruum must contain a minimum of 25 percent alcohol. For health and economic reasons, when making tinctures, always use as little alcohol as possible.

There is no agreed-upon standard for the ratio of alcohol and water used to make a menstruum. An analysis of each plant's chemical constituents reveals how many of them are soluble in either water or alcohol. Using chemical analysis, commercial tincture manufacturers develop custom menstruums for each herb. Determining the perfect menstruum ratio for each herb is like asking if there is one way to make soup; recipes will vary according to the ingredients used and the cook's preferences. What matters is that the final product — the soup — is delicious and nourishing or the tincture is an effective medicine. In this book, the menstruum recommendations for each herb monograph are based on my experience and information from other experienced herbal medicine makers and should be considered a jumping-off point for you to use in developing your own preferences.

A simple method to start with is using a standard menstruum or a mixture of 50 percent alcohol and 50 percent water for all herbs. Standard menstruums result in good tinctures for most herbs. However, if you want to make the strongest tincture possible and get the most tincture from your herbs, making a custom menstruum requires a little more math, as you must determine the amount of alcohol and water needed for each herb. But the extra time needed to research and blend custom menstruums is well worth the effort.

If you don't know how much alcohol to use, start with a standard menstruum or a mixture of 50% alcohol and 50% water. Any 100-proof liquor has this ratio of alcohol to water as the proof of liquor, divided by two, tells you how much alcohol it contains. So, 100-proof liquor is 50 percent alcohol and 50 percent water, and 80-proof liquor is 40 percent alcohol and 60 percent water. Use any liquor with the correct proof, although vodka is often preferred because it has fewer additives and little flavor.

If the recommended menstruum calls for anything other than 40 percent or 50 percent alcohol, you must use grain alcohol or ethanol and dilute it with water to create a custom menstruum. Grain alcohol is typically 190 proof or 95 percent alcohol and 5 percent water.

Grain alcohol is a distilled spirit made from fermenting grains like wheat, corn, rice, rye and sometimes sugar cane. In 2020, the FDA ruled that "distillation removes gluten because gluten does not vaporize," so grain alcohol can be labeled gluten-free even if made from gluten-containing grains.

The chart on page 22 shows you how to calculate the amount of grain alcohol and water needed to make custom menstruums. For best results, first make up a quantity of menstruum in a container and then add it as needed to the herbs. Mix up about two ounces more of the custom menstruum than you need, so you can add a little more if needed as the herbs absorb the liquid or if working with fluffy herbs.

Making Tinctures: Folk and Weight-to-Volume Methods

There are two methods of making tinctures by extraction: the folk method and the weight-to-volume method. The folk method is one of the oldest ways to preserve herbs. The weight-to-volume method is more scientific and uses weights and measures.

The folk method is easy but not cost-effective, as it produces less tincture for the quantity of herbs used. Based on international pharmaceutical standards for tincture making, the weight-to-volume method results in more tincture for the quantity of herbs used. For this reason, all commercial tincture makers use the weight-to-volume method and create custom menstruums for each herb. However, herbalists have used the folk method to make medicine in their kitchens for generations with good results, you may want to try both methods yourself.

Tinctures: The Folk Method

Place chopped fresh or ground dry herbs in a one-quart canning jar, leaving at least 2 inches at the top. Fill the jar snugly but not tightly packed. Mark the level of the herbs on the outside of the jar and then add the menstruum — standard 50:50 or custom — until about two inches above the level of the mark on the jar. Cover the jar with a piece of wax paper and recap; the wax paper keeps the alcohol from corroding the metal of the canning jar lid. Shake it well. Label the jar (not the lid) with the name of the herb used, where it came from, the menstruum type and ratio, and the date. Store the jar in a cool, dark place for two weeks or longer. Once or twice a day, give the jar a good, energetic shake so that the herbs really dance around in the menstruum.

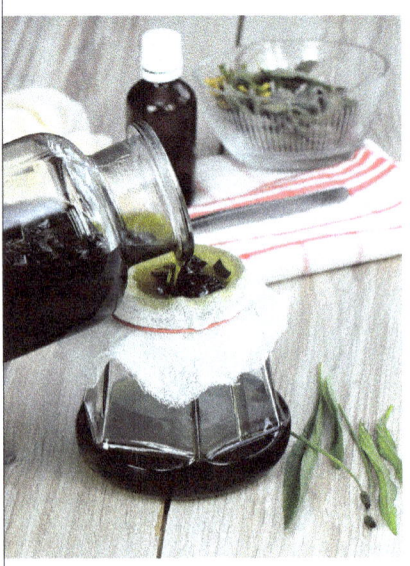

After two weeks, the tincture is ready. Cut a piece of cotton muslin large enough to hang over the sides of a stainless steel colander generously. Place the muslin-lined colander in a large bowl. Strain the entire contents of the jar through the colander. Allow the tincture to drain through the fabric-lined colander for a few minutes, then gather the edges of the muslin together to form a pouch of wet herbs. Remove the colander and, holding the pouch over the bowl, use one hand to firmly hold the pouch closed while you squeeze the liquid out of the herbs with your other hand. When it feels like you've gotten every drop of liquid, discard the spent herbs, pour the tincture into a clean glass jar, cap it, and apply the label. Store in a cool, dark place. Wash the muslin and use it again to make your next tincture.

If bits of herb have escaped the muslin, the best way to remove them is with a paper coffee filter in a freestanding coffee filter holder (the kind used to make pour-over coffee) placed over a clean quart jar. Before you begin, pour a cup of boiling water through the filter. The hot water causes the filter to expand so the tincture flows through. Empty the boiling water from the quart jar. Pour the tincture through the filter, a little at a time.

It is fine to leave the herbs in the menstruum for longer than two weeks or until you are ready to use the tincture. After two weeks, all active compounds in the herbs have been extracted completely, and the potency will not increase.

Tinctures: The Weight-to-Volume Method

To make a tincture using the weight-to-volume method, you must first calculate the weight of your herbs. This determines the amount of menstruum needed, which, being liquid, is measured by volume using a measuring cup or beaker.

WEIGHT-TO-VOLUME METHOD Ratio of Herb to Menstruum	1 part herb to 2 parts menstruum (herb weight x 2 = volume of menstruum)	1 part herb to 5 parts menstruum (herb weight x 5 = volume of menstruum)	1 part herb to 10 parts menstruum (herb weight x 10 = volume of menstruum)
	1:2	1:5	1:10
	fresh herbs	dry herbs	low-dose herbs

Fresh herbs are tinctured at a ratio of one part herb to two parts menstruum, while dry herbs are tinctured at a ratio of one part herb to five parts menstruum. The exception to this is when working with herbs categorized as low-dose botanicals. To be used safely, these herbs require precise dosing with tinctures made at a ratio of one part herb to 10 parts menstruum. Several herbs in this book should be made using the 1:10 ratio; see individual herb monographs for details. Because it is impossible to calculate a safe dose if low-dose botanicals are made using the folk method, tinctures of these herbs must be made using the weight-to-volume method.

Before weighing, fresh herbs should be completely clean and cut into small pieces or chopped finely, and dried herbs should be ground into a coarse powder. To grind dried herbs, use an electric coffee mill (reserved only for use with herbs), a sturdy mortar and pestle or a commercial-grade blender. Vitamix and Ninja are two brands that are strong enough to break down roots, barks and seeds. When herbs are ready, place them in a quart canning jar or other glass container if making a larger quantity.

Use the Weight-to-Volume Chart above to calculate the amount of menstruum needed based on the weight of the herbs. If using a custom menstruum, make the quantity needed for the correct ratio of water to alcohol (see the Custom Menstruum Chart on page 22). Make several ounces more than you think you'll need, as you may have to top off the jar as the herbs absorb the liquid. If using a standard menstruum (50% alcohol to 50% water), simply measure the total volume needed.

TOTAL MENSTRUUM QUANTITY NEEDED	Alcohol to Water Ratios for Custom Menstruums (in milliliters – mL) ☐ Alcohol ☐ Water					
	30%	40%	50%	60%	70%	80%
120 mL (4 ounces)	36	48	60	72	84	96
	84	72	60	48	36	24
240 mL (8 ounces)	72	96	120	144	168	192
	168	144	120	96	72	48
360 mL (12 ounces)	108	144	180	216	252	288
	252	216	180	144	108	72
480 mL (16 ounces)	144	192	240	288	336	384
	336	288	288	192	144	96

Use a measuring cup or glass beaker to measure the amount of prepared menstruum needed and pour the menstruum over the herbs. If you are working with fresh herbs, especially fluffy ones, and the menstruum doesn't completely cover the herbs, pour everything into a blender or food processor and process until the herbs are completely submerged in the menstruum. If using fresh herbs that are not completely submerged, check the jar after a day or two, as the herbs tend to collapse into the menstruum after a while. Whether using fresh or dry herbs, the menstruum should completely cover them. Cut a piece of wax paper big enough to completely cover the top of the jar and then screw on the cap; the wax paper keeps the alcohol from corroding the metal of the canning jar lid. Shake it well. Label the jar (not the lid) with the name of the herb used, the type of menstruum, and the date. Store the jar in a cool, dark place for two weeks or longer. Once or twice a day, give the jar a good, energetic shake so that the herbs really dance around in the menstruum.

After two weeks, follow the steps for straining tinctures described in the Folk Method section. It is fine to leave the herbs in the menstruum for longer than two weeks or until you are ready to use the tincture. After two weeks, all active compounds in the herbs have been extracted completely, and the potency will not increase.

Herbal Syrup

An herbal syrup is simply a concentrated herbal infusion combined with honey. Do not make syrups using refined sugar or artificial sweeteners. Honey enhances the effectiveness of the herbs and acts as a preservative. Syrups are used for coughs, colds, and other respiratory symptoms; they can also make bitter herbs, like boneset, palatable.

First, make a strong herbal infusion. Use a single herb or a combination. For each quart of water, use two ounces of dry herb or four ounces by weight of fresh herb. Grind dry herbs and chop fresh herbs before weighing them. Measure cold water in the amount needed and pour it into a pot with a tight-fitting lid; add the herbs. Bring the water to a boil and remove from heat, cover and infuse for six hours or overnight. Strain out and discard the herbs. Measure the infusion and pour it back into the clean pot. Bring to a boil and then lower heat to a simmer. Simmer uncovered until the volume is reduced by half.

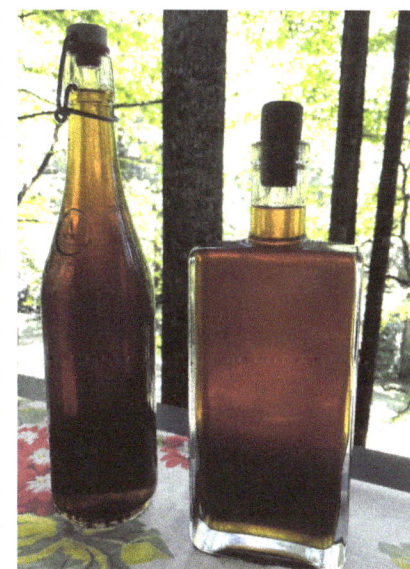

While still warm, measure the concentrated infusion and return to the pot. Take the total volume of liquid and divide by two; this is the amount of honey you will add to make the syrup. Add the honey and stir until completely dissolved. Your herb mixture must be warm when you add the honey. After the mixture cools, pour it into sterile jars or bottles and add a label. You can customize your syrup by adding some brandy or an herbal tincture, a bit of lemon or lime juice, or a few drops of any essential oil used to treat respiratory symptoms, like thyme or eucalyptus. Store syrups in the refrigerator. If properly stored, syrups have a shelf life of one to two years. Check for spoilage and discard if moldy.

Compress

A compress is a moist cloth soaked in a hot or cold herbal infusion or decoction and applied to the skin.

Use a compress to increase blood circulation, warm stiff muscles and joints, break up congestion in the lungs or sinuses, relieve back pain, muscle spasms or inflammation, cool a fever, bring boils to a head, or dissolve cysts or benign tumors.

To make a compress, brew a standard infusion or decoction using one or more herbs. Strain and discard the herbs. To make a hot compress, soak a washcloth, towel or other soft absorbent cloth in the hot herb mixture for a few minutes. You may need to use tongs to do this safely. Lift the towel out of the water, let the water drip a little, and wring it out and fold it to cover the affected area completely when the towel has cooled enough to handle. Apply to the skin and cover the compress with a dry towel to keep it warm. You can also place a hot water bottle on the compress if the weight does not cause discomfort. When the compress begins to cool, replace it with a fresh, hot towel and repeat as needed.

To make a cool compress, make an infusion or decoction as described above, then allow the herb mixture to cool completely or refrigerate briefly to expedite cooling. Soak a washcloth, small towel or other soft, absorbent cloth in the mixture. Wring out the cloth and fold it to completely cover the affected area. Apply the compress to the skin and cover the area with a dry towel to prevent a chill. When the compress gets warm, replace it with a fresh, cool one and repeat several times. Cool compresses are usually used to reduce fevers or to relieve a headache. Compress treatment time should be at least 20 minutes. Repeat as needed.

Poultice

A poultice is a messy but effective way to use herbs topically to heal the skin, relieve inflammation, or stimulate circulation. To make a poultice of fresh herbs, pound herbs in a mortar and pestle or in a bowl with a wooden spoon until they form a juicy pulp. Place dry herbs in a small bowl and add hot water a little at a time until the herbs stick together. If the fresh or dry herbs need more juice, add aloe vera gel a little at a time until they hold together.

To make the poultice easier to handle, loosely wrap the moistened herbs in cheesecloth to make a little packet. Apply the poultice to the affected area and cover with a small piece of a plastic bag or something similar. Place a dry towel on top of the plastic and put a hot water bottle over everything. You can apply a poultice without adding the hot water bottle, but it does increase the absorption of herbs into the skin. Rub some olive oil on the skin before applying the poultice to avoid irritation when using harsh or stimulating herbs. Treatment time should be at least 20 minutes. Repeat as needed.

Herbal Baths

Freshly brewed herbal infusions and decoctions added to a bath are a gentle yet effective way to administer herbs. They may also be used to administer herbal therapies that would otherwise be given orally to someone who is too weak to drink or unable to hold down fluids. Herbal baths can relieve symptoms such as nausea or vomiting, insomnia, anxiety, and itchy, inflamed skin. They are an excellent, non-invasive way to administer herbs to babies and young children.

Make at least one quart of a standard herbal infusion or decoction. Strain out the herbs and discard them. Pour into a warm or hot bath and soak for 20 minutes. Prepare foot and hand baths in the same way.

Enema

Enemas are used sparingly to treat acute symptoms and may provide immediate relief for constipation caused by illness, travel or medications. They may also be used to administer herbal therapies that would otherwise be given orally to someone who is too weak to drink or unable to hold down fluids. Prepared with relaxing herbs, enemas may help to relieve pain, muscle spasms, anxiety and insomnia. Long-term use of enemas to treat constipation is not recommended and always avoid using any herb that might irritate mucus membranes.

Prepare a standard infusion or decoction and allow it to cool to body temperature before using. For best results, follow the directions included with enema bags.

Vaginal Douche

Herbal douches are used to treat vaginal irritation, inflammation or infection. Prepare a standard infusion or decoction and cool to body temperature before using. For best results, follow the directions included with a douche bag. Avoid using any herb that might irritate mucus membranes. Long-term use of douches is not recommended.

Infused Herbal Oil

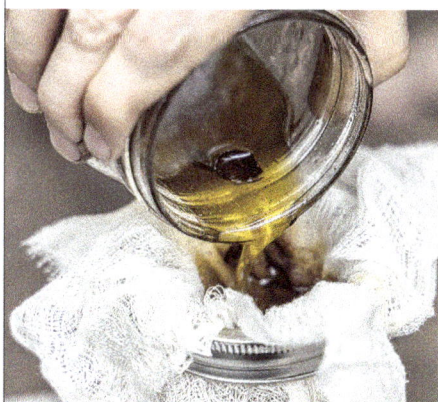

Herbs can be infused into vegetable oils, or animal fats, and use externally. Infused herbal oils made with aromatic herbs can be used in cooking. In both cases, combine fresh or dry herbs with vegetable oil and heat the mixture to make an infused herbal oil. Here are two methods for making infused oils. The first, the solar infusion method, uses heat from the sun over several days to extract the herbs into vegetable oil. Obviously, high temperatures and direct sunlight are needed to make a solar infusion. The second, an infused oil made by the oven method, is ready in only a few hours.

Infused oil may be made using any quality vegetable oil, preferably organic. Some oils, such as olive or almond, are best for treating wounds, rashes, dryness, and other skin problems. Due to their larger molecular structure, these oils stay on the surface longer, allowing the herbs to come in contact with the skin and provide some protection. Other oils, like grapeseed, with their smaller molecular structure, are quickly absorbed into the skin and are often recommended to treat dry skin, bruises and sore muscles.

Infused oils can be made with fresh or dry herbs. If using fresh herbs, you must take extra care to ensure they are completely dry. To reduce moisture content, you can also allow fresh herbs to wilt for a few hours or overnight before making an oil. Fresh roots should be sliced thinly and dried for a few hours. If using dry herbs, grind them into a coarse powder.

Because infused oils are very susceptible to bacterial growth that causes rancidity, they should be stored in sterile jars. Choose a jar that will be completely filled with oil and little or no air space between the oil and the lid. If necessary, divide a larger batch of oil between several smaller jars. Store oils in the refrigerator or a cool, dark cupboard. Check them frequently and discard them if they become cloudy or develop a rancid odor.

Solar-Infused Oil

Place chopped, slightly wilted, fresh or powered dry herbs in a sterile glass jar. Add vegetable oil to cover the herbs with little or no air space between the herb and oil mixture and the top of the jar. The herbs should not be tightly packed; they must be able to move around freely in the oil.

Use a chopstick or butter knife to poke the herbs to release any air bubbles. Cap tightly and shake well. Place the jar in a brown paper bag and set it outside in direct sunlight; the oil needs five or more hours of sunlight each day. Another method that I use is to put the jar (in the paper bag) in my car. In summer, the heat in the car, along with the shaking the jar gets driving on mountain roads, is the perfect combination. Shake the jar well at least once daily for three to five days. When the oil has a deep, rich color, it is ready. Strain the oil through a muslin cloth draped over a metal colander placed over a bowl. The process will be easier if your oil is warm when you strain it.

Follow the directions for tinctures to squeeze the oil out of the herbs. Pour the strained oil into a sterile jar, screw on the cap and add the label. Allow the jar of oil to sit undisturbed overnight. In the morning, slowly pour the oil into another sterile jar, taking care not to stir up any plant residue that will have settled to the bottom of the first jar. Discard the leftover plant matter. Store the infused oil in a cool, dark place or in the refrigerator. Check them frequently and discard them if they become cloudy or develop a rancid odor. Herbal oils have a shelf life of one year.

Oven Method Infused Oil

The oven method is a fast, fool-proof way to make infused oils. You don't have to worry about moisture because it takes just a few hours from start to finish. Place chopped fresh or powdered dry herbs in a two-quart (or larger if needed) oven-safe casserole dish with a lid.

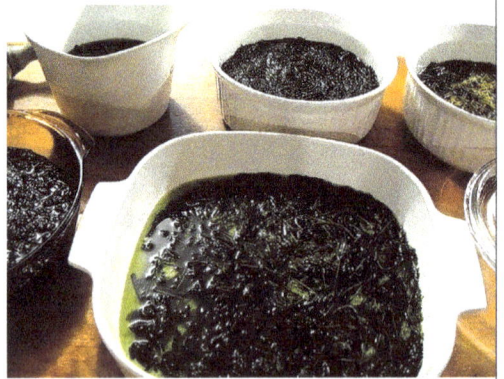

Slowly add enough oil to cover the herbs completely. Cover the dish, and bake at 250 degrees Fahrenheit (176 degrees Celsius) for two to three hours. Every 20 minutes or so, remove the lid from the dish and stir the mixture with a clean spoon. Oils made with dry herbs require less cooking time than fresh ones. Remove the oil from the oven when it has a rich green color, cool for about 20 minutes and strain while still warm.

Follow the directions for tinctures to squeeze the oil out of the herbs. Pour the strained oil into a sterile jar, screw on the cap and add the label. Allow the jar to sit undisturbed overnight. In the morning, slowly pour the oil into another sterile jar, careful not to stir up any plant residue that will have settled to the bottom of the first jar. Discard the spent herbs. Store the infused oil in a cool, dark place or in the refrigerator. Check them frequently and discard them if they become cloudy or develop a rancid odor. Herbal oils have a shelf life of one year.

Herbal Salves

Salves are infused herbal oils thickened with beeswax and used topically to heal wounds, skin abrasions, dry skin or rashes. Combining herbal oils and beeswax promotes healing by holding the herbs' medicinal properties on the skin's surface and adding a protective layer of infused oil and beeswax.

To make an herbal salve, assemble your salve jars and sterilize them. Measure enough herbal oil to fill your salve jars into a non-aluminum pan. Warm the oil over low heat for several minutes, being careful not to leave it unattended or overheat it.

Add one tablespoon of grated beeswax for each ounce of oil and stir the oil with a metal spoon until the wax completely dissolves. Remove the pan from the heat and test the consistency of the mixture by putting a spoonful on a saucer and allowing it to cool completely for about five to ten minutes. A faster method for testing salve consistency is to place the spoonful of the warm mixture on a saucer and cool it in the freezer for five minutes.

If the balance of oil and wax is correct, when completely cool, the salve should be easy to scoop up with your finger but not runny or oily. If the salve is too soft, add a little more grated beeswax to the oil in the pan. If it is too hard, add a little more oil. Test the consistency again. Once you have the proper consistency, pour the warm salve mixture into sterile wide-mouth jars and cool completely. A few drops of skin-soothing essential oils may be stirred into the salve jars before the mixture has cooled completely; consider lavender to soothe inflammation and itching, tea tree for infections or fungal growths, or eucalyptus for sore muscles. Don't move the jars until they are completely cooled and the salve has set.

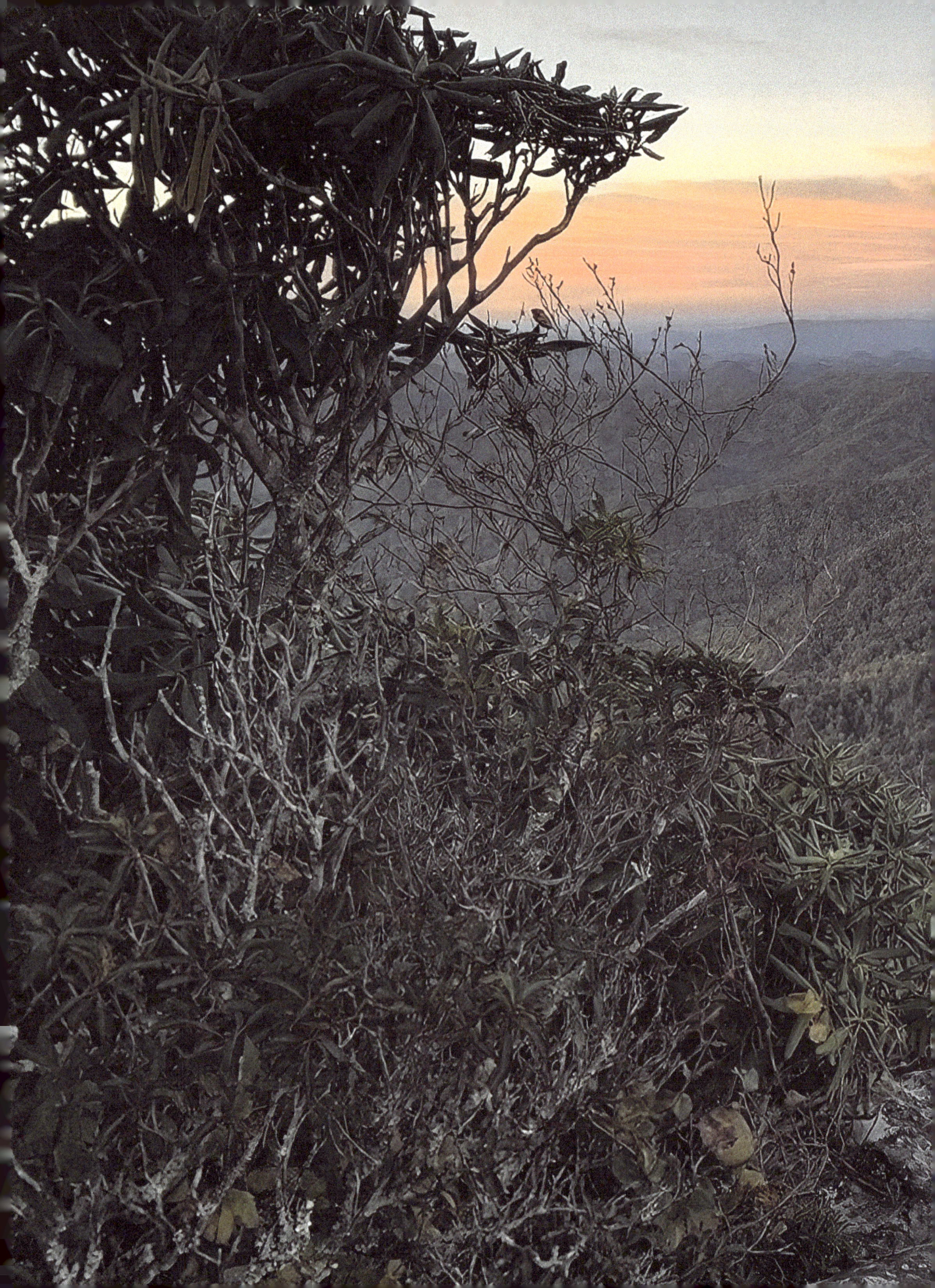

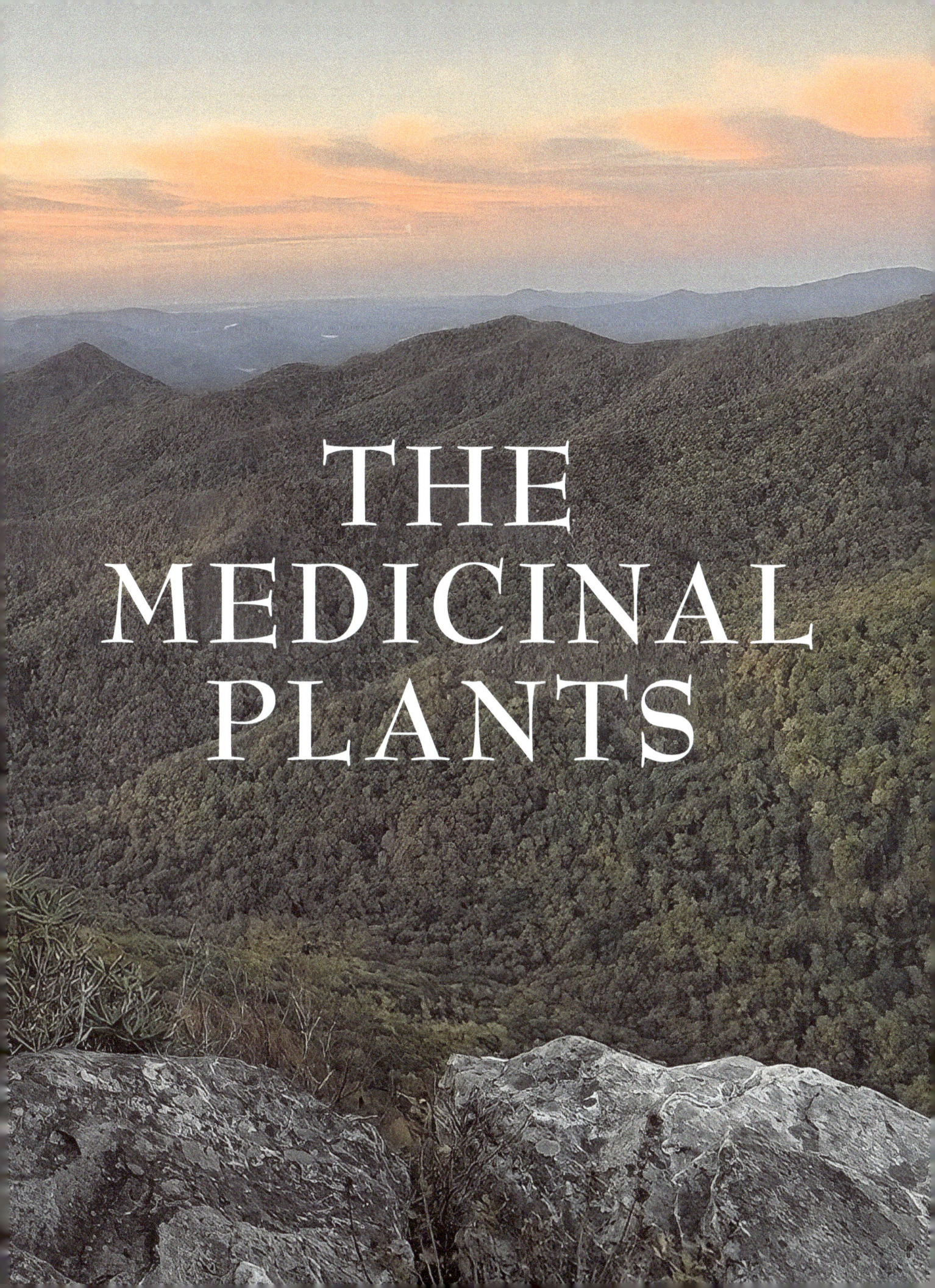
THE MEDICINAL PLANTS

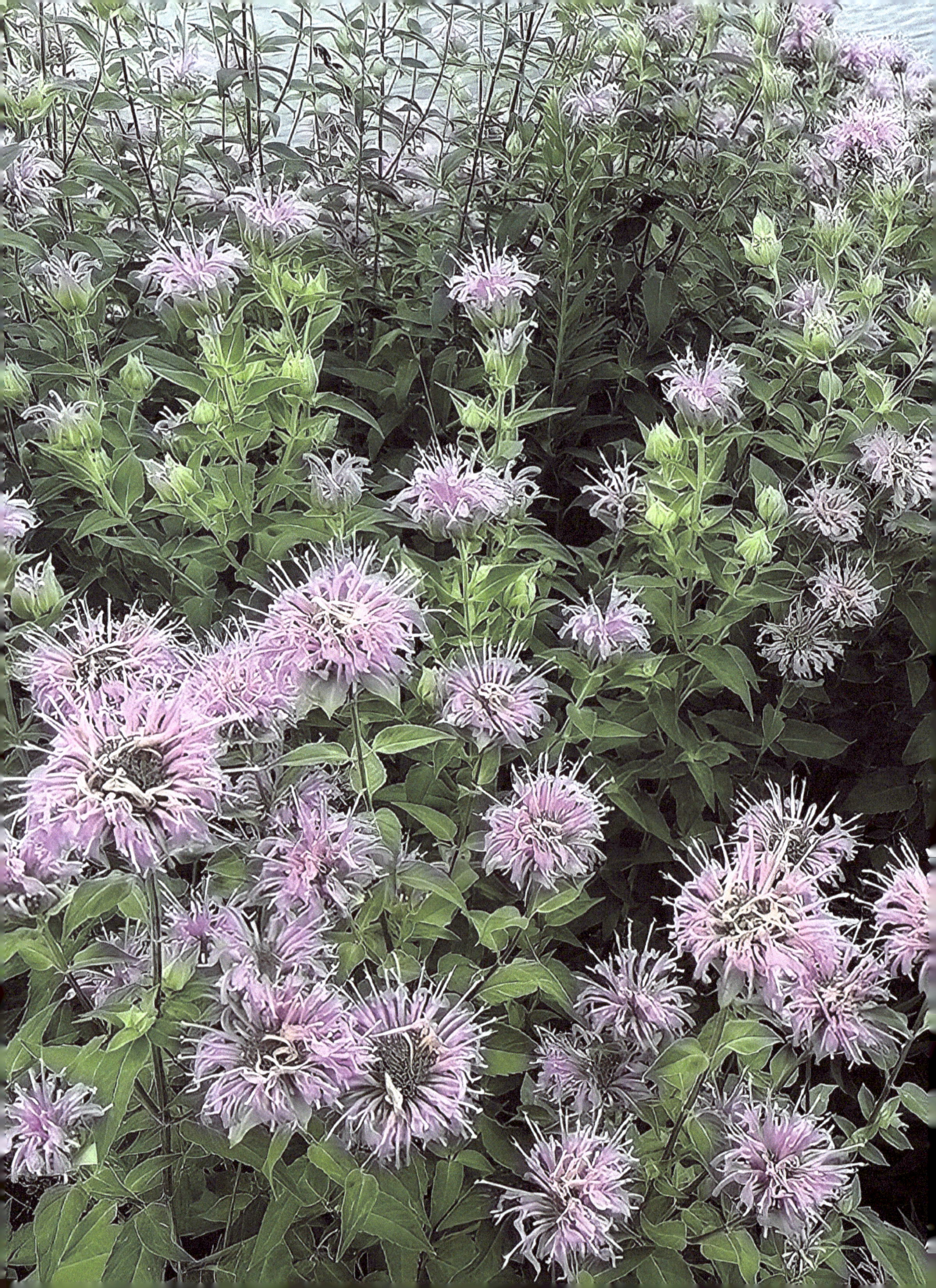

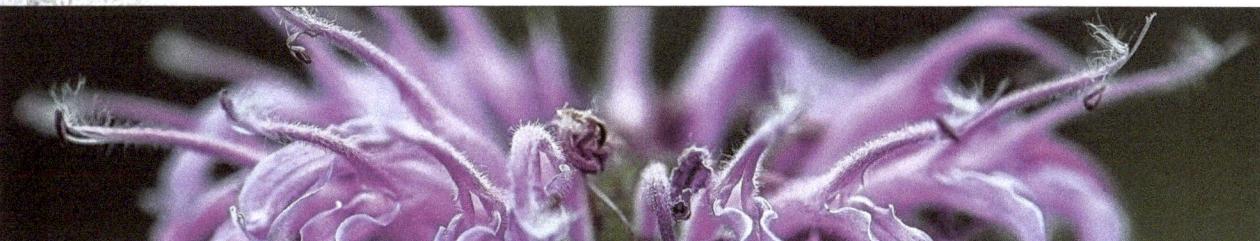

Bee Balm

COMMON NAME: Bee Balm

BOTANICAL NAME: *Monarda species*

FAMILY: *Lamiaceae* (Mint)

OTHER NAMES: Oswego tea, Scarlet Monarda, Scarlet Bee Balm

RELATED SPECIES: There are three species of Monarda in the Southern Appalachians: *Monarda didyma* with red flowers, *M. fistulosa* with lavender flowers, and *M. clinopodia* with white or pinkish flowers with dots. All have similar actions and can be used interchangeably.

DESCRIPTION: Perennial mint, one to three feet tall, with classic mint characteristics: square stems, opposite leaves, terminal flowers, irregular flowers with protruding stamen and very aromatic. Flowers midsummer through fall. Common but not abundant.

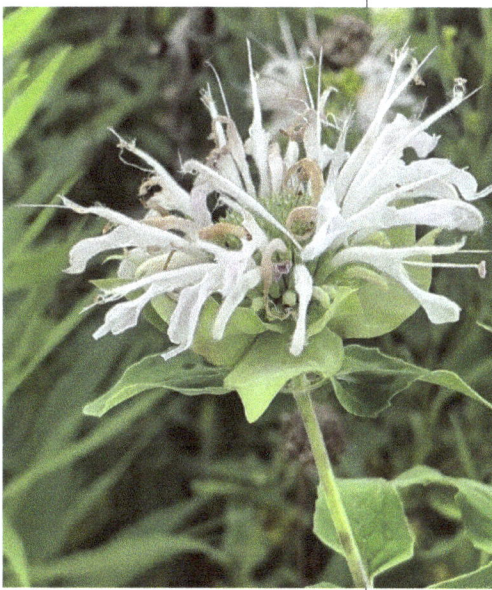

HABITAT: Found in partial shade in wet places, often along waterways and in ditches. All the *Monarda* species are popular garden plants, especially *M. didyma* with its brilliant red flower. Though, like most Mint family plants, they would like to take over your garden.

KEY ACTIONS: Carminative, diaphoretic, anti-inflammatory, analgesic, emmenagogue

PART USED: Aerial parts (in flower)

TRADITIONAL USES: The Cherokee used the entire fresh plant as poultice for colic, bloating and headaches, and as a diaphoretic to "bring out the measles." They also considered it a sedative.[1] Tommie Bass also used bee balm "for the nerves."[2]

---

[1] Moerman, *Native American Ethnobotany*, 346–347

[2] Crellin and Philpott, *A Reference Guide to Medicinal Plants*, 79–80

CURRENT USES: Hot infusions are diaphoretic and may help reduce fevers and relieve bronchial inflammation, coughs and lung congestion. Bee balm also settles the stomach and relieves nausea, stomach cramps, and gas. It is a mild antispasmodic but helpful for menstrual cramps. A liniment can be used topically for sore muscles and rheumatic pain. Because bee balm is a wonderfully aromatic mint, it can be added to tea blends that contain other less flavorful herbs. Its warm energy seems to activate other herbs, especially when used to treat symptoms of coldness in the digestive tract, such as gas, bloating, loose stools and belching.

CAUTIONS: None known.

TIP: MAKING TEA WITH AROMATIC HERBS

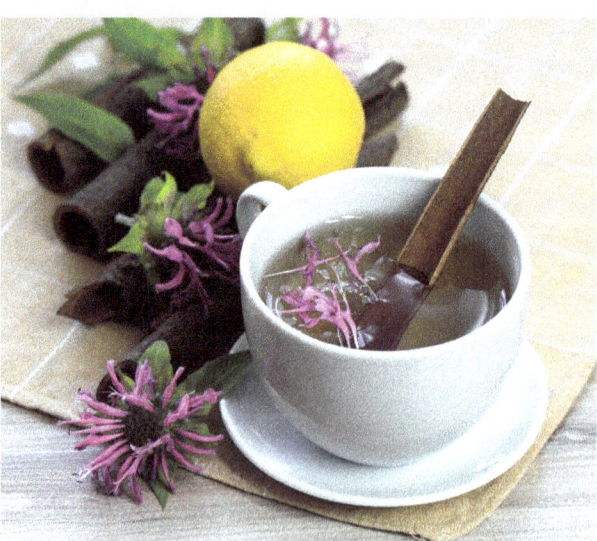

The flavor of aromatic herbs, like bee balm and mountain mint, comes from their fragrant essential oils. Many of the compounds in these essential oils evaporate when heated, leaving only harsh menthol compounds behind. When preparing teas from aromatic herbs, try preserving their complex, delicate flavors with a cold infusion. To make, combine one cup of chopped fresh herb or three tablespoons dried with four cups of cool water. Cover and steep for one hour or overnight. For best results, slightly bruise fresh leaves with a mortar and pestle or a wooden spoon before infusing.

PREPARATIONS

INFUSIONS: Prepare a standard infusion using fresh or dried herbs. Infusions prepared with cold water contain more volatile oils and should be used when addressing digestive system symptoms; steep for one hour or overnight. Infusions prepared using hot water are best suited for fevers and cough symptoms and as antispasmodic: steep for fifteen to twenty minutes. Cover infusions while steeping to keep the volatile oils from escaping.

LINIMENT: See Lobelia Liniment recipe on page 105.

DOSAGES

INFUSIONS: Drink one cup as needed to relieve symptoms. Repeat as needed.

LINIMENT: Apply to sore muscles and bruises as needed.

HARVESTING

Collect aerial parts in flower.

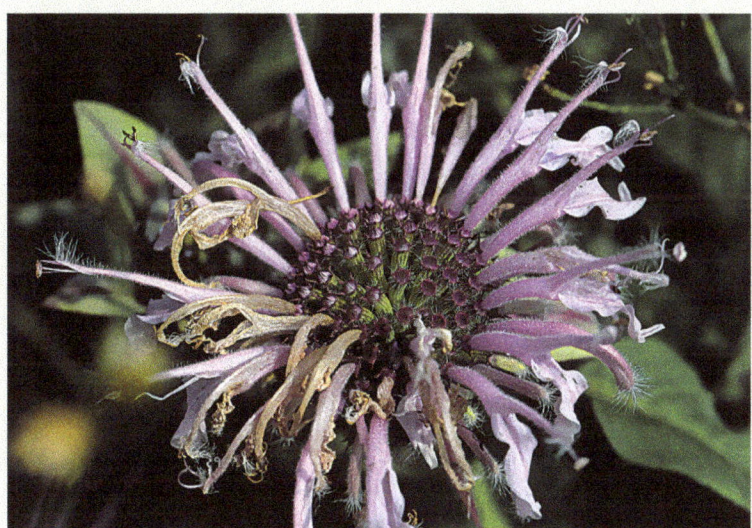

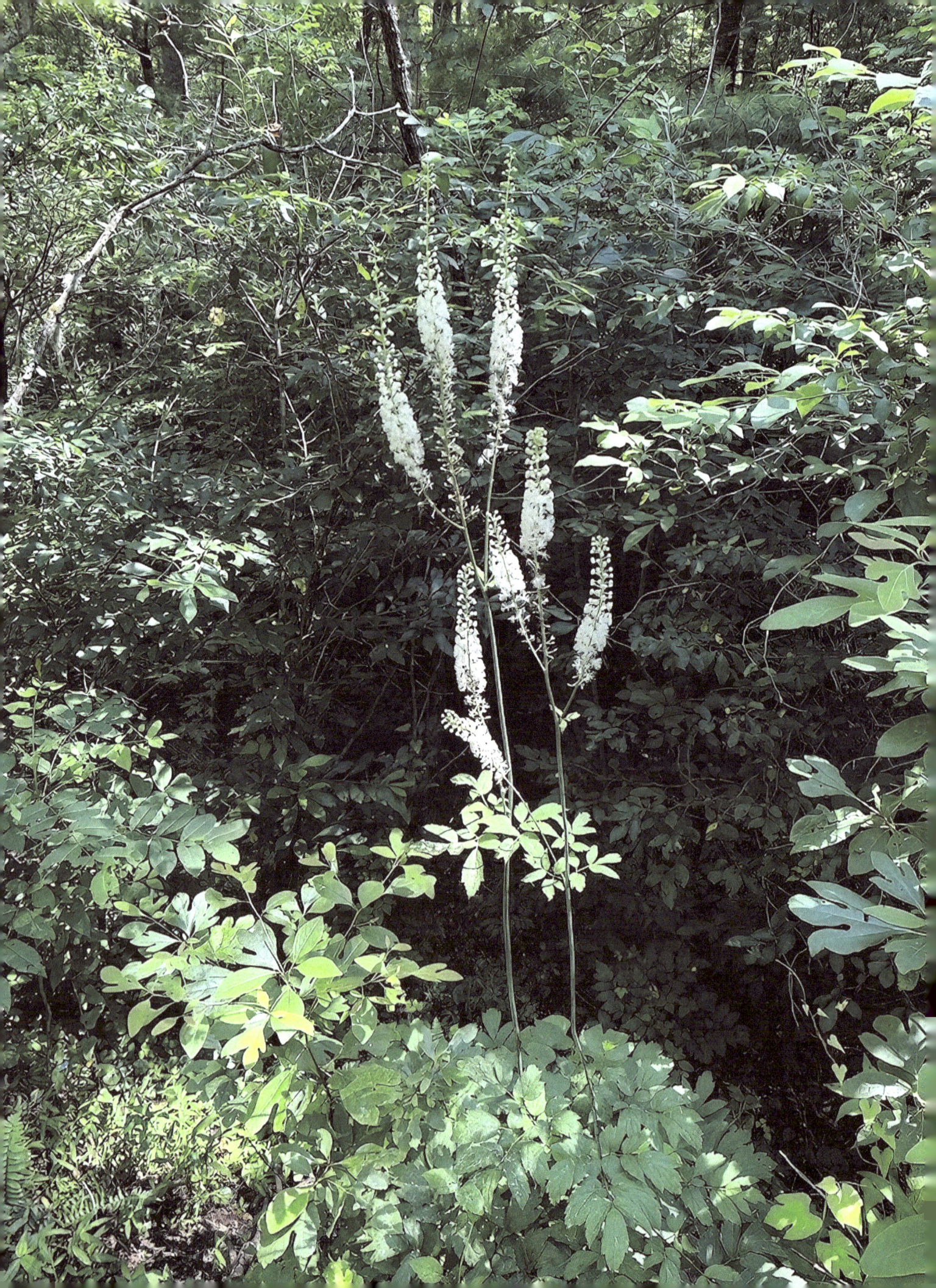

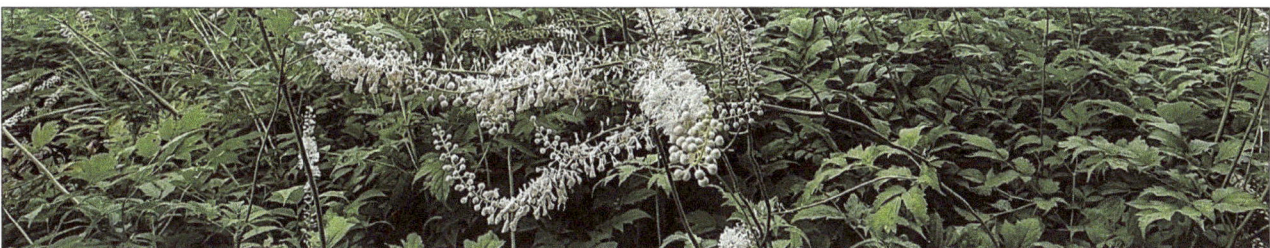

Black Cohosh

COMMON NAME: Black Cohosh

BOTANICAL NAME: *Actaea racemosa* (formerly *Cimicifuga racemosa*)

FAMILY: *Ranunculaceae* (Buttercup)

OTHER NAMES: Black Snakeroot, Bugbane, Bugwort, Rattlewort, Fairy Torches

DESCRIPTION: A two to three feet tall perennial plant with dark green foliage and an overall appearance of airy grace. Three large compound leaves with sharply toothed leaflets on each stem. Notice the black mark on the stem where it forks into three branches.

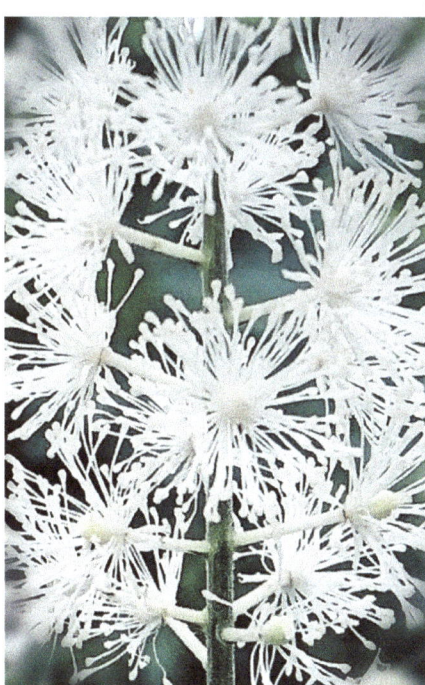

In mid-summer, the stately flower stalk, which may be solitary or branched, rises three or more feet above the foliage. Evenly spaced buds that resemble small green peas remain unopened for a month or more. The blooms open at the flower stalk's lower end in late June or early July. The tiny sepals fall off as the flower begins to bloom, and what appears to be a delicate, fluffy white flower is a cluster of stamens surrounding a rather fat, short stigma. The disagreeable odor of the flowers attracts flies and beetles, the most common pollinators of black cohosh. In the deep shade of the forest, the common name, fairy torches, aptly describes the blooms that seem to emit a glowing, luminous light.

HABITAT: Common in woodlands of eastern North America. It is found on moist slopes in the deep shade of deciduous forests, often with blue cohosh.

KEY ACTIONS: Antispasmodic, nervine, anti-rheumatic, analgesic, anti-inflammatory, emmenagogue

PART USED: Rhizome, roots

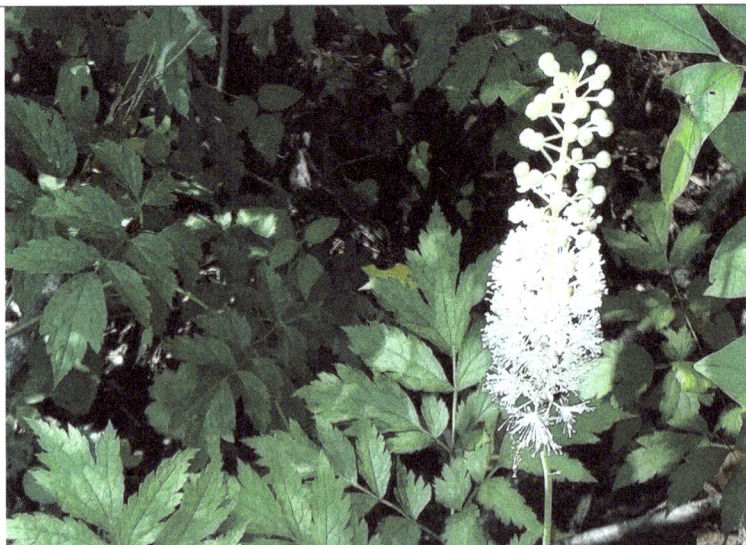

TRADITIONAL USES: American Indians steeped black cohosh roots in alcohol to create a simple tincture for rheumatic pain.[1] Roots were decocted as a wash to clean wounds and to make a salve. The decoction was drunk as a tea to treat colds and relieve coughs, for general pain relief and as a gargle for sore throats. It has been used to relieve a wide range of symptoms caused by hormonal fluctuations such as delayed menses and menstrual cramps, menopausal mood swings, hot flashes and insomnia, and in pregnancy to promote contractions in labor. Flowers were rubbed on the skin as an insect repellent.

CURRENT USES: Black cohosh is strongly associated with the female generative system. It is effective in relieving menstrual and menopausal symptoms, and long-term use tonifies the uterus. As an antispasmodic, it relieves menstrual cramps, uterine pain, and discomfort caused by endometriosis.

In menopause, nervine properties ease insomnia, anxiety, mood swings, and depression, and with regular use, may reduce the severity and frequency of hot flashes.

Black cohosh relieves pain and inflammation caused by arthritis, rheumatism, and fibromyalgia.

Add black cohosh to cough syrups or use it as a tea or tincture to relax spasmodic coughs caused by colds, bronchitis, asthma and whooping cough.

CAUTIONS: Contraindicated in pregnancy and when nursing. Skilled midwives often use black cohosh to promote contractions in labor if they have training in its safe use. If frequent or high doses of black cohosh are used, dizziness, frontal headache, nausea, and even vomiting are possible; discontinue use, and the symptoms will subside.

---

[1] Banks, *Plants of the Cherokee*, 48

PREPARATIONS

DECOCTION: One teaspoon dry or two teaspoons chopped fresh root for each cup of water. Cover and decoct for ten minutes. Strain.

TINCTURE: Fresh root – 1:2, 60%. Dried root – 1:5, 60%.

DOSAGES

DECOCTION: Drink a half cup of decoction every one to two hours as needed.

TINCTURE: Take one-fourth teaspoon in a small amount of water every one to two hours as needed.

HARVESTING

Dig black cohosh roots in early fall before the first frost, as the foliage seems to die back suddenly around this time. To positively identify black cohosh in the fall and avoid harvesting toxic look-alikes (see below), only harvest roots from plants where dried flower stalks are evident. Carefully loosen soil from the base of the plant to determine the shape and size of the root before digging.

Black cohosh rhizomes and rootlets form a thick, twisted bundle that is challenging to clean. Cut rhizomes and rootlets apart to loosen dirt and soak them in water briefly. If there is a nearby stream, I like to toss my roots in a shallow area to let the current do the rinsing while I continue to harvest. Scrub roots with a small brush and lots of patience. Sort through cleaned roots and discard any woody or blackened parts.

If possible, tincture fresh roots immediately. Cut the roots into slices about ¼" thick and completely dry before storing them in glass jars to prevent molding.

Black cohosh is considered At Risk by UpS. Carefully replant the white 'buds' at the tip, along with a few inches of the rhizome to generate a new plant.

Black cohosh may be confused with white baneberry or doll's eyes *(Actaea pachypoda)*. Check the flowers, fruits or seed heads for positive identification. Black cohosh has three to five foot tall flower stalks, and flowers in racemes; white baneberry flowers and fruits are in compact racemes just above the leaves. The berries of black cohosh are dark purple, while those of baneberry are white with a dark purple mark; they resemble small eyes, hence the common name, doll's eyes.

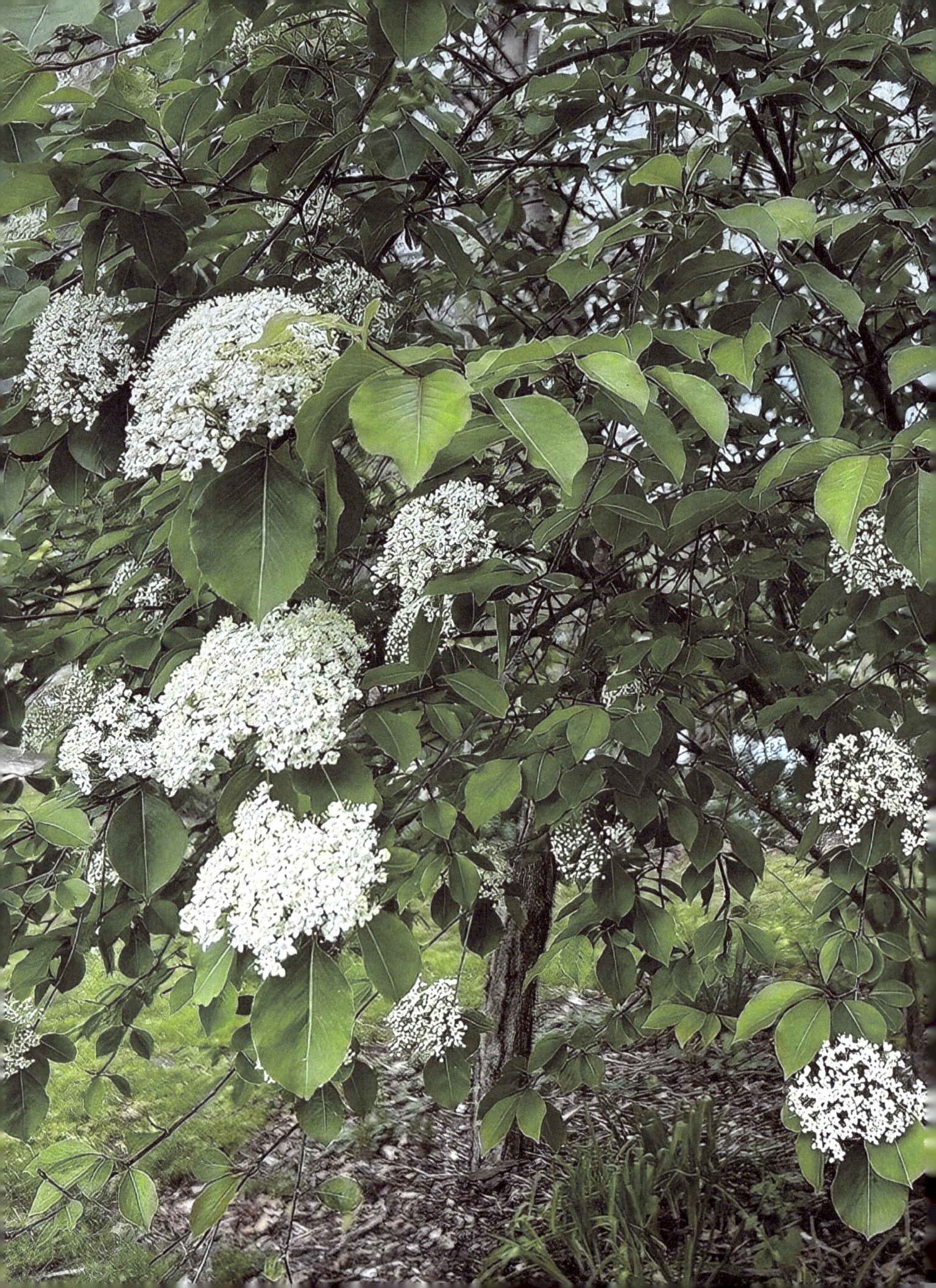

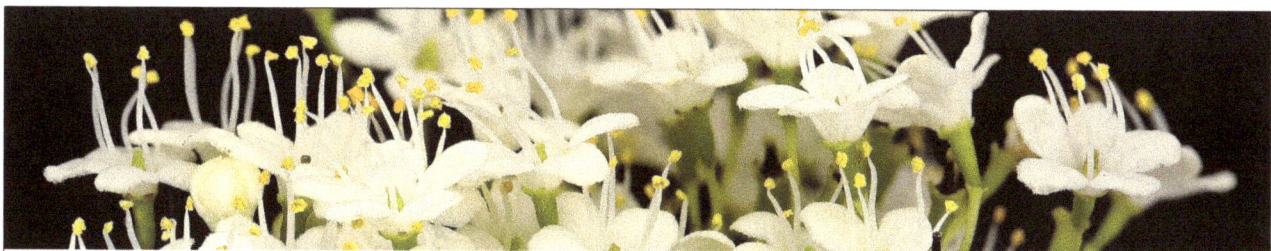

Black Haw

COMMON NAME: Black Haw

BOTANICAL NAME: *Viburnum prunifolium*

FAMILY: *Caprifoliaceae* (Honeysuckle)

OTHER NAMES: Crampbark, Arrow-wood, Snowball Plant

RELATED SPECIES: Possum Haw *(V. nudum)*, Crampbark *(V. opulus)*

DESCRIPTION: Black haw is a small, deciduous shrub or tree, six to twenty feet tall, with finely serrated, oval, opposite leaves and bunches of small white flowers that bloom in flat clusters during April and May. Historically, the straight, smooth branches were used to make arrows, hence the common name, arrow-wood. Small green or dark blue-black berries or "haws" appear in the late summer.

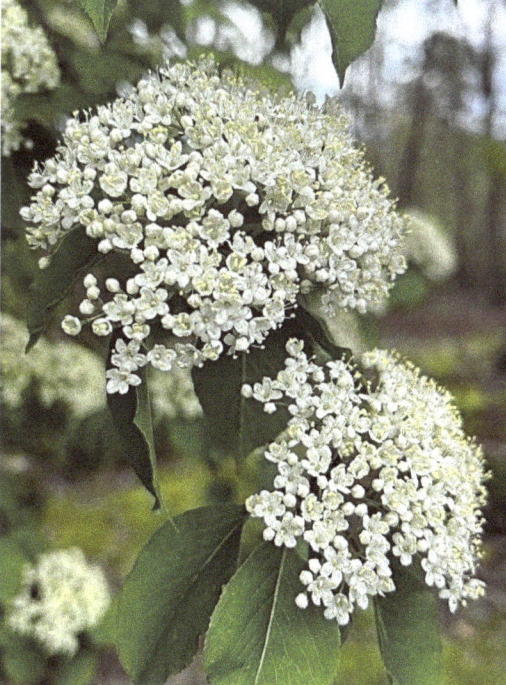

HABITAT: Commonly found in the understory of deciduous forests, along creek banks and at the edges of open, sunny areas.

KEY ACTIONS: Antispasmodic, anti-inflammatory, astringent

PART USED: Bark

TRADITIONAL USES: Black haw was a common ingredient in formulas for women's "monthly troubles" and was used to relieve menstrual cramps, prevent miscarriage and as a labor tonic during the last few weeks of pregnancy. It was an ingredient in one of the best-selling herbal remedies of all times, "Lydia Pinkham's Vegetable Compound for Females." Black haw was also used to relieve nervousness, stomach cramps, and tics or spasms.

CURRENT USES: Black haw is a reliable remedy to relieve cramps and spasms anywhere in the body. Because it works without causing drowsiness, it helps treat a wide range of symptoms without sedation. It is a specific remedy for menstrual cramps, ovarian pain, and excessive menstrual

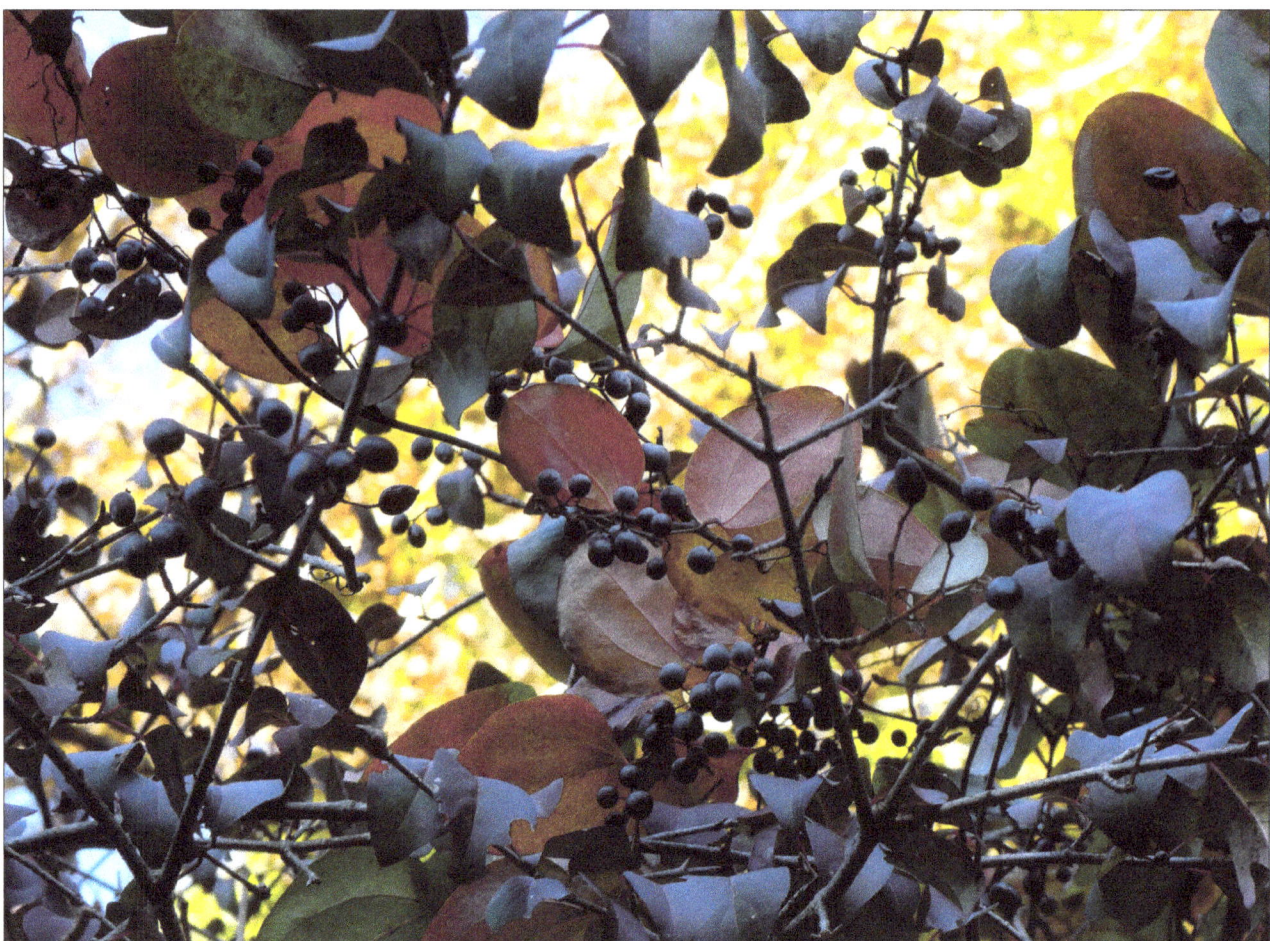

bleeding. Frequent small doses relieve heart palpitations, arthritic, rheumatic or sciatic pain, asthmatic breathing difficulties and wheezing, and intestinal cramps caused by irritable bowel syndrome and Crohn's disease. It is also effective for chronic or acute back pain. During labor, black haw helps to regulate uterine contractions and may reduce post-partum bleeding.

The actions of black haw are similar to those of another *Viburnum* species, crampbark *(Viburnum opulus),* a European native widely available on the commercial herb market. Black haw may require slightly higher dosing to be used as a substitute for crampbark.

CAUTIONS: None known.

PREPARATIONS

DECOCTION: Use two teaspoons of dried or one teaspoon of fresh bark, chopped) for each cup of water. Bring to a boil; cover and simmer for fifteen minutes. Remove from heat and steep for another thirty minutes.

TINCTURE: Fresh bark – 1:2. Dried bark – 1:5, 50%.

DOSAGES

For the fastest results when treating acute symptoms, use small, frequent doses until symptoms improve. After this, reduce dosage frequency to every hour or more as needed.

DECOCTION: Drink one-half cup of warm black haw decoction every twenty minutes until symptoms improve, then as needed.

TINCTURE: Put one teaspoon of tincture in one ounce of warm water; take every twenty minutes. Repeat until symptoms improve. Increase dosage to two teaspoons every twenty minutes if symptoms fail to improve after two to three doses. Adding tincture to warm tea, especially ginger, enhances black haw's antispasmodic action.

HARVESTING

The best way to harvest black haw is to prune the outer branches of this shrub in early spring as soon as the leaves emerge. If you harvest several branches each spring, one or two plants are enough to provide an abundant source of medicine for a home apothecary. And the good news is that black haw thrives when pruned in the spring. Strip leaves off the cut branches. Cut them into foot-long pieces and use a sharp knife to peel the bark into strips; discard the inner pith. Thin twigs, smaller than one-half inch in diameter, may be cut into thin slices and used without separating the bark from the pith. Tincture the fresh bark or dry completely for future use.

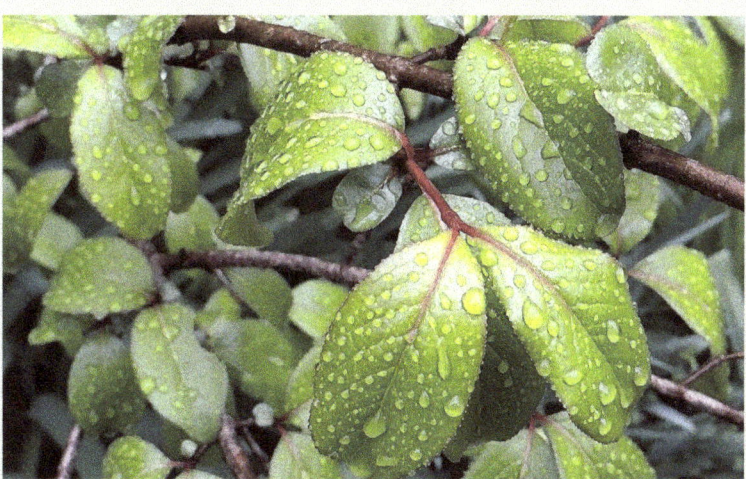

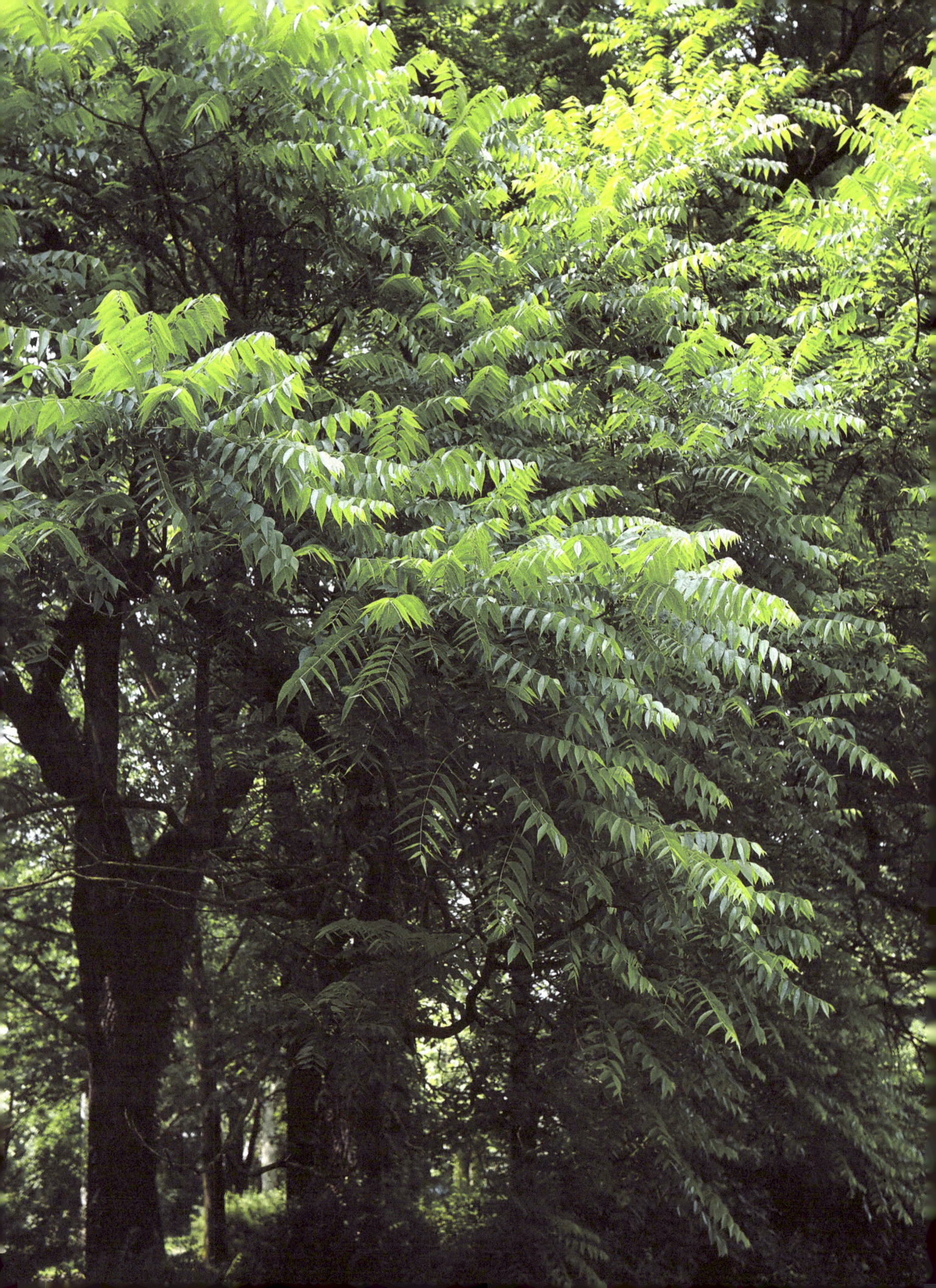

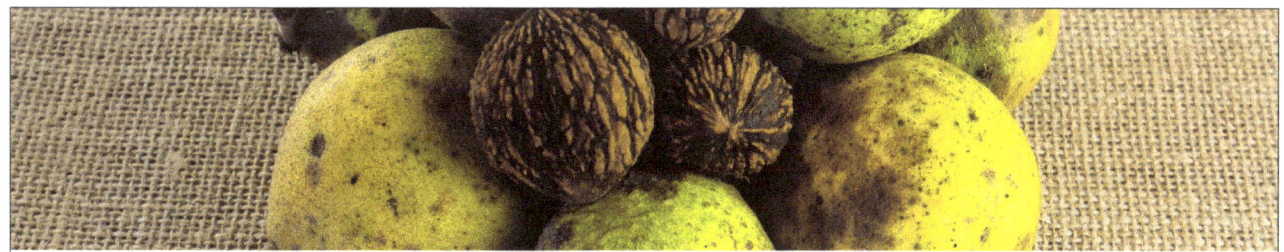

Black Walnut

COMMON NAME: Black Walnut

BOTANICAL NAME: *Juglans nigra*

FAMILY: *Juglandaceae* (Walnut)

OTHER NAMES: American Walnut

DESCRIPTION: A large, deciduous tree, twenty to a hundred feet tall, with deeply ridged, gray-black bark. Leaves appear late in the spring and are reddish-pink when they first emerge, followed by catkins (male flowers) and inconspicuous female flowers. The pinnately compound leaves of alternate leaflets, usually twelve to twenty-four per stem, are finely toothed and about three inches long. The green fruit is about the size of a tennis ball, grows singly or in clusters, and the thick outer hull becomes blackened and furrowed with age. When green, the hull has a pungent odor and is used to make a dye in shades of tan and brown. Be aware that anything that touches the hulls, like your hands, will be stained brown for weeks or longer. Within the hull is a brown, hard-shelled nut that contains delicious oil-rich black walnut meat. The tree secretes juglone, a chemical that prevents most other plants from growing within its drip line.

HABITAT: Throughout the region.

PART USED: Leaf, green hull

KEY ACTIONS: Anti-fungal, astringent, antiseptic, bitter, purgative, vermifuge

TRADITIONAL USES: In Native American and local folk medicine, black walnut leaves were decocted, and the extract was used topically as an antiseptic wash for skin infections and applied to the skin of horses and other animals to repel fleas.[1]

The leaves were also dried, powdered and mixed with table salt and applied to skin infections.[2] The juice of the black hull was said to cure

---

[1] Porcher, *Resources of the Southern Fields and Forests,* 155

[2] Wiggington and Bennett, *Foxfire 9,* 132

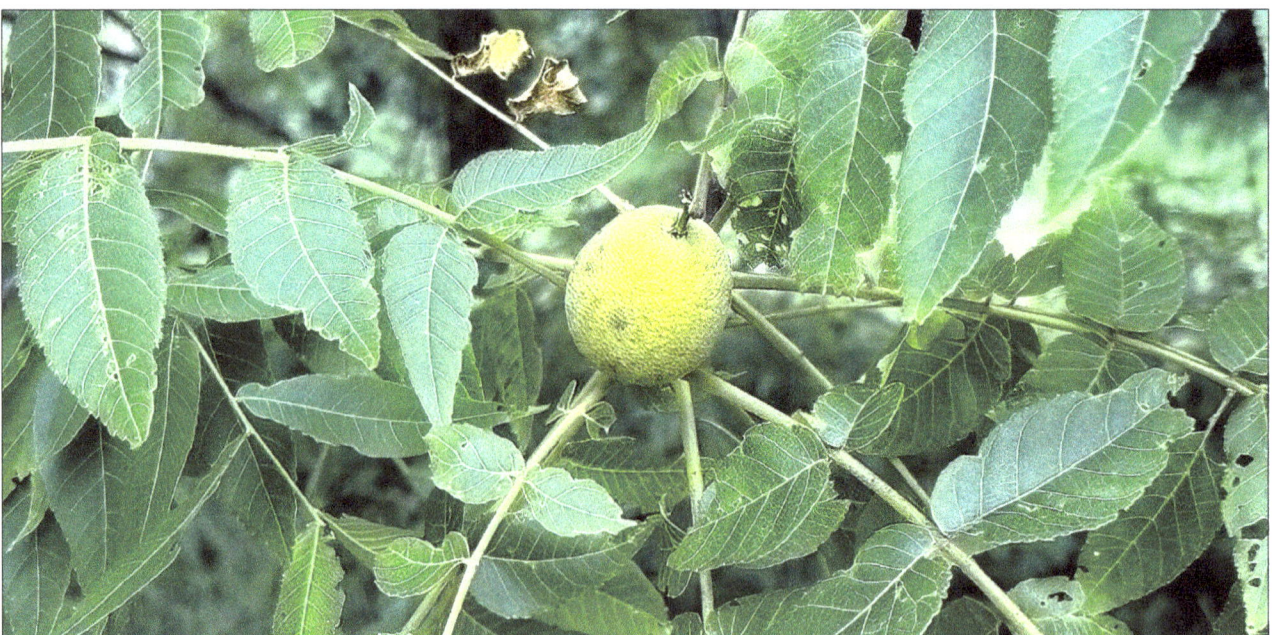

herpes and eczema. In the 1800s, Eclectic practitioners used black walnut root bark internally to relieve intestinal irritation and inflammation that resulted in diarrhea. During the Civil War, black walnut leaves and bergamot oil were combined in skin salves used to treat infected sores.

Black walnut meat is a delicacy, though extracting them from their shells is serious work. The unripe fruit was pickled. Nocino, a traditional Italian liqueur, is made with green walnuts harvested at the summer solstice. An important dye plant, the hulls produce a beautiful chocolate brown color while the leaves produce a green dye.

CURRENT USES: Black walnut leaf and hull are still used in herbal practice, though when taken internally, they are potent, somewhat harsh remedies that should be used cautiously. For this reason, black walnut hull tincture is usually a small part of a larger tincture formula. Black walnut hull tincture or decoction treats systemic yeast infections (candidiasis) and may eliminate intestinal worms and parasites. In large doses, it acts as a strong laxative. Black walnut hulls and leaves are used as a wash or salve for ringworm, scabies, cradle cap and athlete's foot. It is also used as a douche to relieve vaginal discharge (leucorrhea) and itching (vaginitis).

CAUTIONS: Internal use is contraindicated in pregnancy, while nursing or for babies and young children. Used internally, black walnut leaves and hulls can have a powerful purgative action, causing severe diarrhea or vomiting. Start with the lowest dose recommended. Use freely as a topical skin preparation.

PREPARATIONS

DECOCTION: Decoct one tablespoon of dried leaves for each cup of boiling water. Cover and steep for fifteen minutes. Strain. To decoct green hulls, place them in a pot, cover them with water, bring to a boil and simmer for twenty minutes. Strain.

TINCTURE: Fresh leaves – 1:2, 95%. Dried leaves – 1:5, 80%. Green hulls – 1:5, 95%.

SALVE: To make a salve, infuse fresh or dry black walnut leaves and green hulls in vegetable oil. Traditional folk recipes recommend boiling black walnut hulls in hog lard if you happen to have some on hand.

DOSAGES

Careful attention to dosing is essential for safe internal use.

DECOCTION: Use decoctions to wash the skin or as a compress. Apply once or twice a day until symptoms improve.

TINCTURE: Take one-fourth teaspoon in water once a day. Along with diet changes and other anti-fungal protocols, long-term use (several weeks) may be needed for systemic yeast infections.

SALVE: Apply once or twice a day as needed.

HARVESTING

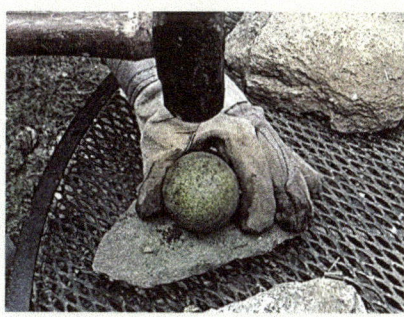

Collect black walnut leaves in early summer before the fruits fully form.

Walnuts fall to the ground while still green in early autumn. I have always used green hulls but some only use them when they turn black.

With green hulls, crack them open with a hammer and use a sturdy, sharp knife to separate the hull from the nut. With black hulls, place them in a burlap bag on a paved surface, then drive a car over it several times. Remove the bag and, wearing gloves, separate the hulls from the nuts. To eat the nuts, let them age for a few months in a cool, dry place (out of reach of squirrels and chipmunks) before cracking them open and picking out nut meats.

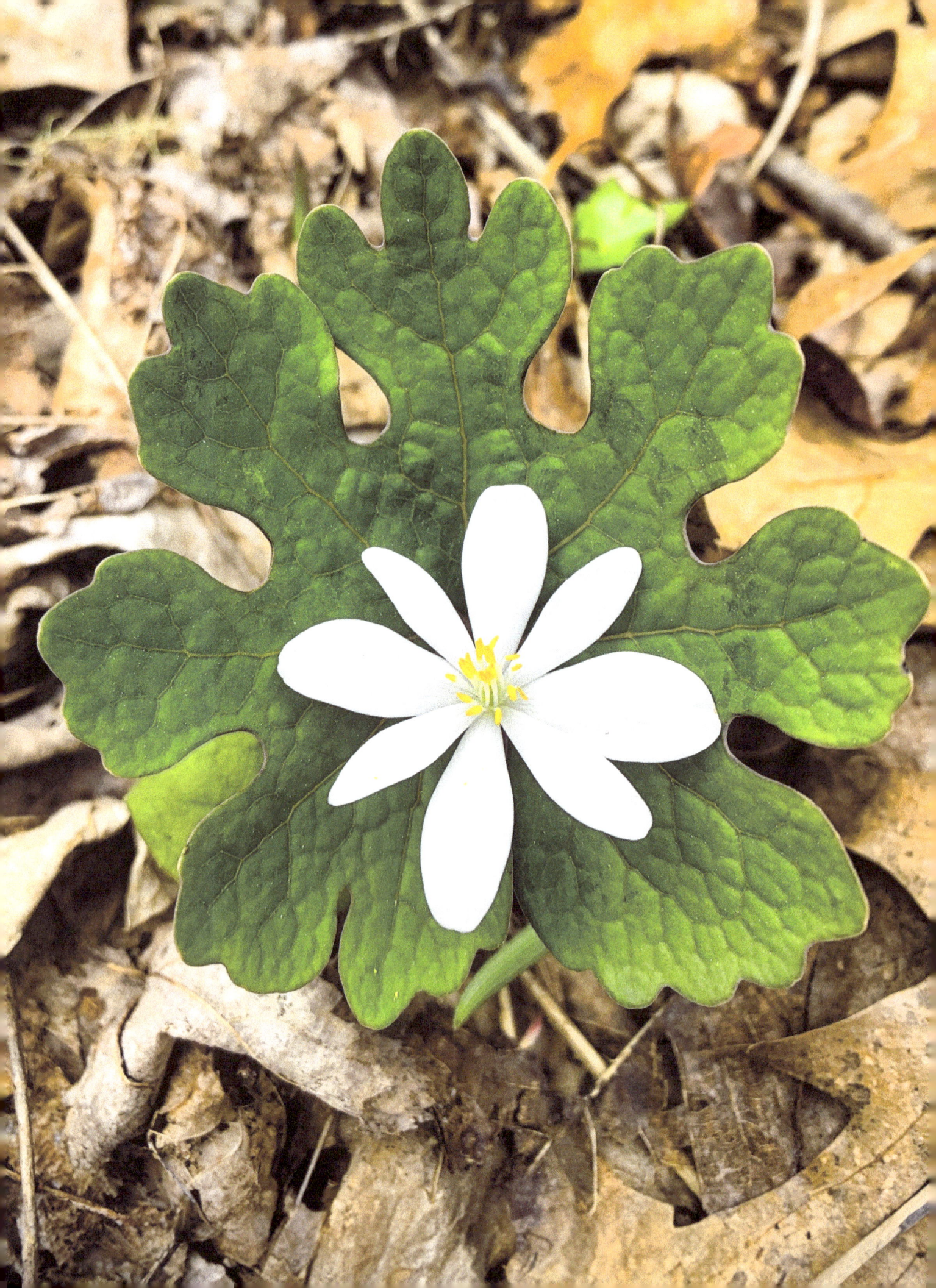

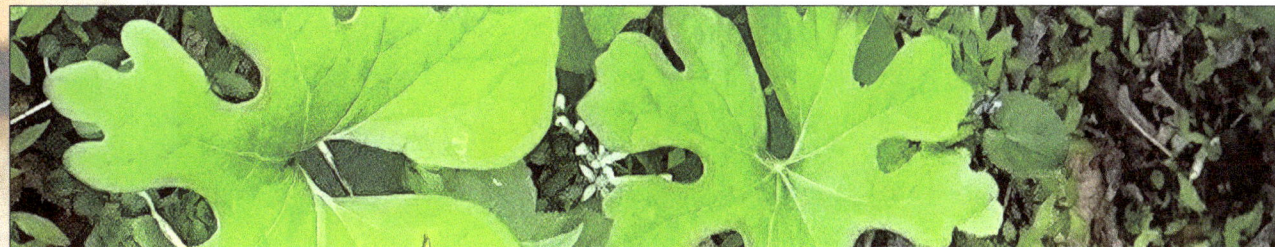

Bloodroot

COMMON NAME: Bloodroot

BOTANICAL NAME: *Sanguinaria canadensis*

FAMILY: *Papaveraceae* (Poppy)

OTHER NAMES: Puccoon, Red Puccoon, Indian Paint

DESCRIPTION: Bloodroot is one of the earliest spring ephemerals that blooms before the leaf canopy fully emerges. The leaf appears as a vertical tube, and the flower rises on a separate stalk, moving through the vertical leaf and blooming above the foliage. The solitary white flower has golden yellow stamens; it blooms briefly, and as the flowers fade, the leaf unfurls. Bloodroot leaf has a unique palmate shape described as 'irregularly lobed.' It reminds me of a large green jigsaw puzzle piece. The entire plant ranges from four to six inches tall. The root is thick and fleshy, about the size and shape of a little finger, and when cut, secretes a bright red-orange juice. This juice is caustic and may cause skin irritation.

Small, lipid-rich nubs, known as elaiosomes, attached to bloodroot seeds attract ants who carry seeds back to their nest, where they eat the elaiosomes and discard the seeds, which then germinate.

HABITAT: Deciduous hardwood forests

KEY ACTIONS: Stimulating expectorant, antispasmodic, anti-inflammatory, cathartic, emetic, escharotic, emmenagogue

PART USED: Rhizome

TRADITIONAL USES: Bloodroot is one of the best-known indigenous remedies in the Appalachians and throughout the Eastern States, and it has a long history of use. It was reputed to be an effective external treatment for malignant and benign skin conditions. A paste of the fresh root, combined with zinc chloride and other herbs, sometimes referred to as black salve, was repeatedly applied to the skin. The result was necrosis, as the salve burned away the healthy skin and, hopefully, the skin growth;

this treatment was also used to remove warts, skin tags, and fungal infections. Native Americans used bloodroot as a basketry dye.[1]

In the 19th century, a physician noted that bloodroot "cures or relieves pneumonic inflammation, while it checks or suppresses expectoration."[2] It was combined with wild ginger, rabbit tobacco, wild cherry, and lobelia, as a cough remedy. The powdered root was inhaled as a snuff and thought to act as a tonic stimulant to reduce mucus in the lungs and sinuses. Bloodroot was carried as a love charm and believed to have aphrodisiac properties. Tommie Bass noted that African Americans drank bloodroot-infused whiskey to "build a nature" or increase sex drive.[3]

CURRENT USES: Bloodroot is a low-dose botanical. Small doses relax the bronchioles to ease breathing difficulties. At the same time, it acts as a stimulating expectorant to clear congestion from the lungs. The tincture is used in formulas with other expectorant and demulcent herbs to relieve bronchitis, coughs, and lung congestion. It also reduces inflammation in the throat and lungs. Bloodroot tincture warms the stomach to relieve symptoms of dampness such as indigestion, gas and bloating. It also stimulates bile secretions and relieves liver congestion in treating hepatitis and jaundice.

Bloodroot salve is applied to slow-healing sores, ulcerations, eczema, and warts. It is also an ingredient in escharotic cancer salves, which are used to eliminate tumors and basal cell carcinomas. However, evidence of its effectiveness is controversial.[4] Bloodroot reduces gum inflammation and plaque build-up as an ingredient in commercial mouthwash and toothpaste.

CAUTIONS: Tinctures and salves are the most common bloodroot preparations. However, bloodroot is a low-dose botanical, so the tincture is made using a ratio of one part bloodroot to ten parts menstruum. Contraindicated for internal use in pregnancy, when nursing, or for children.

---

[1] Banks, *Plants of the Cherokee*, 54

[2] Moerman, *Native American Ethnobotany*, 83

[3] Crellin and Philpott, *A Reference Guide to Medicinal Plants*, 102

[4] *Int. J. Mol. Sci.* 2016, 17, 1414; doi:10.3390/ijms17091414, *Sanguinaria canadensis:* Traditional Medicine, Phytochemical Composition, Biological Activities and Current Uses.

PREPARATIONS

Bloodroot is a low-dose botanical. Prepare tinctures using a higher ratio of menstruum to herb as indicated. Use fresh root for tinctures and dried root for infused oils.

TINCTURE: Fresh root – 1:10, 50%.

SALVE: Prepare a standard salve with an infused oil made with dried bloodroot. Consider combining with other vulnerary herbs to reduce chances of skin irritation.

DOSAGES

Careful attention to dosage is essential for safe internal use. Tinctures should be accurately measured in drop doses. Traditionally, the tincture is used internally to treat lung congestion and coughs, but always along with other demulcent lung herbs such as the leaves of mullein *(Verbascum thapsus)*, plantain *(Plantago major)*, or coltsfoot *(Tussilago farfara)*. Bloodroot is usually less than one-eighth part of the total formula.

TINCTURE: Take five drops of tincture diluted in one ounce of water three to four times a day. As a mouthwash for gum inflammation or to reduce plaque, add ten drops of tincture to one cup of warm water.

SALVE: Apply daily to the affected area and cover with cotton gauze. Bloodroot salve may cause some degree of skin inflammation.

HARVESTING

Collect the rhizome in early spring after the flower fades or in late summer as the leaves turn yellow. Contact with the fresh root can cause skin irritation; gloves are recommended.

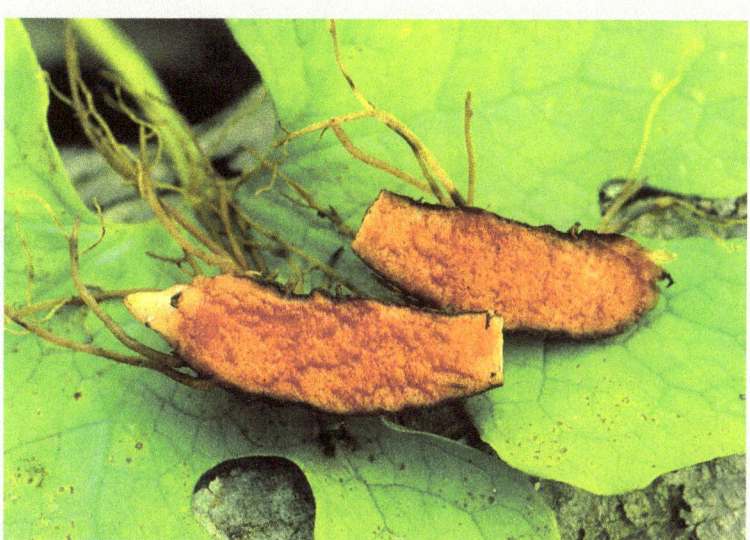

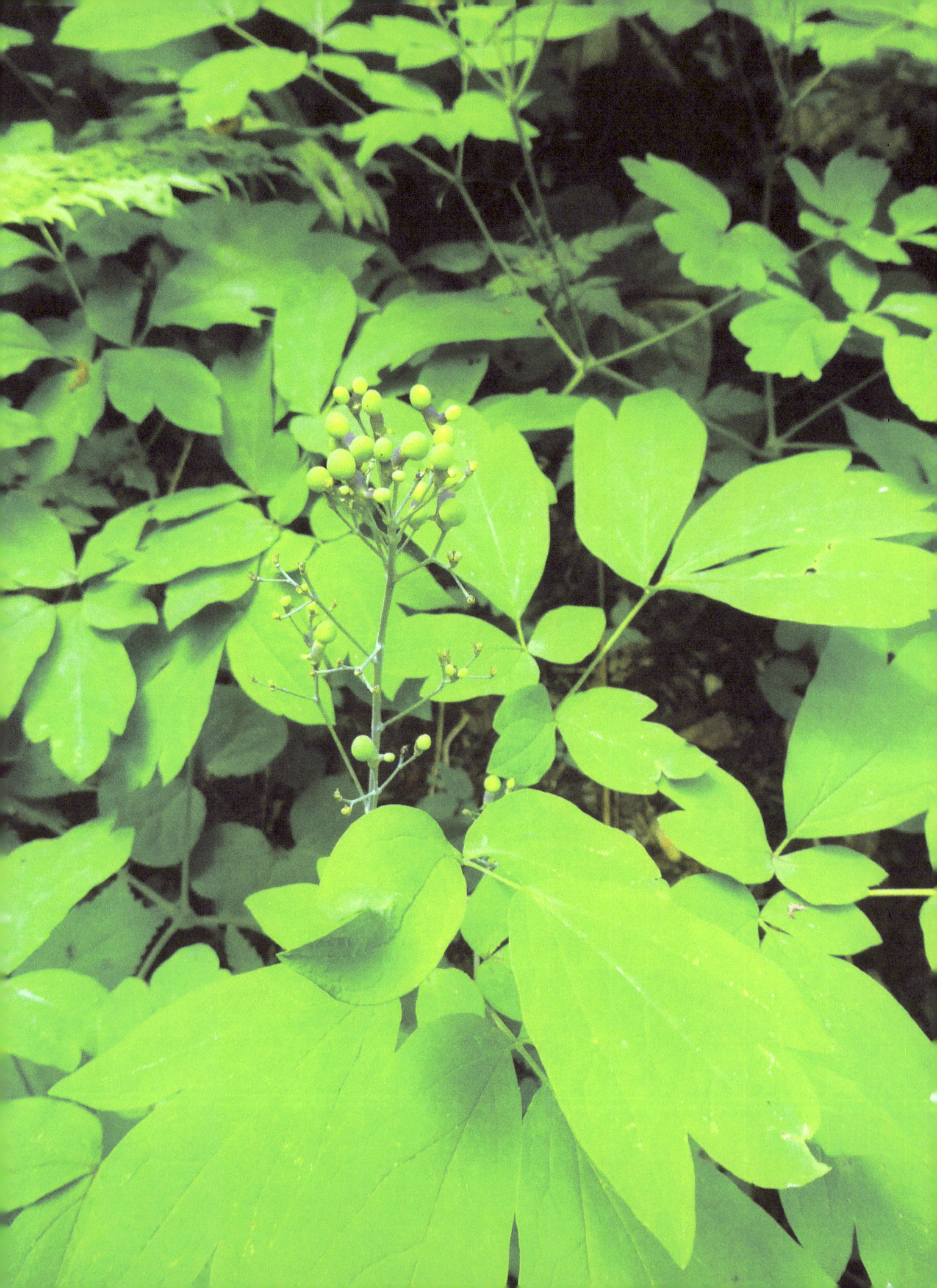

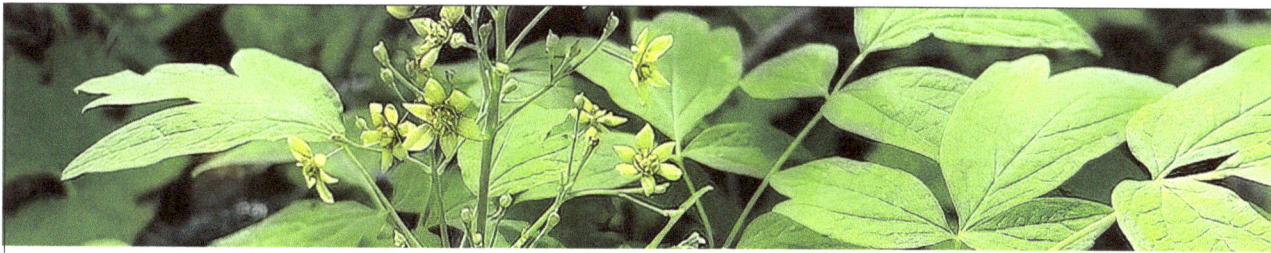

Blue Cohosh

COMMON NAME: Blue Cohosh

BOTANICAL NAME: *Caulophyllum thalictroides*

FAMILY: *Berberidaceae* (Barberry)

DESCRIPTION: An airy, delicate perennial, about two feet tall, blue cohosh has compound leaves, each with two or three delicately lobed leaflets. Leaves are irregular and of various shapes. The underside of the leaf has a blue-green cast that contrasts with the surface color. Small clusters of chartreuse flowers, composed of six tiny sepals with even smaller actual petals at the base, bloom in terminal clusters in early April and turn brown as they age. The fruit, the size and color of a blueberry, is inedible and toxic; it often persists after the foliage yellows and fades in late summer. The leaves of blue cohosh resemble those of meadow rue *(Thalictrum polygamun* or *T. revolutum),* which often grows nearby. Meadow rue is a much taller plant (two to four feet) with tiny white flowers that give off a distinctive sharp odor and is unsafe for internal use.

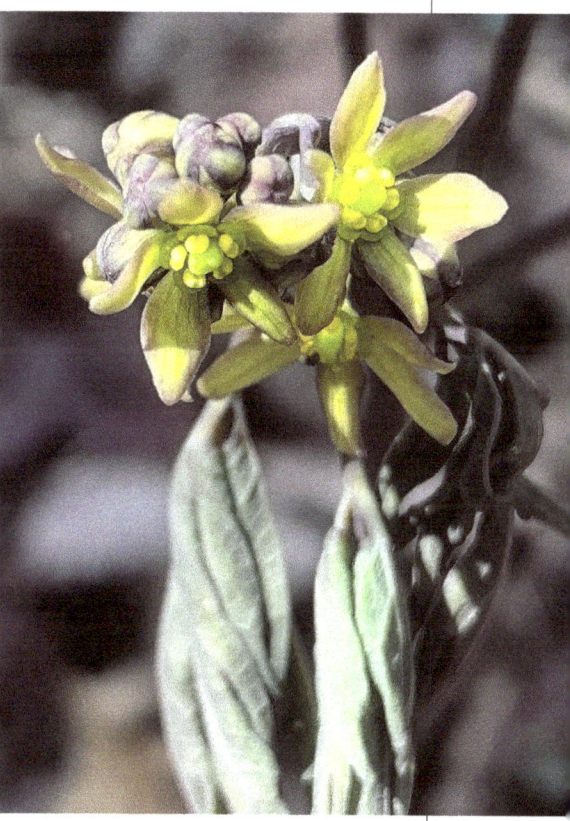

HABITAT: In moist places in deciduous forests. It is found on hillsides in deep shade, often with black cohosh, trillium *(Trillium spp.),* and bloodroot.

KEY ACTIONS: Uterine tonic, oxytocic, antispasmodic, emmenagogue, anodyne

PART USED: Rhizome and root

TRADITIONAL USES: Blue cohosh was used to stimulate and regulate contractions in childbirth and as a general tonic for the female generative system, usually in combination with black cohosh. It was used internally to relieve joint pain from osteoarthritis and rheumatism. As an antispasmodic, it relieved colic, hiccups, muscle cramps and spasms. Blue cohosh was used as a partus preparator during the final weeks of pregnancy to

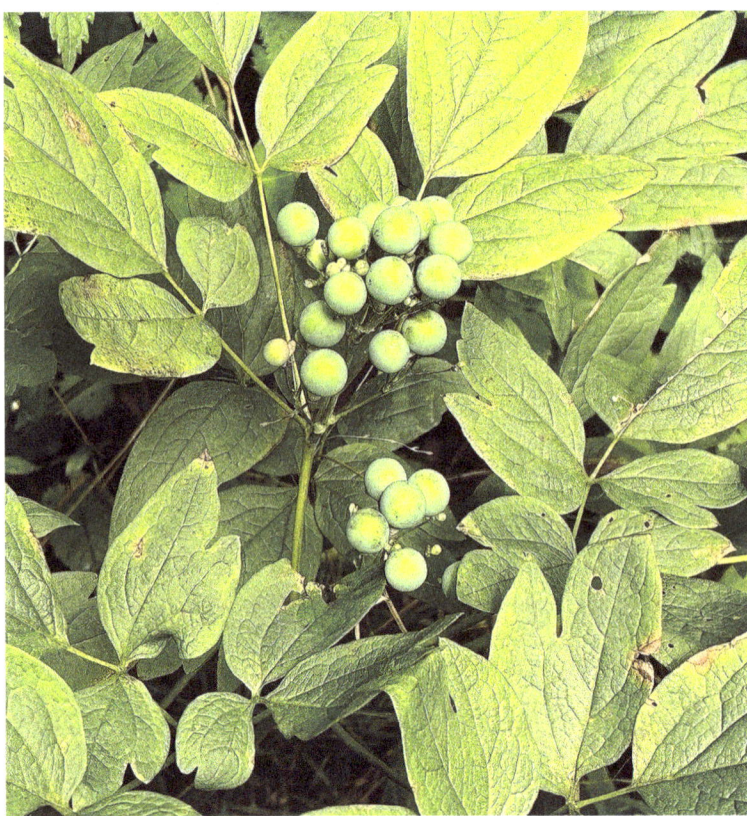

ensure easy labor; however, there are concerns about its safety, and it is no longer used for this purpose.[1]

CURRENT USES: Blue cohosh is a tonic for the female generative system. It strengthens uterine function and is often included in formulas to promote fertility, especially for women with a history of miscarriage. Blue cohosh relieves pain caused by endometriosis, fibroid tumors, polycystic ovaries, menstrual cramps and menopausal headaches. It may bring on delayed menses.

As an antispasmodic, it also eases bronchial spasms and wheezing in asthma and allergic reactions, soothes persistent coughs, and is used to relieve bronchitis symptoms.

CAUTIONS: Contraindicated in pregnancy. There is evidence blue cohosh could harm the fetus,[2] though blue cohosh is sometimes used to facilitate labor by practitioners trained in its safe use. Do not use with medications for cardiovascular disease, blood thinning drugs or if experiencing elevated blood pressure. High doses may cause headaches, nausea, and vomiting.

---

[1] Romm, *Botanical Medicine for Women's Health*, 529

[2] Ibid.

PREPARATIONS

DECOCTION: Use one teaspoon dry or one tablespoon fresh root for each cup of water. Cover and decoct for ten minutes. Strain.

TINCTURE: Fresh – 1:2, 70%. Dried – 1:5, 50%.

DOSAGES

DECOCTION: Drink a half cup three to four times daily to relieve symptoms.

TINCTURE: Take one-half teaspoon in a small amount of water three to four times daily or as needed to relieve symptoms.

HARVESTING

Dig roots in the late summer as the foliage begins to fade. The rhizome and rootlets are difficult to unearth and clean. See black cohosh for more sustainable collection suggestions as blue cohosh is considered At Risk by UpS.

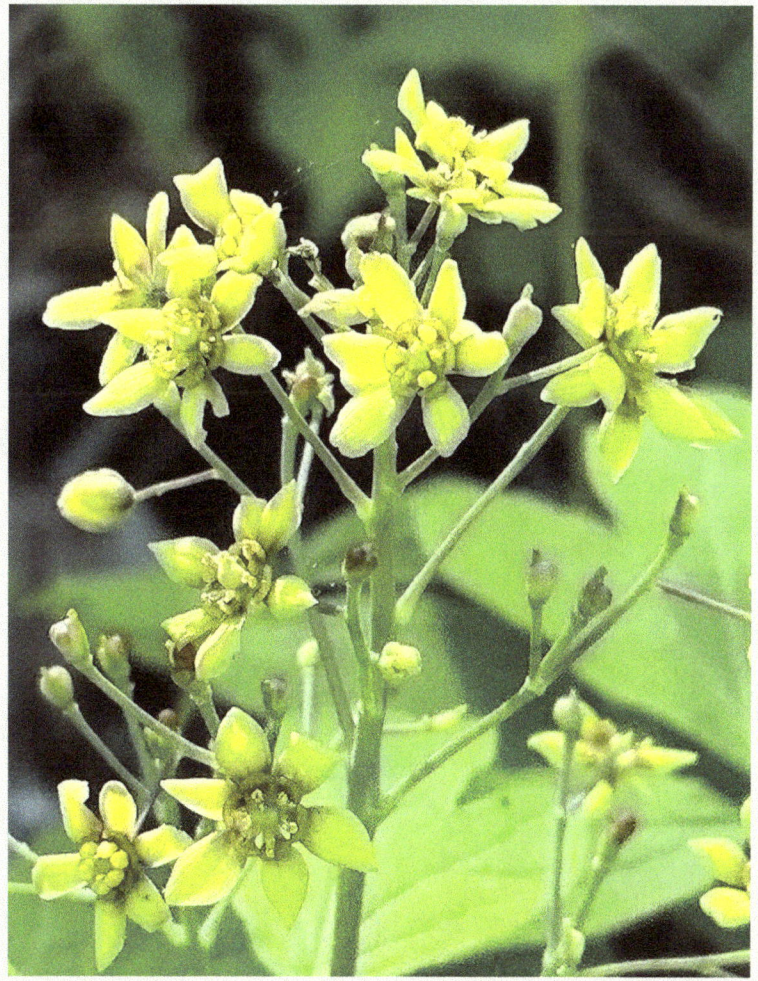

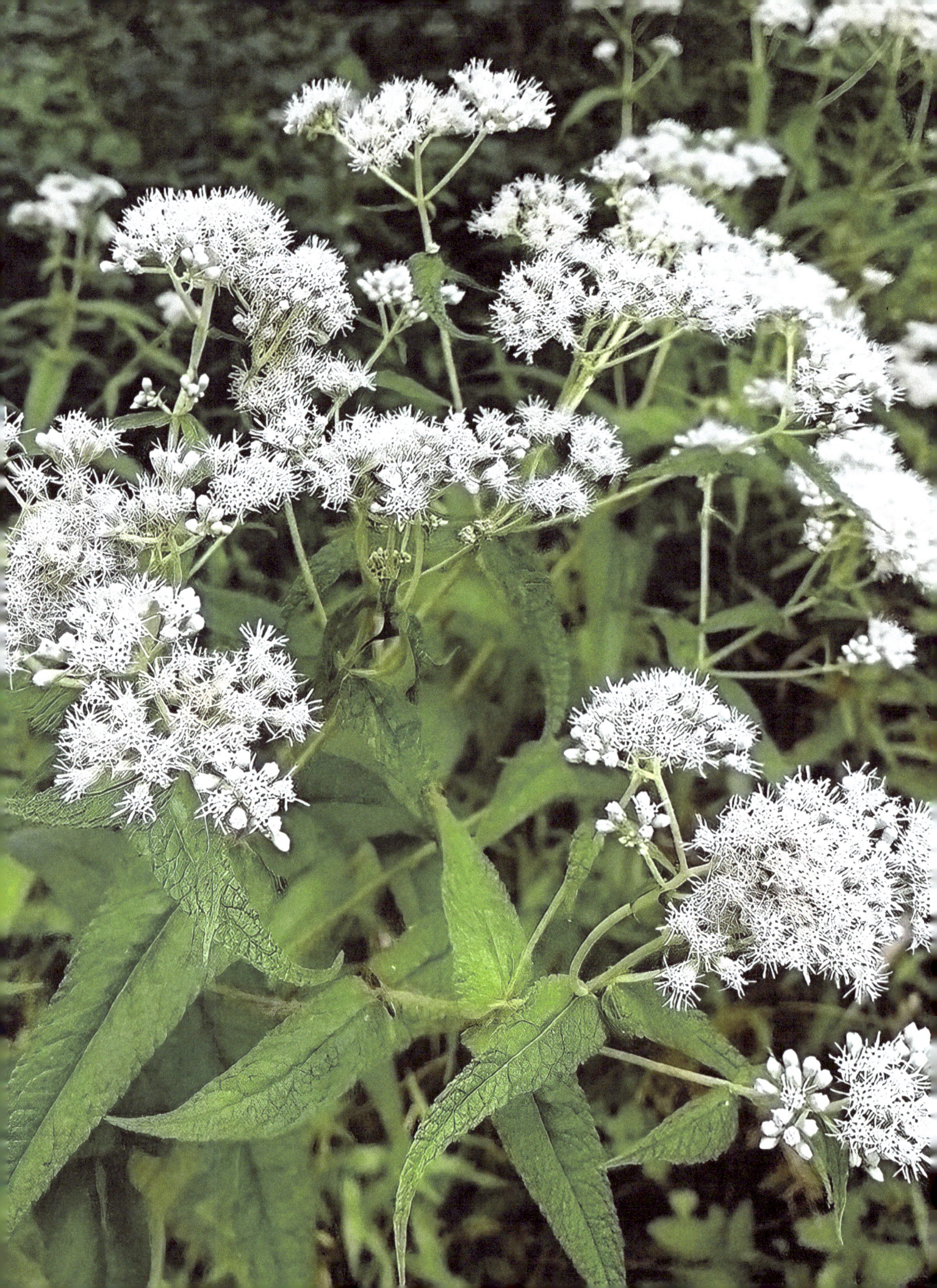

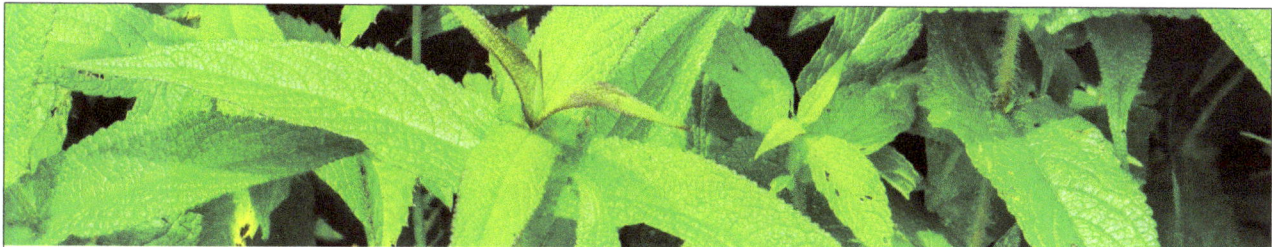

Boneset

COMMON NAME: Boneset

BOTANICAL NAME: *Eupatorium perfoliatum*

FAMILY: *Asteraceae* (Aster)

OTHER NAMES: Thoroughwort, Ague Weed, Indian Sage

DESCRIPTION: Boneset is a perennial herb, one to four feet tall, with a single stem ending in a slightly branched cluster of small, shaggy, white flowers. It blooms from August to October. Boneset has distinctive opposing leaves that are slightly toothed and joined at the base, so the stem appears to perforate the leaves, hence the species name *perfoliatum*. The leaf has a rough texture, and the leaves and stem are covered with soft white hair.

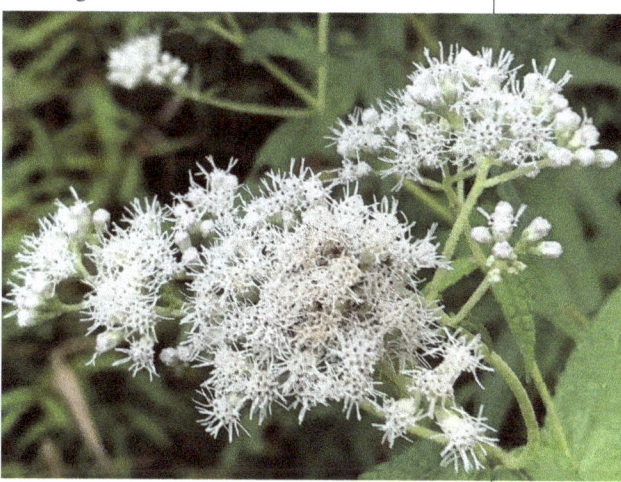

HABITAT: Common in sunny, open fields and partial shade along waterways.

KEY ACTIONS: Expectorant, diaphoretic, immune stimulant, antibiotic, digestive bitter, analgesic, laxative, emetic

PART USED: Aerial (in flower)

TRADITIONAL USES: Boneset was an essential herbal medicine for Native Americans. Enslaved Africans and European colonists also used it. American Indians used the tea to treat colds, flu, respiratory infections and fevers. They consider it a tonic for poor digestion and helpful in relieving rheumatic pain. The common name "boneset" refers to its analgesic properties when used to treat dengue fever, as it relieves the intense muscle pain that feels like bones are breaking. They also soaked broken bones in boneset tea to stimulate bone growth and relieve pain.

During the 1800s, boneset may have been one of the most frequently used household herbs in the eastern United States. Maude Grieve, writing in 1931, noted that "No plant in American domestic practice having more

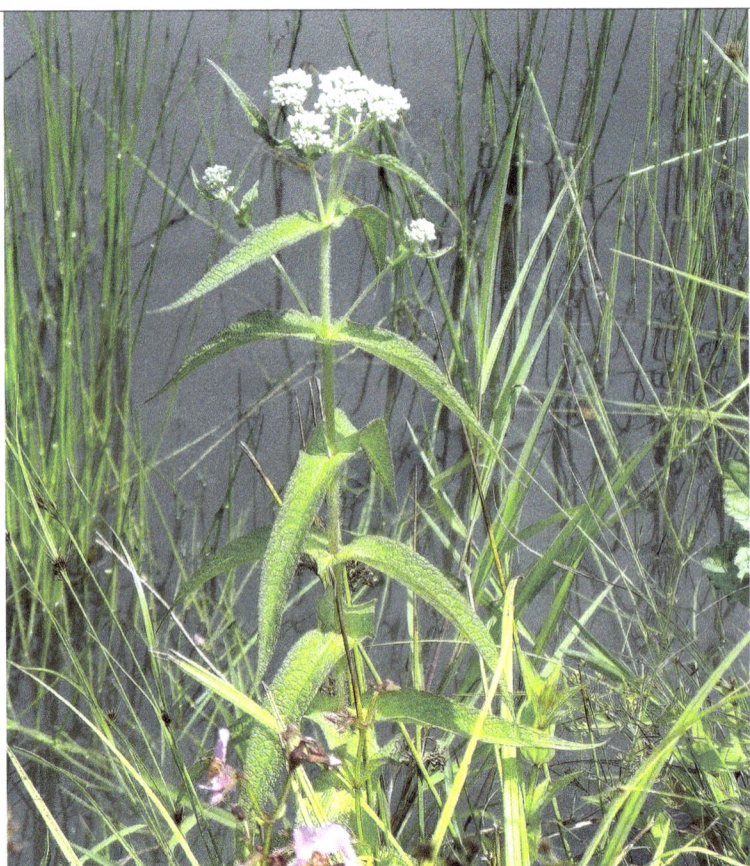

extensive and frequent use."[1] Boneset was used extensively during the Spanish Flu epidemic in 1918 – 1919. Strong infusions relieve fever, calm coughs, stop headaches and reduce rheumatic joint pain. Boneset was also used as an emetic to remove mucus from the stomach. Eclectic physicians strongly promoted it as an immune stimulant and anti-inflammatory agent after it was shown to contain water-soluble polysaccharides.

Herbalist Tommie Bass of Alabama included boneset in almost every liquid medicine he made. He claimed many "old-timers" would make a strong, hot boneset infusion and soak their feet to "steam themselves."[2] Bass regularly made cough syrup with boneset, elder flowers, cherry bark, mullein *(Verbascum thapsus)*, rabbit tobacco and sweetgum.

CURRENT USES: Boneset is one of the most effective herbs for treating colds and influenza. Like echinacea *(Echinacea spp.)*, boneset contains water-soluble polysaccharides that stimulate the immune response. When drunk hot, boneset acts as a diaphoretic to induce sweating and reduce fevers. It also helps break up lung congestion. As an analgesic, it is specific for body aches and pains caused by fever or rheumatism.

An underused tonic for the digestive system, boneset strengthens the entire system. It dispels dampness, stimulates digestion, and supports the

---

[1] Grieve, *A Modern Herbal*, 116

[2] Crellin and Philpott, *A Reference Guide to Medicinal Plants*, 106

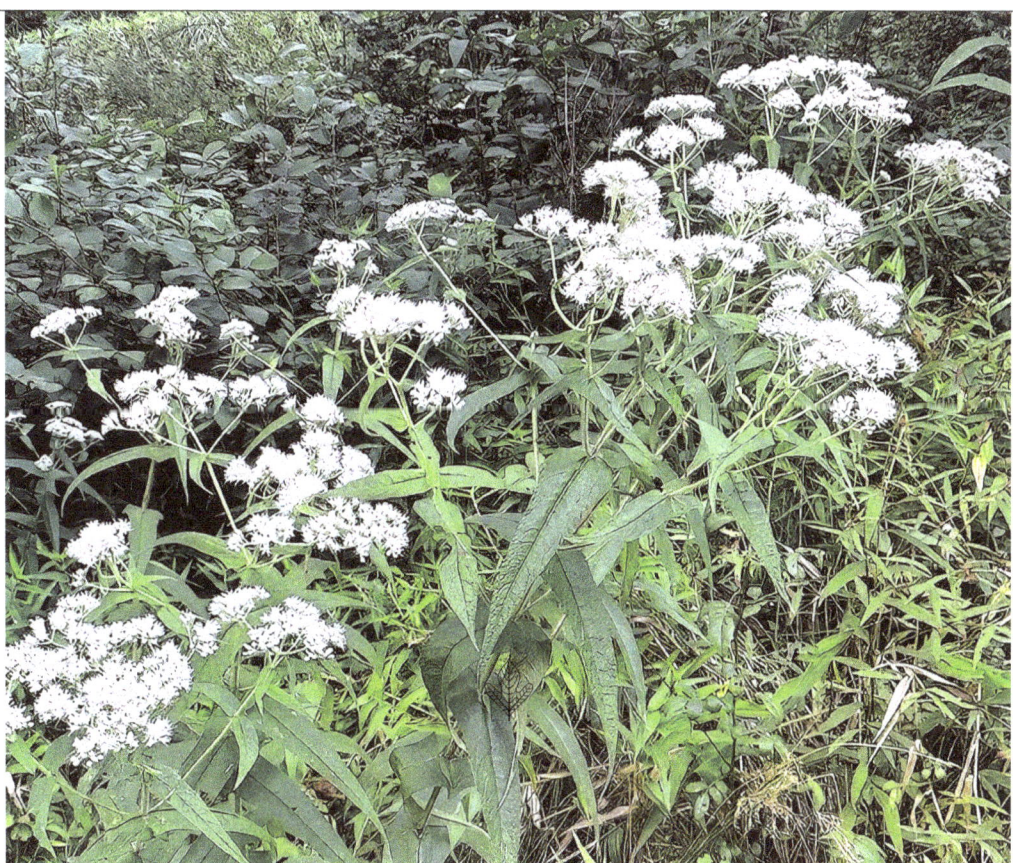

liver. Taking small doses, one-fourth to one-half cup of infusion or one-fourth teaspoon of tincture after meals invigorates digestion and relieves indigestion, gas, belching, bloating, chronic constipation, and lethargy after eating. It also increases appetite, especially among the sick and elderly. Be sure to read CAUTIONS before using boneset.

CAUTIONS: Boneset contains pyrrolizidine alkaloids, potentially harmful to the liver. Do not use the boneset daily for more than two weeks and avoid it entirely if you have a history of liver disease. Boneset is contraindicated in pregnancy and while nursing. Do not give to children under twelve years of age. Doses larger than those recommended here may cause nausea, vomiting, and severe diarrhea; should this occur, discontinue use and symptoms should subside.

"It is just as bitter as all get-out, but when you sweeten it down, it's all right, and so we think it is as good a one as the Lord put out there. Try it to start when you think you're taking a cold, or you're nervous or got rheumatism, why you just make the tea and drink it as hot as you can bear it."

Tommie Bass, (1988) A Reference Guide to Medicinal Plants

PREPARATIONS

Due to its bitterness, boneset needs help to be palatable and frequent or large doses may cause nausea. For this reason, I make boneset syrup (see recipe) to add to hot teas. You can also use fresh or dry boneset to make tinctures.

INFUSION: Add one and one-half teaspoons of dried or one tablespoon of fresh boneset to each cup of water. Steep for fifteen minutes. To counter the bitter taste, sweeten liberally with honey. Boneset infusions may be made with hot or cold water. Hot water infusions relieve cold and flu symptoms, while cold infusions invigorate the digestive system.

TINCTURE: Fresh – 1:2. Dried – 1:5, 50%.

SYRUP: See recipe on page 59.

DOSAGES

Boneset is an intensely bitter herb. It is probably not a remedy for anyone unconvinced of the benefits of herbal healing!

INFUSION: Prepare a standard infusion. Drink one-half cup of hot boneset infusion every two hours to relieve cold and flu symptoms. To reduce fever, repeat every thirty to forty minutes until you experience sweating and your temperature drops. Use cold infusions for sluggish digestion; take one to two tablespoons after meals or as needed.

TINCTURE: Add one-half teaspoon to water or tea every two hours for general cold and flu symptoms. To reduce a fever, add one-half teaspoon of tincture to hot tea and drink every thirty minutes until you experience sweating and a drop in temperature.

SYRUP: Add one tablespoon of boneset syrup (see recipe) to a cup of hot tea and follow the dosing recommendations for teas. Combines well with elderflower, mountain mint (or any other mint like bee balm), mullein *(Verbascum thapsus),* and echinacea *(Echinacea spp.).*

Boneset tincture and infusion may be used interchangeably. Feel free to sweeten boneset infusions with liberal amounts of honey to make the taste bearable. When using boneset as a digestive aid, you must taste the bitter flavor to stimulate gastric secretions and drink small doses without sweeteners if possible.

HARVESTING

Harvest boneset in late summer just as the flowers bloom. Collect the entire plant from the ground up. Discard any yellowed or damaged leaves. Boneset dries quickly, even in humid weather. Bundle four or five stems with a rubber band and put the bundled herbs in a paper bag with the flower end down. Gather the bag around the base of the stems, secure it with a second rubber band and hang it in a cool, dark place to dry. The dry herb is ready when leaves crumble easily. Crumble leaves and flowers into small pieces and store in glass jars.

BONESET SYRUP

This basic syrup recipe can be made with a single herb like boneset or a combination of herbs. Herbal syrups are used for colds, flu, coughs, fevers, and respiratory infections. Other herbs that combine well with boneset include mullein leaf *(V. thapsus),* rabbit tobacco, sumac berries, and mountain mint.

Make a hot infusion using one ounce of dried or two ounces of fresh boneset (leaf and flower) with sixteen ounces of water. Pour boiling water over herbs in a canning jar or teapot; cover and steep for eight hours or overnight. Strain out the spent herb and discard. Return the infusion to a clean pot, bring to a boil and simmer until the total volume of liquid is reduced by half. Allow to cool slightly; measure and combine one part infusion with one-half part honey while still warm. Mix well. Store in a glass bottle in the refrigerator. Take one to two teaspoons as needed, or add syrup to hot tea.

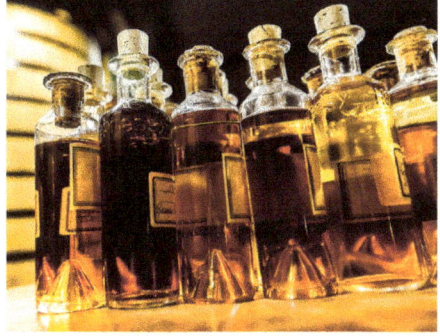

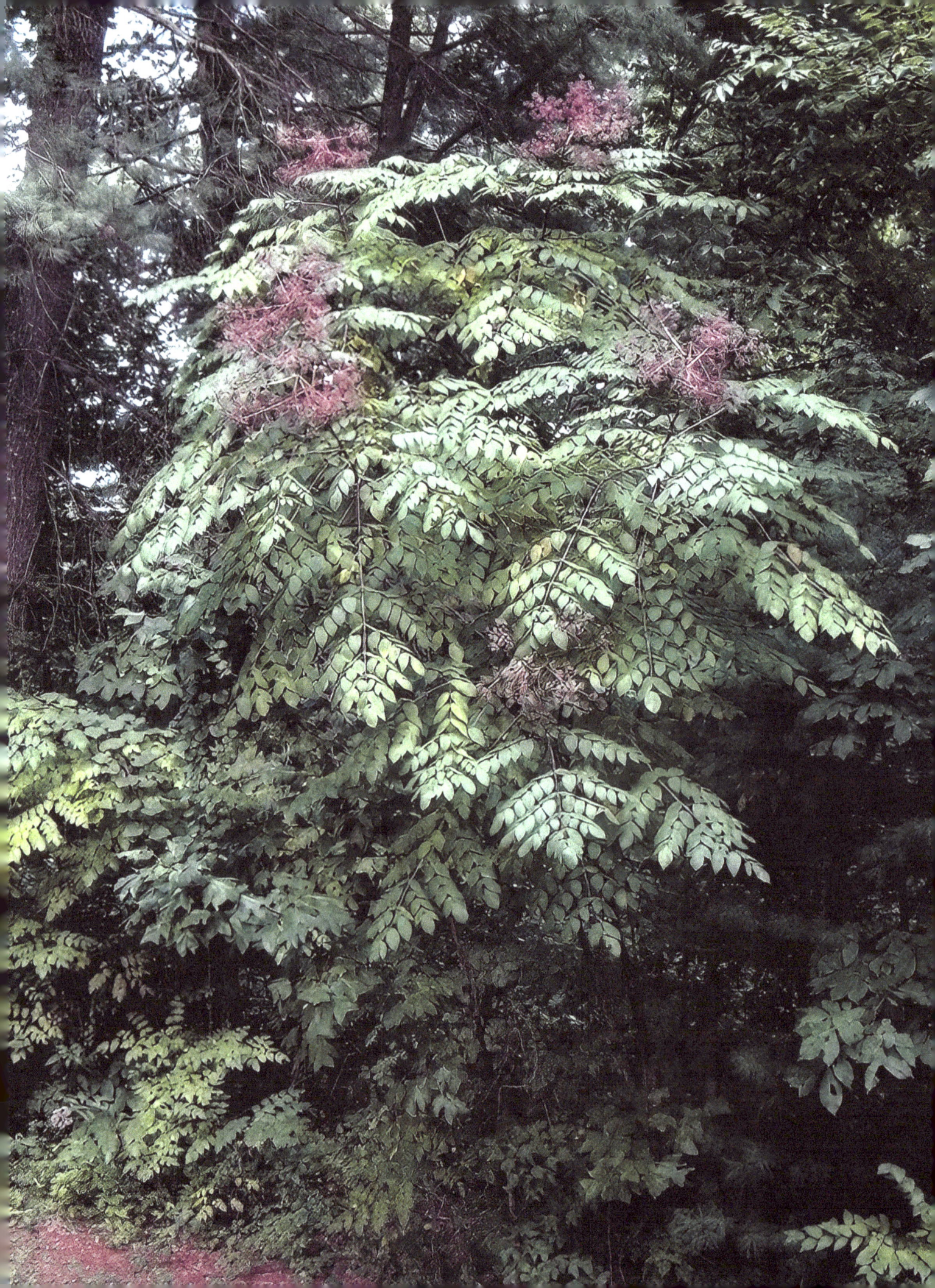

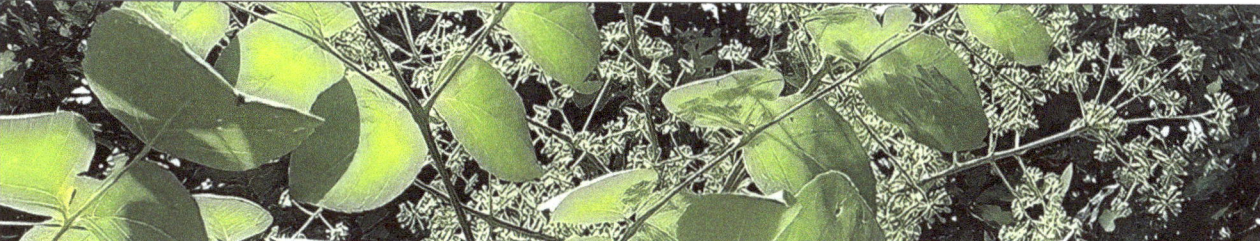

Devil's Walking Stick

COMMON NAME: Devil's Walking Stick

BOTANICAL NAME: *Aralia spinosa*

FAMILY: *Araliaceae* (Ginseng)

OTHER NAMES: Hercules' Club, Angelica Tree, Toothache Tree, Southern Prickly Ash

DESCRIPTION: A shrub or tree, between six and thirty feet tall, with sharp spines along a slender, woody trunk, and to a lesser degree, on stems and leaves, with large compound leaves, often two to four feet in size. Leaves are composed of twice-divided leaflets; the individual leaflets are deep green, smooth and finely toothed. Tiny white flowers bloom in large umbels between July and September, followed by masses of deep purple berries in September and October. Devil's walking stick is robust, growing up to ten feet in a year; it spreads by roots.

HABITAT: Forms thickets often found in transition zones at the edge of forests and open sunny areas.

KEY ACTIONS: Anti-rheumatic, circulatory stimulant, anti-inflammatory, emetic (in large doses)

PART USED: Berry or bark

TRADITIONAL USES: The Cherokee used the berries and bark to treat rheumatic pain. Roasted, pounded roots were decocted to make a powerful emetic. Tommie Bass recommended the berries and bark for rheumatism. Devil's walking stick has been used to treat earaches (drops of infused bark oil) and to relieve toothaches (chewing on strips of inner bark or packing the tooth with powdered bark) and rheumatic pain (berries infused in liquor).

CURRENT USES: Although the devil's walking stick has a long history of use in folk medicine, it is not available commercially. Its actions are

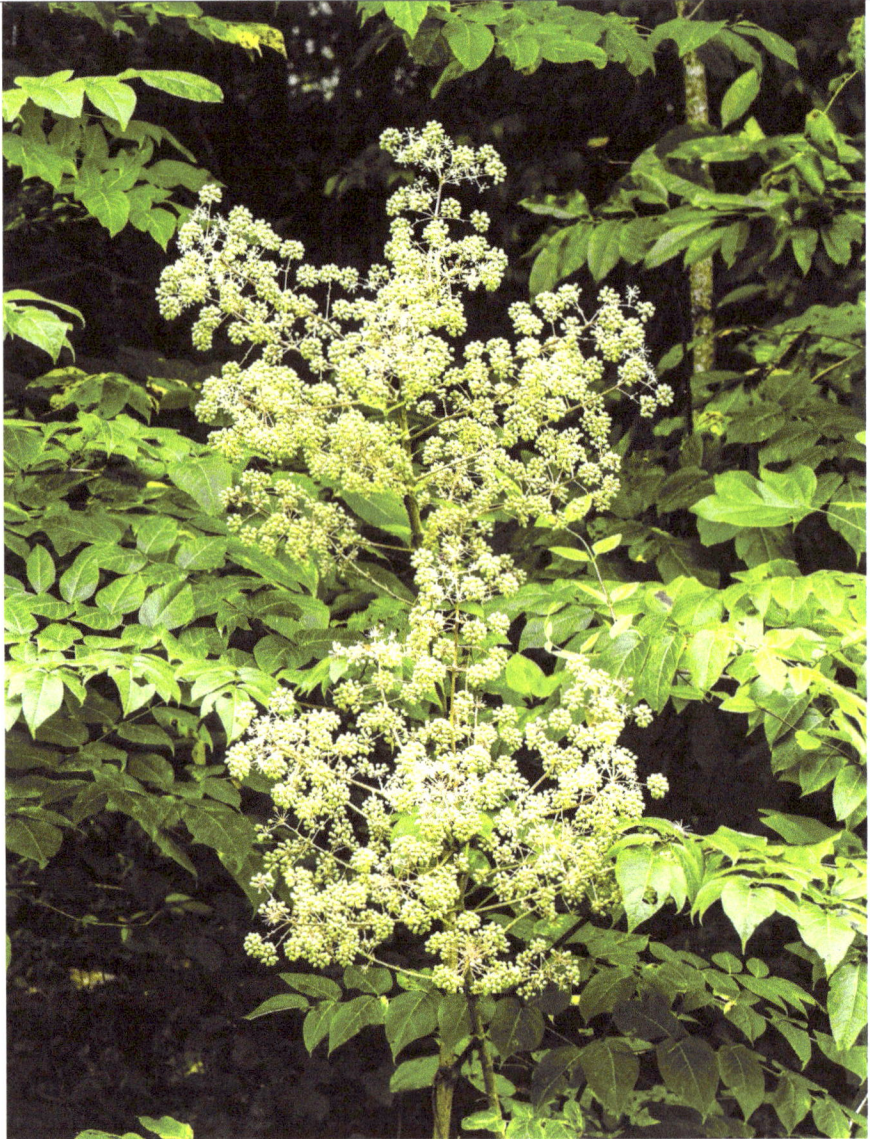

milder than those of prickly ash bark *(Zanthoxylum clava-herculis)*. A simple tincture of fresh berries or a bark decoction relieves rheumatic pain. Use drops of infused oil for earaches and powdered dried bark applied to the gums to relieve toothaches.

CAUTIONS: Although devil's walking stick enjoys a long history of folk use, use it cautiously and in small doses. In large doses, the berries and bark can cause nausea and vomiting. Do not use it internally in pregnancy, while nursing, or with children or babies.

PREPARATIONS

DECOCTION: Use one ounce of bark to one quart of water and decoct for twenty minutes. Strain and use within twenty-four hours.

TINCTURE: Make a simple berry tincture when berries ripen in the fall. Strip the berries from the stem, place them in a quart jar and crush them with a wooden spoon to release their juices. Cover entirely with brandy, whiskey or other liquor. Shake daily for two weeks. Strain and store in a glass bottle. Herbalist Tommie Bass recommended using 1 pint of 100-proof whiskey for every 6 ounces of fresh berries.

INFUSED OIL: Cut fresh bark into thin strips (having removed and discarded the thorns). Place in a heavy cooking pot and cover completely with olive oil. Heat until the oil barely simmers; watch carefully. Use tongs to lift a strip or two of the bark every ten minutes. If they start to stiffen and become rigid (they may even crackle), remove from heat and cool. Strain and store in a glass bottle in the refrigerator.

DOSAGES

DECOCTION: Drink one-half cup of bark decoction two or three times daily to relieve rheumatic pain. If there is no improvement, increase to one cup three times a day.

TINCTURE: Follow the directions above to prepare a simple berry tincture. To relieve rheumatic pain, take one teaspoon twice a day. The tincture can be applied directly to the tooth as needed for toothaches.

INFUSED OIL: Warm the oil and put one or two drops of oil in the ears. Repeat as needed.

HARVESTING

Collect bark in early spring as soon as the plant can be positively identified or in the fall after the leaves begin to fade. Carefully strip the bark from the trunk, avoiding and discarding the spikes. Leather gloves are needed here! Reserve the inner bark. Harvest berries in the fall when they are a deep purple. Devil's walking stick is abundant throughout most of its range, and there are few concerns about its conservation.

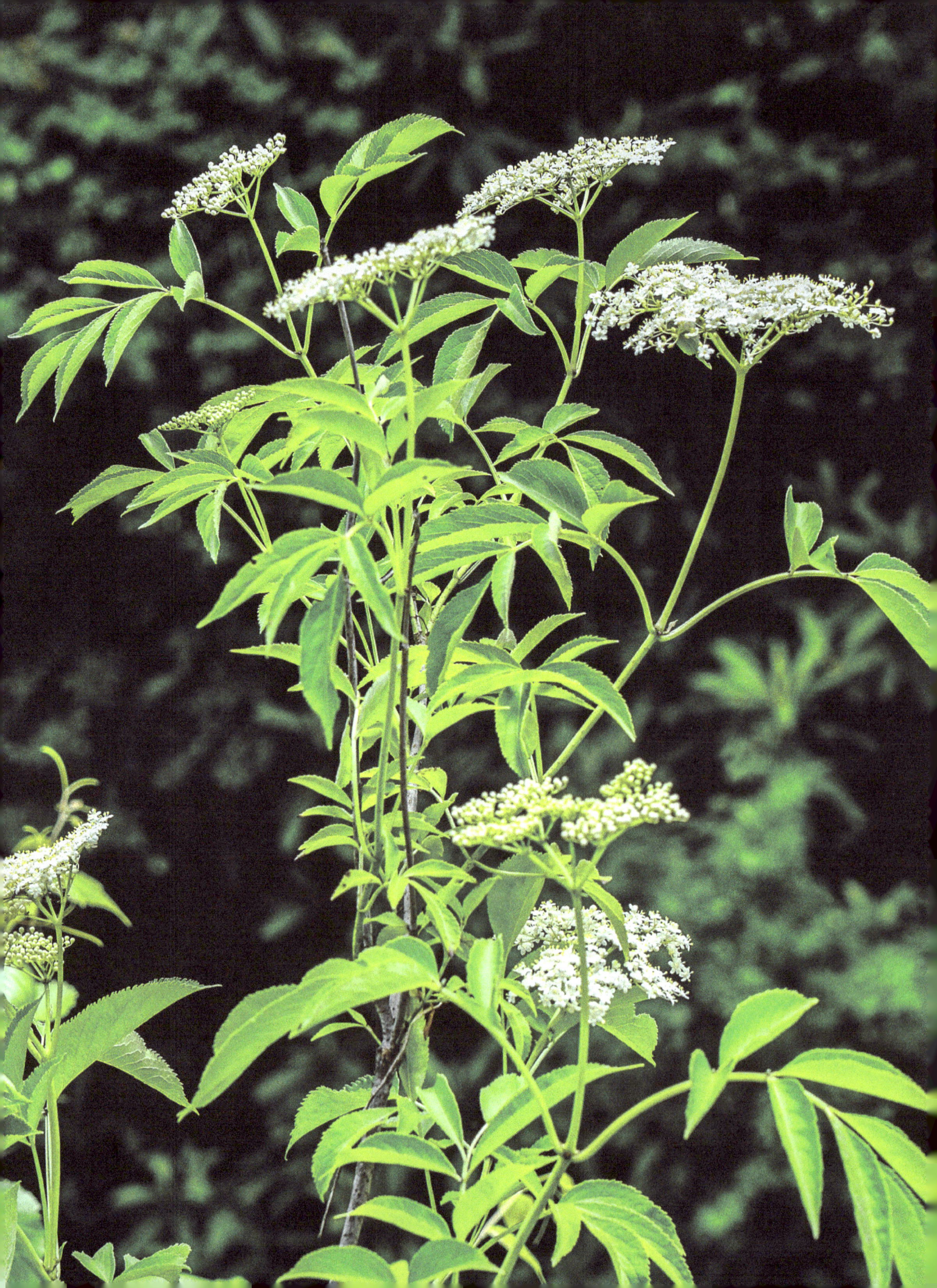

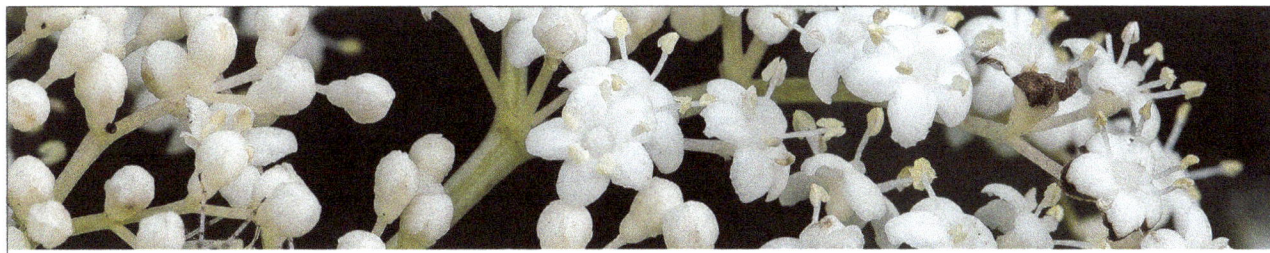

Elder

COMMON NAME: Elder

BOTANICAL NAME: *Sambucus canadensis*

FAMILY: *Caprifoliaceae* (Honeysuckle)

DESCRIPTION: Elder is a deciduous shrub or small tree with multiple stems, fifteen to twenty feet tall, common throughout the eastern woodlands. Pinnately compound leaves are dark green, finely serrated and in pairs. Large clusters of small white, five-petaled flowers in early summer have a slightly cloying fragrance. In late summer, bunches of dark blue-purple berries (or drupes) ripen, often weighing the branches down. The bark of younger branches has spongy ridges (or lenticels) and a soft, cottony pith in the center.

HABITAT: Usually found in damp habitats and along the edges of woodlands, it spreads through rhizomes and often forms thickets.

KEY ACTIONS: Every part of the elder has some medicinal activity, but the actions vary significantly.

Flower: diaphoretic, expectorant, anti-catarrhal, astringent, anti-inflammatory

Leaf: emollient, vulnerary, astringent

Berry: anti-viral, diaphoretic, anti-catarrhal, expectorant, mild laxative, astringent

PART USED: Flower, leaf, berry

TRADITIONAL USES: Elder has a long history of use in North America and Europe. Archaeological evidence suggests that it has been used since Neolithic times. American Indians drank hot elderflower infusions to induce sweating, relieve coughs, treat colds and reduce fevers. Poultices of leaf and bark were used for breast inflammation, burns, wounds, and swellings. Leaves were used as salves to treat skin infections, boils, and other hot eruptive conditions. Cooked or dried berries were used as food.

> *"In Denmark, we come across the old belief that he who stood under an Elder tree on Midsummer Eve would see the King of Fairyland ride by, attended by all his retinue."*
>
> Maude Grieve, (1931) *A Modern Herbal*

CURRENT USES: Although all parts of the elder shrub have medicinal properties, the flower and berry are most commonly used in herbal practice. The leaf is for external use only.

Hot infusions of elderflowers are effective for treating colds and flu as the diaphoretic action of the hot tea stimulates the surface immune system to fight off invading pathogens, induce sweating and reduce fevers. With respiratory infections, elderflower infusions help disperse congestion and soothe coughs. Elderflower also relieves seasonal allergy symptoms such as itchy eyes, runny nose and throat irritation.

Elderberries have little flavor and are toxic when fresh. They address many of the same symptoms as the flower but also have anti-viral properties. Elderberry syrup is a traditional remedy for respiratory infections, relieving coughs and lung congestion.

Elderberry wine or cordial is a traditional digestive aid and is mildly laxative. The berries are used for syrups, wine, jams, and pies but must be sweetened or combined with other fruits like raisins or crabapples.

Salves or infused oils made with elderflowers or leaves are used to heal wounds and relieve dry, irritated skin and itching. Elder leaf infusions are used topically as a wash for cleaning wounds and soothing burns. Apply fresh leaf poultice or salve to painful bruises.

CAUTIONS: Fresh elderberries are toxic and may cause vomiting or diarrhea. Do not eat unripe berries; they should be cooked or dried, and as much of the stem as possible should be removed when preparing them. There are no known safety issues when using dried or cooked elderberries or fresh or dried flowers during pregnancy or while nursing. Berries are mildly laxative; adjust the dosage if needed and use them cautiously in pregnancy.

> *"Now you can see that it is possible for the many products of the elder berry to add to the richness of living… In the future, let's show more appreciation for this common shrub which stands at the roadside, freely offering food and drink, medicine and beauty. It would be churlish indeed to refuse such graciously offered gifts."*
>
> Euell Gibbons, (1962) *Stalking the Wild Asparagus*

PREPARATIONS

All parts of elder are used medicinally; some common preparations are infusions and tinctures made with flowers, infused oil and salve made with flowers or leaves, and berry syrups.

INFUSION: Infuse one tablespoon dry or two tablespoons fresh flowers (from one sizeable fresh flower head) for each cup of boiled water. Cover and steep for twenty minutes. Strain. Reheat before drinking for the diaphoretic actions. Sweeten with honey if desired.

TINCTURE: Fresh flowers – 1:2, 95%. Dried flowers – 1:5, 50%. Fresh berries – 1:3, 50%. Dried berries – 1:5, 50%.

SALVE: Make a standard salve using infused elder leaf or flower oil. See also the Green Elder Ointment recipe. Let the fresh leaves wilt overnight before infusing in oil to make salves for topical use.

SYRUP: See the Elderberry Rob (or Syrup) recipe on page 69.

DOSAGES

Flower or berry tincture, flower infusion and berry syrup can be used interchangeably.

INFUSION: Drink one cup of hot elderflower infusion or elderberry decoction every hour or as needed to relieve congestion and reduce fever.

TINCTURE: Take one-half teaspoon of elderflower or berry tincture every hour or as needed to relieve congestion and reduce fever. For a more significant diaphoretic effect, add the tincture to hot tea.

SALVE: Apply elder leaf and flower salve as needed to heal wounds, soothe itchy, dry skin and treat painful bruises.

SYRUP: Take one teaspoon of elderberry syrup at least four times daily. Reduce the dosage slightly for children between two and six years of age. The syrup makes a lovely addition to tea.

HARVESTING

Elder leaves should be harvested before the flower blooms in late spring or early summer. Harvest the entire flower cluster when in full bloom at midsummer. To dry, place the elderflowers face down on a screen lined with thin cotton cloth or a paper towel (to catch the pollen and smaller petals that will drop off in the drying process). Store the elderflowers carefully in glass jars when they are completely dry.

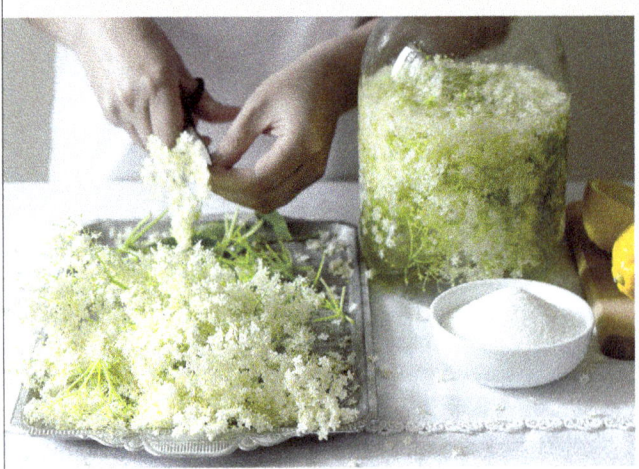

Collect berries in late summer. Remove stems as much as possible. Look for ripe berries that are slightly soft and dark purple. The berries can be used fresh to make syrup, wine, cordial, jam or pie; dried berries can also be used.

Red elder *(Sambucus pubens)* is a toxic species with distinctly red berries. The center (pith) is black. Red elders are rare in our region and easy to identify.

RECIPES

Because every part of the elder has medicinal activity and the plant has such a long history of use, there are endless recipes for using elder as food and medicine. Here are a few that I like to make.

GREEN ELDER OINTMENT (OR SALVE)

In her book, *A Modern Herbal,* published in 1931, Maude Grieve writes, "Here is another recipe, not made from Elder leaves alone, and very much recommended by modern herbalists as being very cooling and softening and excellent for all kinds of tumours, swellings and wounds."[1]

INGREDIENTS

Eight ounces of fresh elder leaves, coarsely chopped
Four ounces of fresh plantain leaves *(Plantago major),* coarsely chopped
Four ounces of fresh wormwood leaves *(Artemisia absinthium),* coarsely chopped
Four ounces of fresh ground ivy *(Glechoma hederacea),* optional
Good quality olive oil
Oven-proof dish with a lid

Follow directions for making a standard salve on page 27.

---

[1] Grieve, *A Modern Herbal,* 270

ELDER ROB (OR SYRUP)

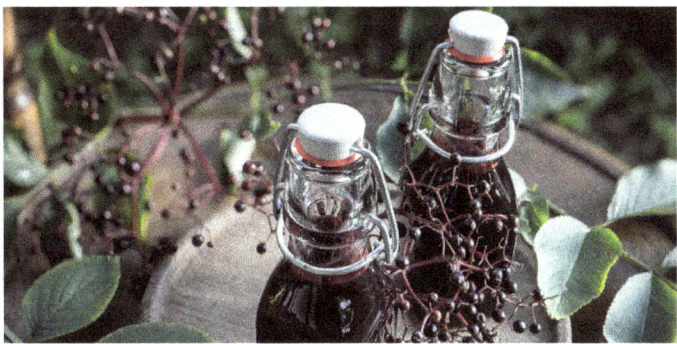

Elder Rob, or syrup, is a traditional preparation in many European herbals. It is a reliable remedy for sore throats, coughs, colds, respiratory infections, and lung congestion and promotes restful sleep. Put two tablespoons of Elder Rob into a cup of hot water or tea and stir well. Add a shot of brandy or other liquor if you like that sort of thing.

INGREDIENTS

Five cups of fresh, ripe berries, stems removed, or four cups of dried berries
Five tablespoons of water (or more if using dried berries)
One cinnamon stick
Ten whole cloves
One thumb-sized piece of ginger root, sliced
Four cups honey (or to taste)

If using fresh berries, rinse them well. Place fresh or dried berries in a large pot with the water and spices. Cook over medium heat until the mixture begins to simmer. After ten minutes, crush the berries with a sturdy wooden spoon or potato masher. Simmer until the berries have given up all their juices, about thirty to forty minutes. While still warm, but not too hot, strain through a colander lined with several layers of cheesecloth. Use a spoon to press out every drop of juice; discard the spent berries and spices. Rinse the pot. Measure the juice and return it to the pot; add an equal amount of honey. Simmer over a very low heat, stirring frequently, until the honey completely dissolves into the berry juice. Skim and discard any foam. Cook for five minutes, but don't let it come to a boil. Cool completely, and pour into sterilized bottles with caps. Store in the refrigerator or a cool, dark place. Shelf life is about one year. Discard if mold appears or the contents become cloudy.

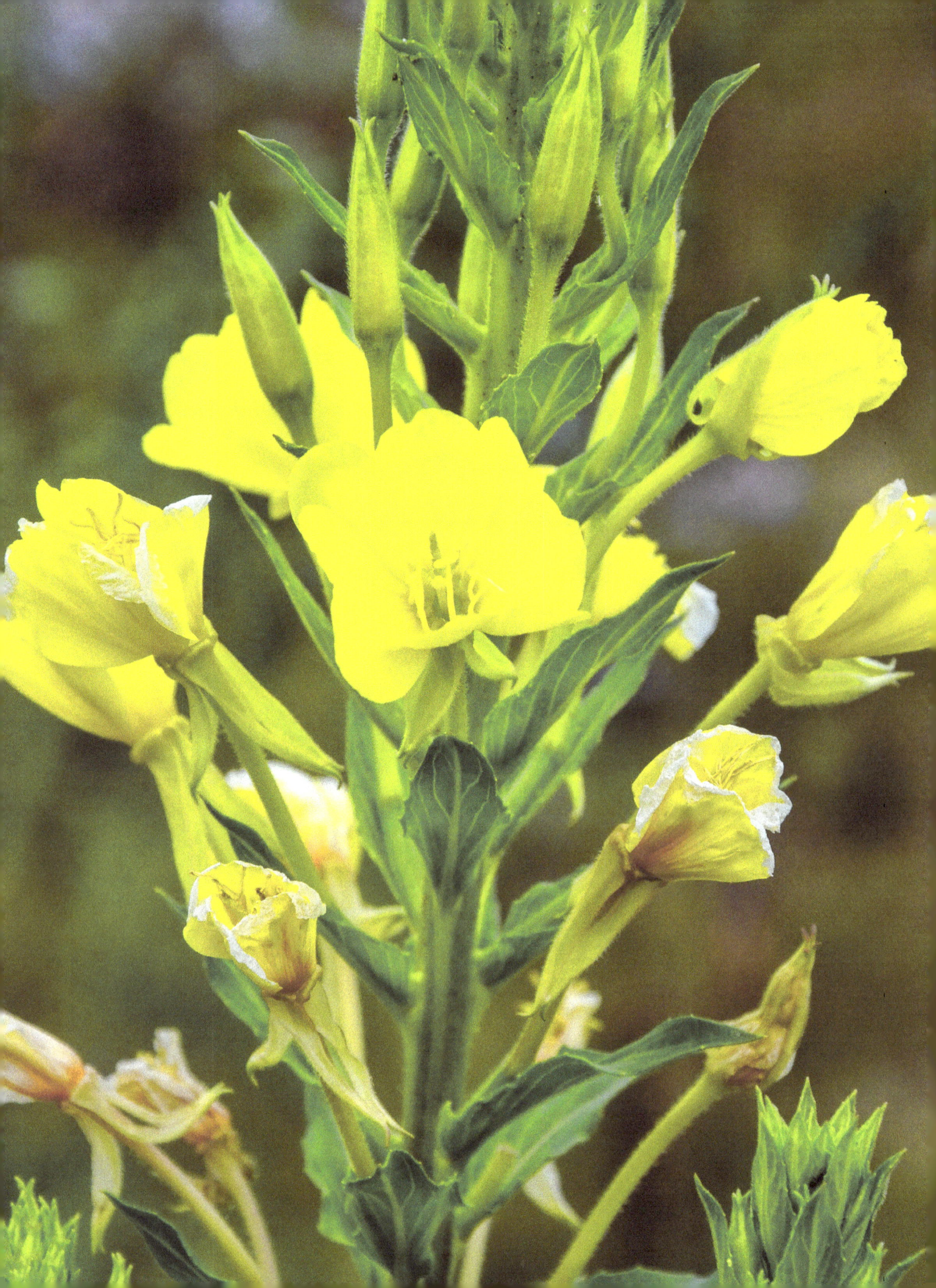

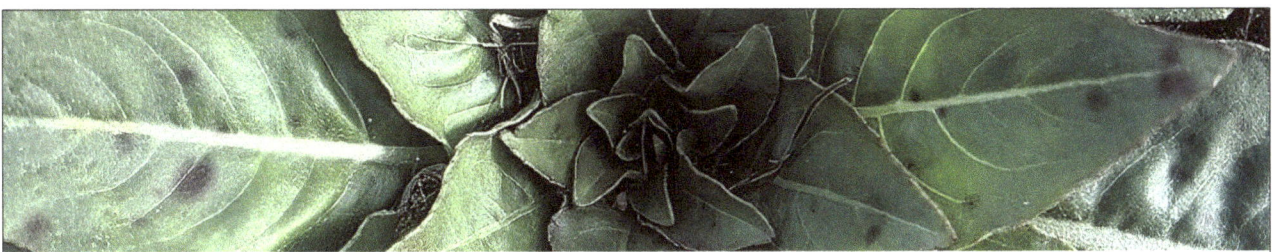

Evening Primrose

COMMON NAME: Evening Primrose

BOTANICAL NAME: *Oenothera biennis*

FAMILY: *Onagraceae* (Evening Primrose)

OTHER NAMES: Sundrops

RELATED SPECIES: *O. fruticosa, O. lacinata*

DESCRIPTION: An herbaceous biennial, one to four feet tall. Leaves are lance-shaped with a rough texture and slightly ragged edges. They form a basal rosette in the first year; during the second year, the flower stalk emerges with alternate leaves and yellow flowers on terminal spikes. The showy yellow flowers have four sepals, four petals, four or eight stamens, and a conspicuous stigma with four lobes. Botanist Tim Spira notes that under poor growing conditions, evening primrose may only produce flowers in the third year, but if growing conditions are good, blooms may appear in the first year. After evening primrose blooms, the plant dies. The flowering period is June until October.

The luminous yellow flowers open at dusk and bloom for one night. Later in the summer, as the days become shorter, the flowers bloom during the day. Moths are the primary pollinators, but with the arrival of daylight, bees may also visit the flowers. The fleshy white taproot may be up to one foot long.

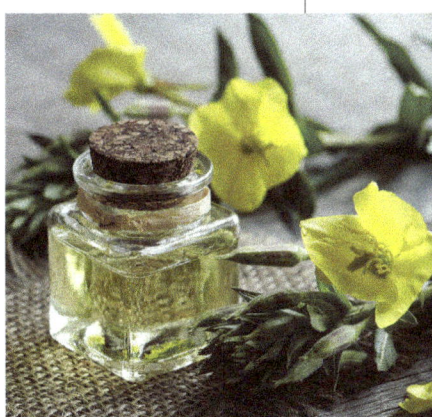

HABITAT: Common along roadsides, fields and open sunny areas, evening primrose tolerates dry, poor soil conditions. Plants are scattered widely and may be difficult to identify until they flower.

KEY ACTIONS: Demulcent, emollient, nervine, antispasmodic

PART USED: Entire plant

TRADITIONAL USES: Evening primrose has a long history of being used as a medicine and food in North America and Europe. American Indians made poultices of the fresh plant to treat bruises, wounds, ulcers, and other inflammatory conditions. Evening primrose has been used as

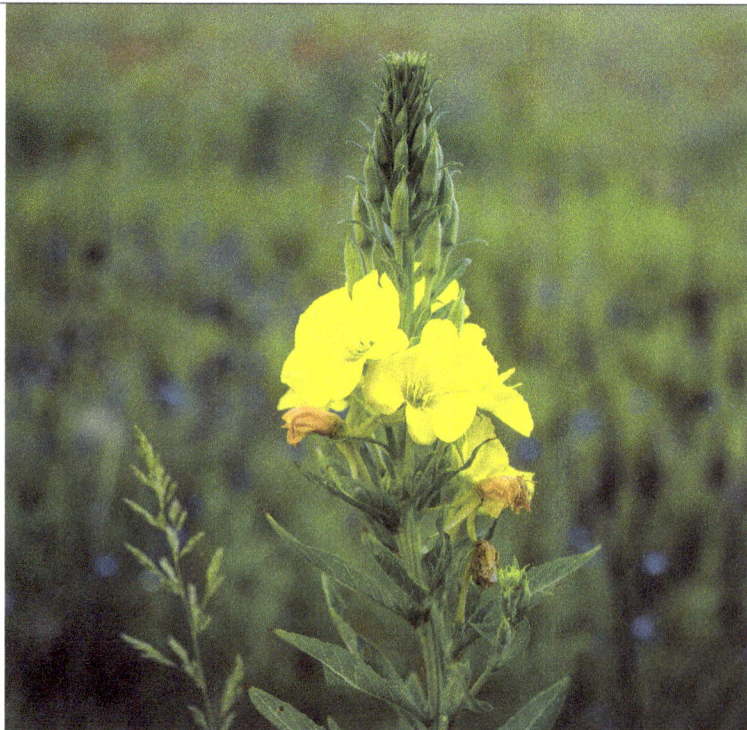

a folk remedy for symptoms such as sore throat, cough, upset stomach, urinary tract infection, and skin problems. In the Southern United States, evening primrose was a well-known remedy for nervousness.

CURRENT USES: Evening primrose is a mild, underused medicine, but because it is so abundant, I encourage everyone to use it when a soothing demulcent is needed. Spring-harvested leaves, roots collected from the first-year plant, flowers, and seeds are all edible and continue to be enjoyed as wild foods.

Use the demulcent leaves in salves and poultices to relieve inflammation, infections, itching, hemorrhoids, and other hot eruptive skin conditions. They can also be used on painful, swollen bruises. Add the leaves to any skin preparations, use infusions in baths, and consider tossing a few leaves into teas or syrups for cough and sore throats. Evening primrose leaf is a mild nervine relaxant.

Commercially extracted evening primrose seed oil is a source of omega-6 essential fatty acids. Research has shown that evening primrose seed oil contains two important essential fatty acids, gamma-linolenic (GLA) and linoleic acid (LA). These fatty acids play a role in treating pre-menstrual syndrome, eczema, psoriasis, high cholesterol, arthritis, migraines and asthma. Research also indicates that in high doses (five to eight grams a day), evening primrose oil may be helpful for ADD and ADHD.[1]

CAUTIONS: None known.

---

[1] Kuhn and Winston, *Herbal Therapies and Supplements*, 124

PREPARATIONS

INFUSION: Infuse one heaping handful of fresh or dried evening primrose herb (leaf, flower, root and stem) in one pint of boiling hot water. Add boiling water, steep for ten minutes and strain. Evening primrose has a mild flavor.

POULTICE: When in flower, gather fresh plants along with the roots. Rinse off any dirt, chop finely, then crush or bruise the herb using a mortar and pestle or a bowl and wooden spoon. The crushed plant will produce sticky juices. If there is not enough juice to hold the mass together, add a small amount of aloe vera gel or warm water to the mixture and mix well. Apply the poultice directly on the skin and cover it entirely with gauze or a cotton cloth. Put a thick towel on top and consider topping it off with a hot water bottle. Leave the poultice on for twenty minutes and repeat as needed, using fresh herbs each time.

SYRUP: Follow the directions on page 22 for making syrup. Use the entire plant, including the roots, or only the leaves.

SALVE: Make a standard salve with infused oil using all parts of the plant or only the leaves.

DOSAGES

INFUSION: Drink one cup of evening primrose infusion two to three times a day or as needed. Combine evening primrose with other nervines, like passionflower and skullcap.

POULTICE/SALVE: Use a fresh herb poultice or salve to relieve inflamed and itchy skin conditions.

SYRUP: Take one tablespoon of evening primrose syrup every half-hour or as needed to relieve coughs and soothe throat irritation.

HARVESTING

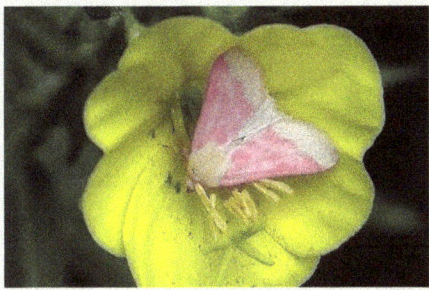

Harvest the entire plant as the first flowers open in mid-summer. Young leaves are edible (when cooked) in the spring and harvested for medicinal use anytime they appear healthy. Rinse leaves before use. Dig roots in the fall of the first year (before it produces a flower stalk) before the first frost or in the spring of the second year just as the flower stalk emerges. The roots of first-year plants are edible.

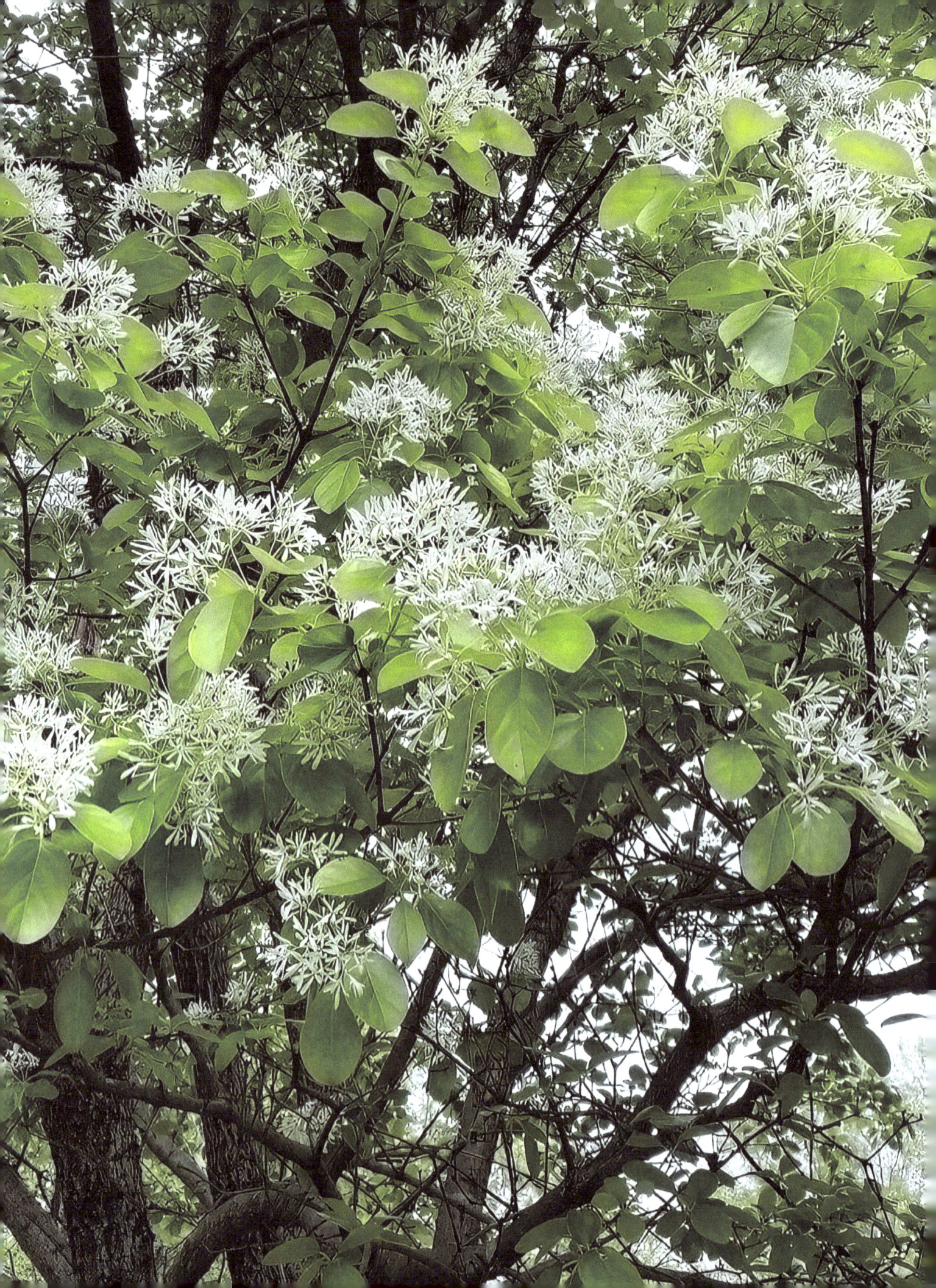

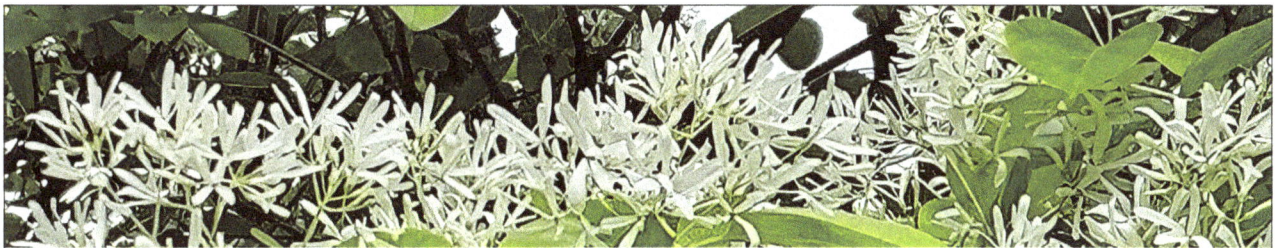

Fringetree

COMMON NAME: Fringetree

BOTANICAL NAME: *Chionanthus virginica*

FAMILY: *Oleaceae* (Olive)

OTHER NAMES: White Ash, Old Man's Beard, Granddad's Beard

DESCRIPTION: A small tree, twenty feet tall, leaves are opposite, oval with smooth edges. The distinctive fragrant white flowers have four fringe-like, drooping petals that bloom in late spring. Male and female flowers are typically on separate trees, but sometimes both are found on the same tree. In late summer, female trees produce an oval fruit that resembles a small blue-black olive

HABITAT: Found in various habitats, both moist and dry deciduous forests and in the partial shade at the edge of woodlands.

KEY ACTIONS: Hepatic, cholagogue, diuretic, aperient, anti-inflammatory

PART USED: Dried root bark

TRADITIONAL USES: American Indians used a decoction prepared with dried root bark to clean infected wounds. As a regional folk remedy, fringetree was used to treat various symptoms, including indigestion, poor appetite and diabetes.

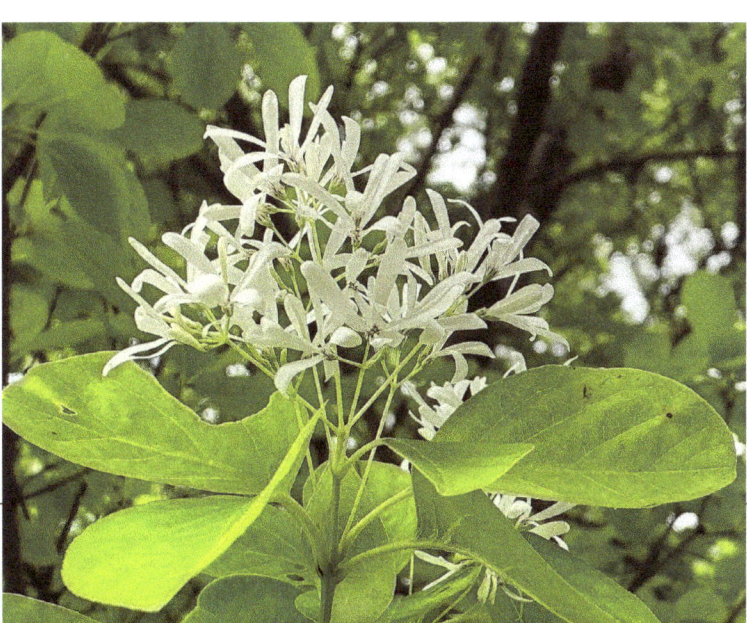

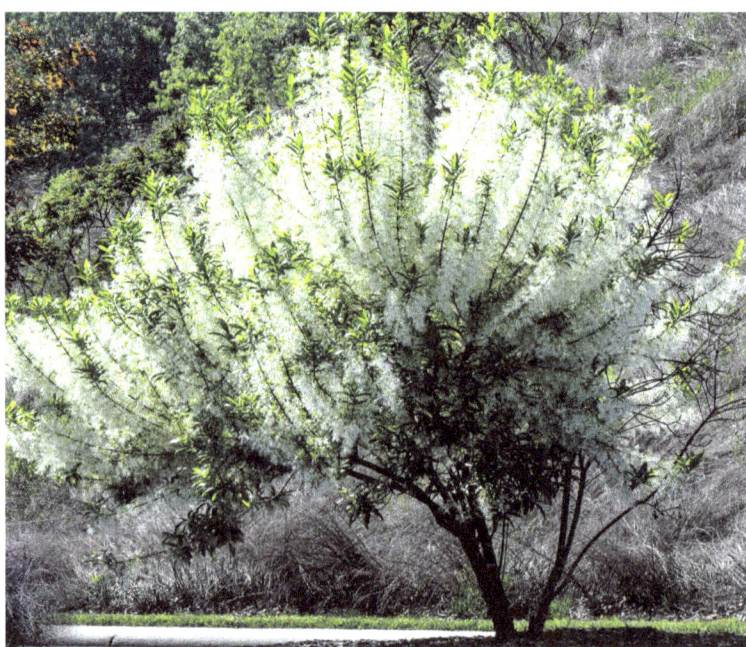

Writing in the 19th century, Eclectic physicians praised fringetree as one of the most valuable remedies for liver disease. Considered a cure for jaundice, it was also used to treat gallstones, kidney stones, poor liver function, and pelvic congestion.

CURRENT USES: Fringetree is a gentle but effective tonic that improves liver and gallbladder function. It gently stimulates bile secretions, increases appetite, and regulates digestion and elimination. It is a specific remedy for treating jaundice, reducing gallbladder inflammation, and preventing the formation of gallstones. Herbalist CoreyPine Shane combines fringetree with black haw and wild yam to relax the common bile duct and minimize pain when passing gallstones.[1]

To address the underlying cause of most chronic eruptive skin conditions like acne, eczema, cysts, and itchy rashes from unknown causes, fringetree supports liver detoxification without increasing the overall toxic load. It is also a regenerative liver tonic to be used after taking pharmaceuticals, recreational drugs and other substances that impair liver function.

CAUTIONS: Fringetree is a safe herb for general use and can be used with children and the elderly. There have been no reports of safety concerns in pregnancy or while nursing.

---

[1] Shane, *Southeast Medicinal Plants*, 116

PREPARATIONS

DECOCTION: Use one heaping tablespoon of dried root bark for each pint of cold water. Bring to a boil over high heat, then low heat to simmer, covered, for thirty minutes. Strain.

TINCTURE: Dried root bark – 1:5, 60%.

DOSAGES

Fringetree is a mild bitter that is often easier to tolerate than other intensely bitter hepatic herbs. Combining all bitter herbs with an aromatic herb, like bee balm or mountain mint, may be helpful.

DECOCTION: Take one-half cup of the decoction every thirty minutes for acute symptoms. As a tonic, drink four ounces of warm decoction twice daily, ideally with meals.

TINCTURE: Take one-half teaspoon every thirty minutes or every two hours for acute symptoms. Ten drops of tincture in a small amount of warm water with meals improves digestion and elimination. As a general tonic for the liver and gallbladder, take one-half teaspoon in a small amount of water twice daily.

HARVESTING

Harvest root bark in early spring just as leaves emerge or in the fall as the first frost approaches. Dig straight down at the tree's drip line (directly below the outermost tips of the leaves) to locate surface roots. Immediately after harvesting, wash the root and peel off the outer bark. Dry the bark entirely before using it.

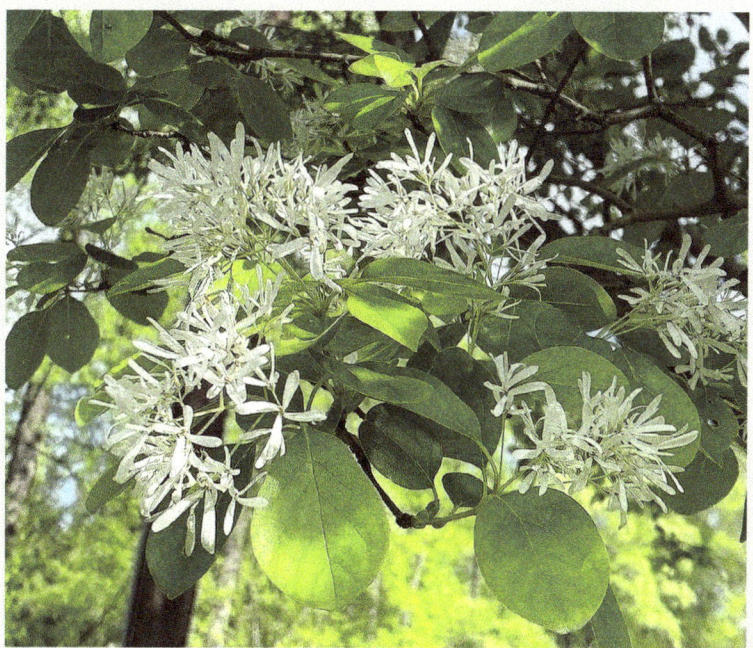

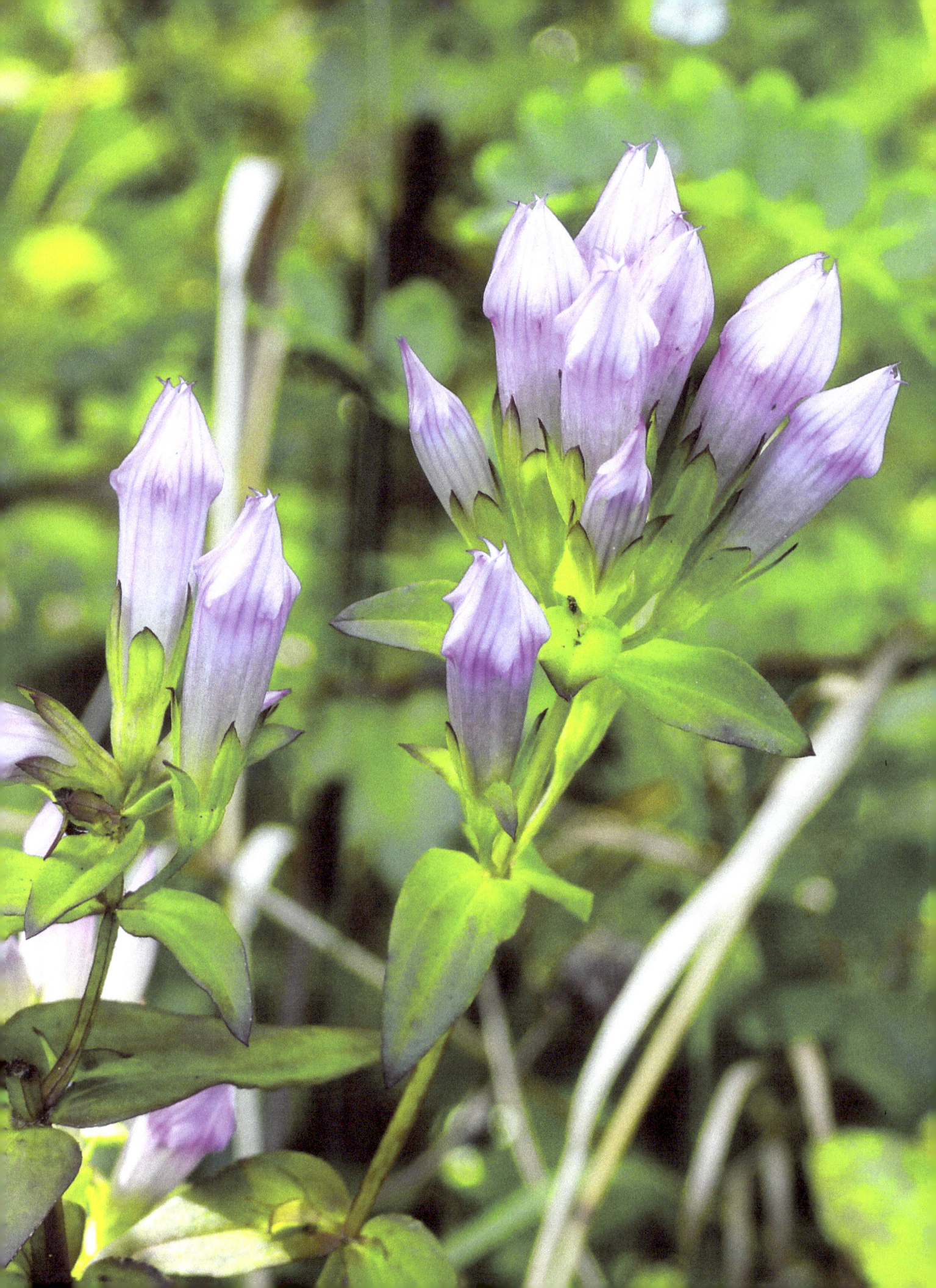

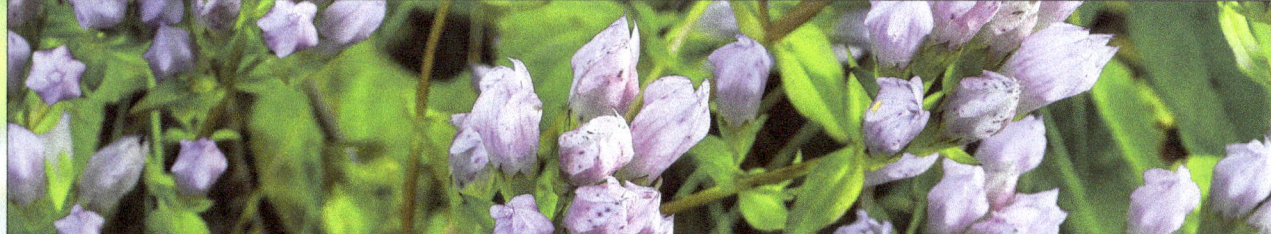

Gentian

COMMON NAME: Gentian

BOTANICAL NAME: *Gentiana quinquefolia*

FAMILY: *Gentianae* (Gentian)

OTHER NAMES: Ague Weed, Stiff Gentian, American Gentian

RELATED SPECIES: Around eight species of *Gentiana* grow in the region, including soapwort gentian *(G. saponaria)* and closed or bottle gentian *(G. clausa),* which have similar properties. Most of the gentian sold commercially are the roots of European yellow gentian *(G. lutea)* and can be used similarly. However, it is a much stronger bitter than local *Gentiana* species, so dosing should be reduced.

DESCRIPTION: An annual herb, one to two feet tall, with narrow oval leaves in pairs. Branched stems have five or more flowers in clusters at the terminal end. The small, upright, tubular gentian flowers vary in color from deep purple to pale blue and appear between July and October. The flower petals remain tightly closed until opened by a pollinator, usually a bumblebee.

HABITAT: Grows along streams and ponds in partial shade in damp areas.

KEY ACTIONS: Bitter, stomachic

PART USED: Entire plant (aerial parts and root) or aerial parts only

TRADITIONAL USES: In Europe, the root of yellow gentian, *Gentiana lutea*, is a traditional digestive bitter used to stimulate digestion, especially after a rich meal. While the actions of the European species are similar, our local gentian species, sometimes referred to as American gentian, are milder. A common folk remedy was gentian and other bitter herbs steeped in brandy or other liquor to create a simple bitter tonic. Chewing on the root was said to numb the gums. Gentian was a specific remedy for headaches, poor liver function, jaundice, weak digestion, and gallstones.

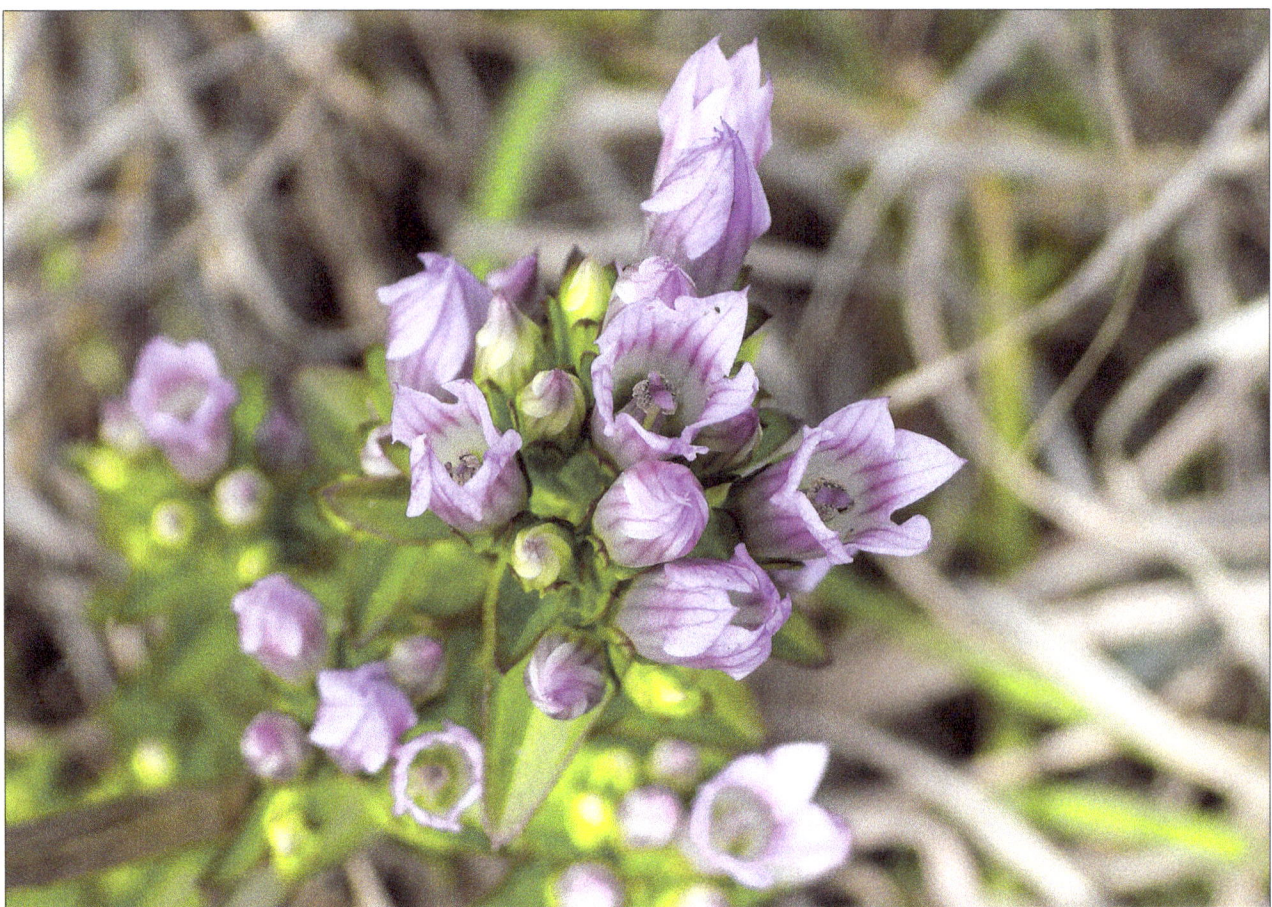

CURRENT USES: Gentian relieves chronic and acute digestive system symptoms such as bloating, gas, belching, constipation, and headaches. Used regularly as a digestive bitter taken with meals, gentian improves digestion, assimilation and elimination. A general tonic for weakness and fatigue, especially when digestion and appetite are diminished.

CAUTIONS: In large doses, higher than those recommended here, gentian can irritate the stomach and cause nausea, vomiting or even diarrhea. Start with a low dose and increase slowly as needed. Do not use gentian with stomach (gastric) ulcers or inflammation. Like all intensely bitter herbs, gentian should be avoided during pregnancy and while nursing, and it is not safe for babies and children.

"Use gentian where the powers of life are depressed, and recovery depends on the ability to assimilate food."

Felter and Lloyd, (1808) King's American Dispensatory

PREPARATIONS

Due to their bitter flavor, gentians are traditionally made into simple tinctures combined with other aromatic herbs such as cardamom, ginger, and fennel seed or root.

TINCTURE: Fresh – 1:2, 95%. Dried – 1:5, 50%.

GENTIAN DIGESTIVE BITTERS: See the recipe below.

DOSAGES

TINCTURE: Take one-half teaspoon in a small amount of warm water with meals or as needed.

GENTIAN DIGESTIVE BITTERS: Take ten to fifteen drops in warm water with meals or as needed. See the recipe below.

HARVESTING

Aerial parts (in flower).

GENTIAN DIGESTIVE BITTERS RECIPE

Put three ounces of dried or five ounces of fresh gentian into a quart jar with the peel of two organic oranges (thinly sliced), one tablespoon of ground cardamom seed, one teaspoon of whole fennel seed and 16 ounces of good brandy or apple cider vinegar. Replace the jar lid and shake well. Store in a cool place for one month, shaking well every few days.

After one month, strain out the spent herbs and discard them. Add one-fourth cup of honey and mix well. Store in a glass bottle. Gentian bitters do not need to be refrigerated.

Take 10 to 15 drops in a small amount of warm water with meals. Add one tablespoon of bitters to eight ounces of sparkling mineral water for an energizing drink.

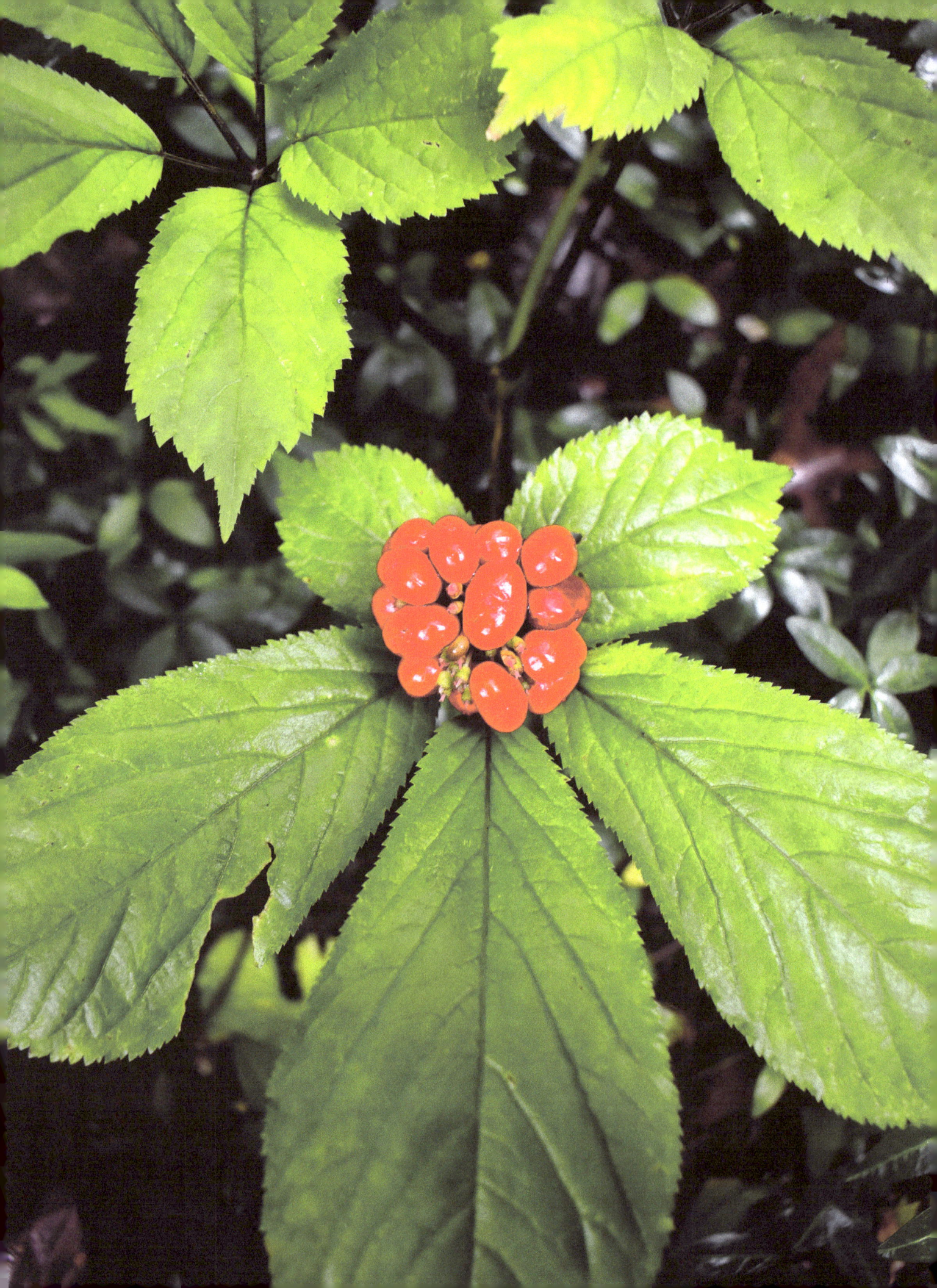

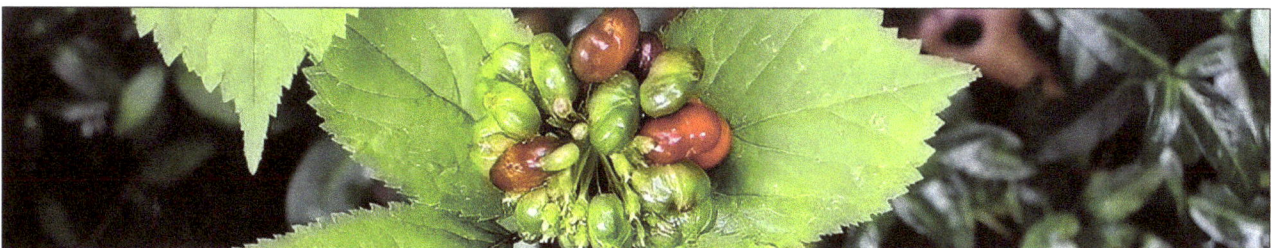

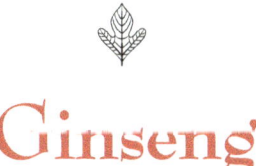

Ginseng

COMMON NAME: Ginseng (American)

BOTANICAL NAME: *Panax quinquefolius*

FAMILY: *Araliaceae* (Ginseng)

OTHER NAMES: American Ginseng, Sang

RELATED SPECIES: Dwarf ginseng (*Panax trifolius*)

DESCRIPTION: Ginseng is a low-growing perennial, eight to twelve inches tall, found in the deep shade of deciduous forests, often on north-facing slopes. Plants emerge in late spring as the tree canopy completely shades the forest floor. Each plant has two to four palmately compound leaves, or prongs, each with five sharply toothed leaflets; the three center leaflets are larger than the outer two. The compound leaves on younger plants may have only three leaflets. The flower head is a single terminal rounded umbel composed of small, inconspicuous green flowers that bloom midsummer. The fruit forms a cluster of green berries (drupes) that turn brilliant red when ripe. Ginseng has a single fleshy, white and fragrant taproot. As the plant ages, the roots tend to fork and sometimes resemble a human body, hence the origins of the name ginseng, which means man root.

HABITAT: North-facing slopes in deciduous hardwood forests. Ginseng prefers rich soil in moist areas and is often found in plant communities that include bloodroot, black cohosh and wild ginger. Ginseng was once very common in the forests of Eastern North America. However, it has been overharvested for the past three hundred years, and wild stands are now rare. Fortunately, more cultivated ginseng, either woods-grown or field-cultivated, is now available on the commercial market.

KEY ACTIONS: Adaptogen, lung tonic, carminative, immune stimulant

PART USED: Root, leaf

TRADITIONAL USES: Ginseng is one of the most prized herbs in China and other parts of Asia, where it has been used for thousands of years as a longevity tonic. American Indians considered it a restorative

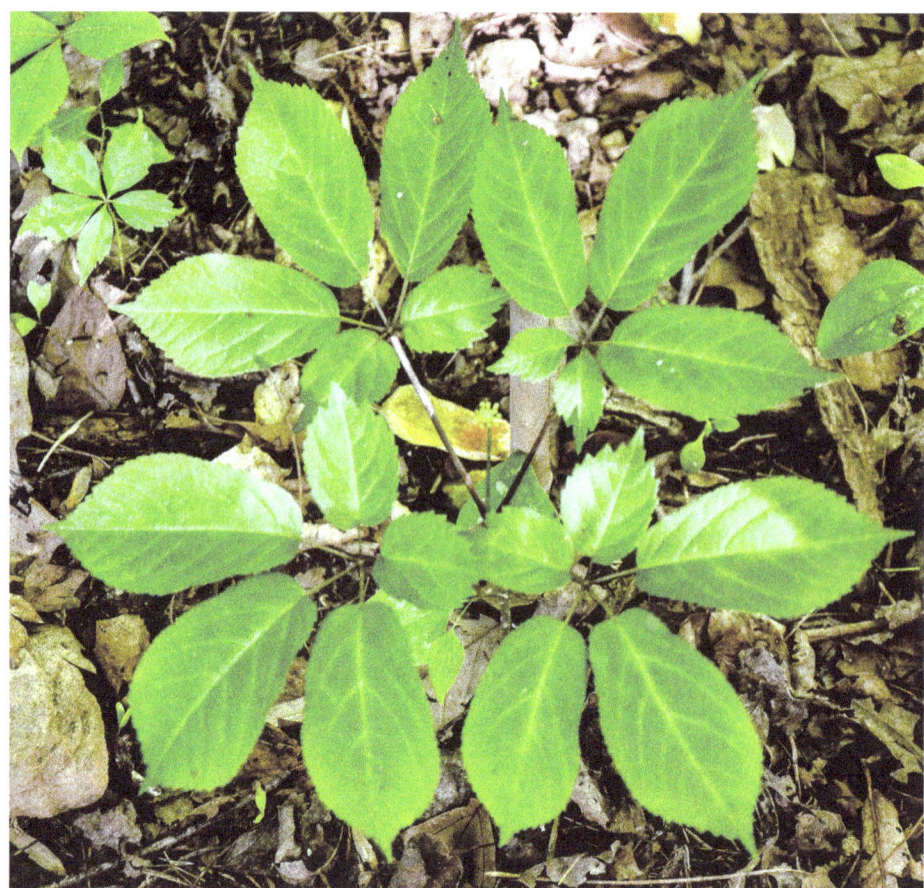

tonic to relieve fatigue, lung weakness, shortness of breath, fainting, and nervous debility. It was also used to ease colic in children and as a general tonic.

CURRENT USES: In modern herbal practice, ginseng is still an exalted tonic. It regulates and nourishes the entire body, improving digestion and respiration to increase energy reserves. Use for all symptoms of weakness and frailty, especially after illness, physical trauma and long periods of stress.

Ginseng nourishes all body fluids to restore flexibility in the ligaments and tendons, lubricate the mucus membranes, and replenish the blood. The cumulative effect of daily use is a sense of calm that improves concentration and sleep quality, enhances digestion and elimination, and regulates immune function.

Ginseng regulates and strengthens the heart. Long-term use may relieve cardiac symptoms, such as high or low blood pressure, arrhythmia, restless sleep patterns, disturbing dreams or nightmares, depression and poor concentration.

Recommended as a tonic for stress, overwork, poor diet, sleep difficulties, traumatic injuries, and aging. Ginseng is an excellent seasonal tonic for the winter months.

CAUTIONS: Although side effects are rare, discontinue use or reduce dosage if heart palpitations, headaches, insomnia or elevated blood pressure occur. Taking ginseng late in the day may disrupt sleep. Ginseng is contraindicated in pregnancy and while nursing.

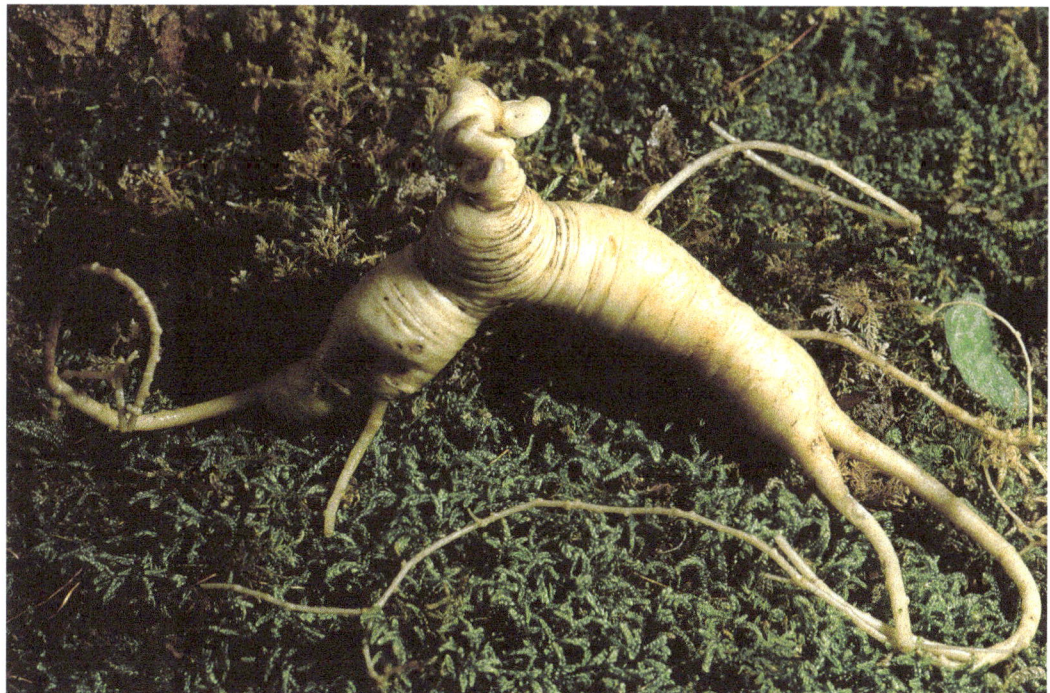

PREPARATIONS

Traditionally, ginseng roots are prepared as decoctions. Whole steamed roots can be chewed. Alcohol tinctures and powder (capsules) are also used. Only purchase ginseng roots from reputable sources; if possible, buy woods-cultivated ginseng, as conventionally farmed ginseng crops are treated with herbicides and pesticides. Be forewarned that good quality ginseng is costly, and you should be prepared to pay dearly for woods-cultivated roots.

DECOCTION: Due to the high cost of quality ginseng root, use the recommended ratios of herb to water and the preparation method described here. You can use each ginseng root to make three or four batches of decoction before discarding. Weigh your roots and use four to five grams of dried root for every eight ounces of water. Add roots and cold water to a pot with a lid. Simmer over medium heat, covered, for about twenty minutes. Strain. After making a batch, allow the roots to dry for an hour or so on an absorbent cloth, then store them in a loosely capped, clean glass jar in the refrigerator. Use the same roots three or four times before discarding.

TINCTURE: Fresh root – 1:2, 50%. Dried root – 1:5, 60%.

GINSENG COOKER: These small ceramic crocks cook the roots without exposing them to water. The ginseng cooker is filled with dried roots, covered and placed in a large pot with enough water to reach halfway up its sides. Bring the water to a boil and simmer for twenty to thirty minutes; keep an eye on the water and add more if necessary. When done, the cooked ginseng roots will be soft and chewy. Be sure to collect the juice from the bottom of the cooker (not the pot) and dilute it with water for a potent tea. Cut the cooked roots into one-inch pieces and store them in a jar in the refrigerator. Chew one piece daily.

DOSAGES

American ginseng works slowly and deeply in the body, tonifying, regulating and strengthening organs and tissues. Long-term use, three to six months of daily use, is recommended for best outcomes.

DECOCTION: Drink a half cup of decoction three times a day.

TINCTURE: Take one-half to one teaspoon in a small amount of water three times a day.

COOKED ROOTS: Chew a one-inch piece of root daily.

HARVESTING

Wild ginseng should only be harvested after checking the laws governing ginseng harvesting in your state and using sustainable practices.

If you live in an area that provides the necessary growing conditions for ginseng, consider growing your own from roots or seeds, and prepare to be patient as germination is slow.

Harvest ginseng roots that are at least three years old; these plants will have three or more compound leaves or prongs. The number of leaf scars on the rhizome indicates the plant's precise age.

Harvest mature plants in the fall when the seeds are red. Pull the seed heads apart and bury them under about one inch of soil. Break the stems of any remaining plants so that no one else harvests from that patch.

All states with ginseng populations have enacted laws regulating when ginseng can be harvested, and permits are needed to sell or purchase wildcrafted roots. Of course, there is still a robust underground market for ginseng, so it is frequently poached from private property.

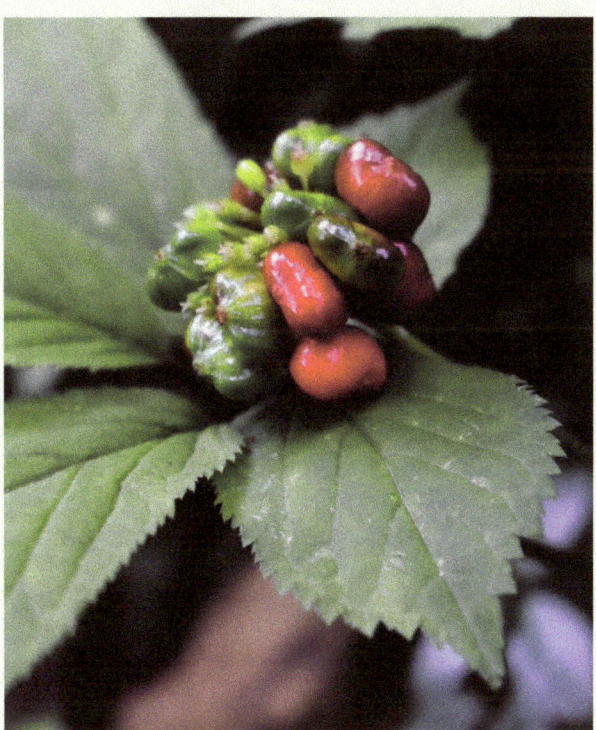

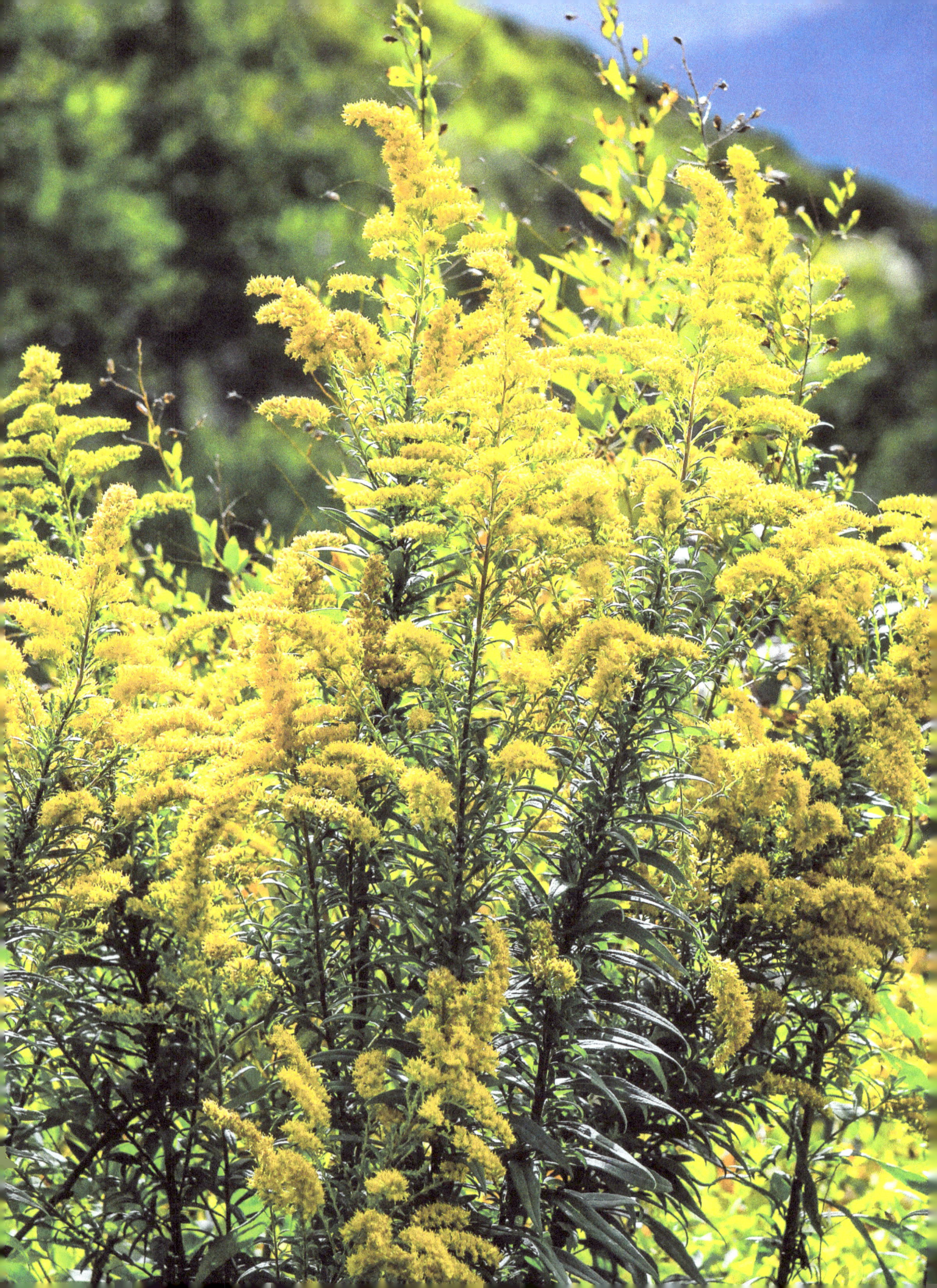

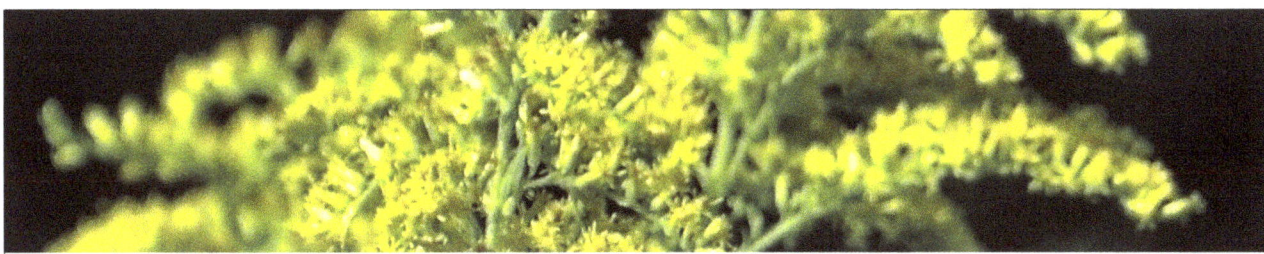

Goldenrod

COMMON NAME: Goldenrod

BOTANICAL NAME: *Solidago spp.*

FAMILY: *Asteraceae* (Aster)

OTHER NAMES: Aaron's Rod, Woundwort, Sweet Goldenrod, Anise-Scented Goldenrod, Farewell-to-Summer

RELATED SPECIES: The two species of goldenrod with the most documented use in the region are the sweet or anise-scented goldenrod *(Solidago odora)* and the Canadian goldenrod *(S. canadensis)*. With more than thirty-eight species of goldenrod growing in the Appalachian Mountains, identification is difficult for even the most exacting botanist. Fortunately, the medicinal properties of most species are similar.

DESCRIPTION: An erect perennial, two to four feet tall, with a solitary stem, sometimes with branched or arching flower stalks. Lance-shaped leaves, two to four inches long, most with a roughly textured surface, are more prominent at the plant's base, becoming smaller towards the top of the stem. Leaf margins vary according to species; *S. odora* has smooth edges, while *S. canadensis* is toothed.

The arrangement of the small, ragged clusters of golden-yellow flowers also differs based on species; bloom time is from late summer until the first frost. *S. odora* flowers grow only on one side of the stalk; the leaves smell like anise when crushed. The flowers of *S. canadensis* form a triangular plume. Goldenrod spreads by underground rhizomes.

HABITAT: Goldenrod grows in dry, open, sunny areas. Common and abundant.

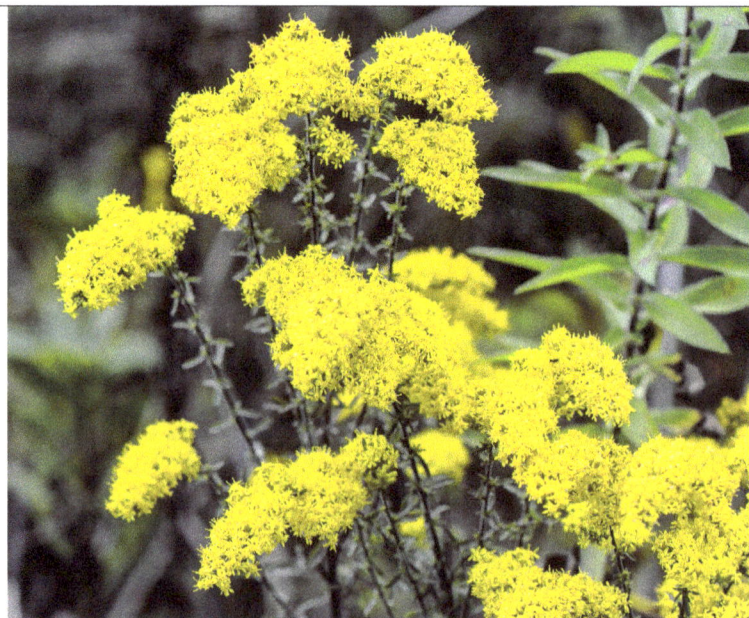

KEY ACTIONS: Anti-inflammatory, vulnerary, astringent, anti-lithic, anti-catarrhal, sedative

PART USED: Aerial parts (in flower)

TRADITIONAL USES: American Indians used goldenrod as a soothing remedy for diarrhea and coughs, to reduce fevers and as a gentle sedative. Fresh leaf poultice was applied to the head to relieve headaches or as a bandage for wounds and burns. Infusions of goldenrod were added to baths to relax women during labor and to calm fussy babies.

In the early 19th century, goldenrod tea was promoted as a popular beverage in the Eastern United States. In the Appalachian Mountains, where it was called 'Blue Mountain Tea,' it was served to tourists and was considered a remedy for exhaustion and fatigue.

In Europe, the endemic *S. virgaurea* treats urinary infections, dissolves or helps eliminate kidney stones, and reduces inflammation and congestion in the upper respiratory system.

CURRENT USES: Goldenrod is underused in modern herbal practice, and commercial sources can be hard to find. Fortunately, it grows abundantly in the wild. Goldenrod soothes inflammation and congestion in the upper respiratory system and can relieve seasonal allergy symptoms, sinus infections, and colds. As an infusion, it soothes inflammation in the digestive system to relieve heartburn, indigestion, and diarrhea. It also calms inflamed tissues in urinary tract infections and may help prevent or dissolve kidney stones. Goldenrod salve and poultices are used to heal wounds and burns.

CAUTIONS: Avoid if allergic to Aster or *Asteraceae* family plants.

PREPARATIONS

INFUSION: Most goldenrod species, especially *S. odora,* make a pleasant tea. Infuse two teaspoons of dry or one tablespoon of fresh leaves and flowers for each cup of water. Cover and steep for twenty minutes. When making infusions with bitter herbs, add some goldenrod to the blend to improve the flavor.

TINCTURE: Fresh – 1:2, 70%. Dried – 1:5, 50%.

SALVES: Prepare a standard infused oil using fresh or dried goldenrod to use in a salve.

POULTICE: Pound fresh leaves in a mortar and pestle to make a paste, adding a little water or aloe vera gel to hold the paste together. Apply to wounds or burns to reduce inflammation and promote healing.

DOSAGES

INFUSION: Drink half a cup warm infusion every hour or as needed.

TINCTURE: Take half to one teaspoon of tincture in water every hour or as needed.

SALVE: Apply to the skin as often as needed.

POULTICE: Apply fresh leaf poultice to burns, wounds, and other inflamed skin conditions. Cover with a towel or cotton cloth. Remove after about ten minutes. Repeat several times.

HARVESTING

Because the leaves are covered with fine hair, harvest on a clear day after a good rainfall has cleaned the plant of dirt and debris. Cut the stem just above any dirty or bug-eaten leaves. Bloom time varies by species. Flowers in full bloom should be tinctured quickly as they will turn to fluff within hours. Choose plants with most of the flowers unopened if you plan to dry them.

Strip leaves and flowers from the stem and process immediately. Bundle four or five goldenrod stems together using a rubber band and hang them in a well-ventilated area to dry. Goldenrod dries quickly, although you may have to break up the flower clusters to keep them from molding.

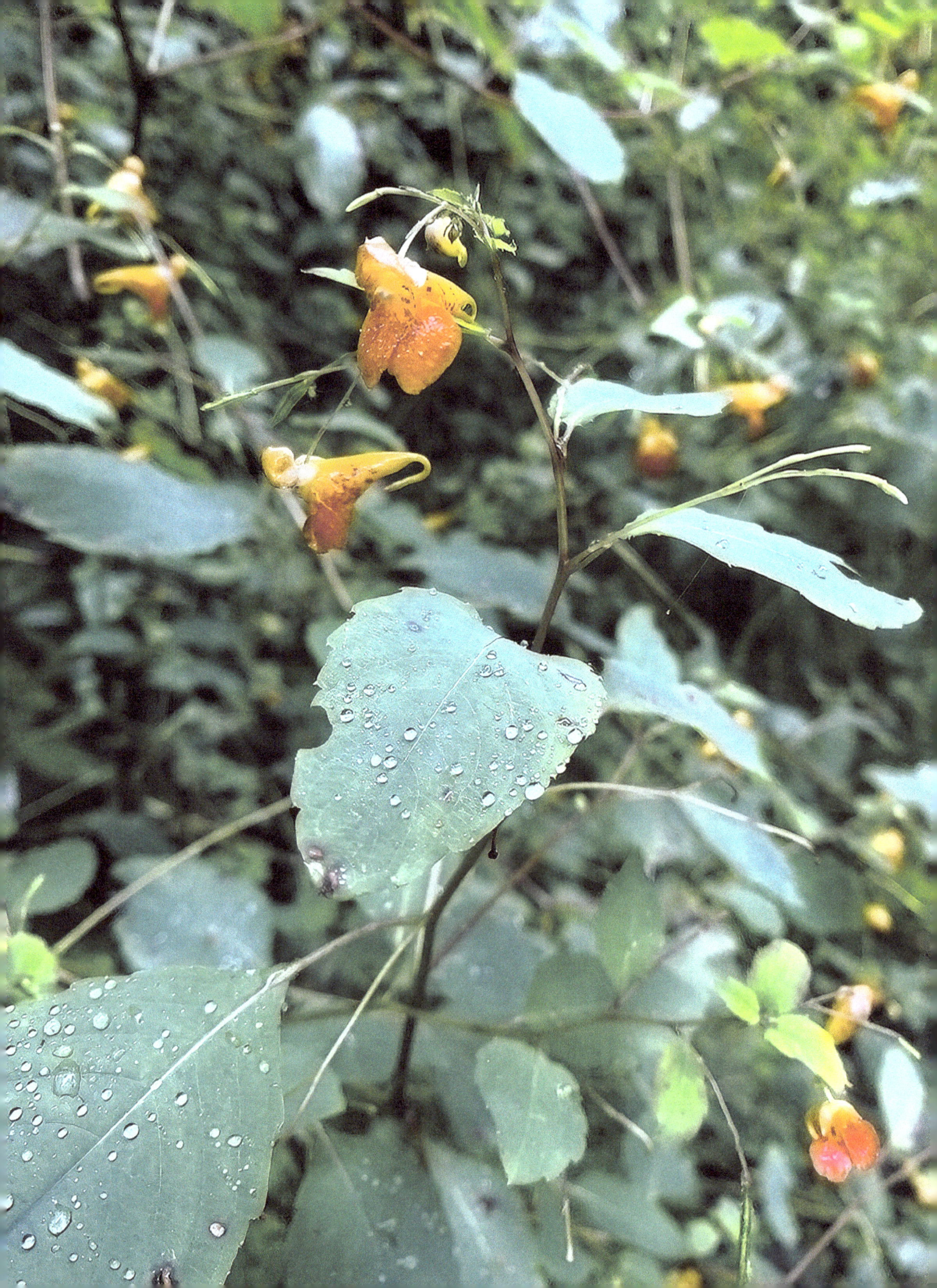

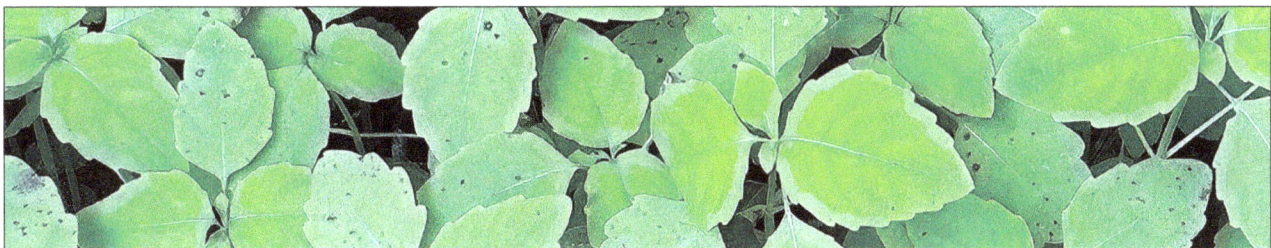

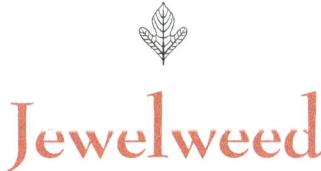

Jewelweed

COMMON NAME: Jewelweed

BOTANICAL NAME: *Impatiens capensis*

FAMILY: *Balsaminaceae* (Touch-Me-Not)

OTHER NAMES: Touch-Me-Not, Spotted Touch-Me-Not

RELATED SPECIES: Yellow Jewelweed or Pale Touch-Me-Not *(Impatiens pallida)*

DESCRIPTION: Both *Impatiens* species are succulent annuals, two to five feet tall, with smooth, slightly translucent stems and leaves. Oval leaves with roundly scalloped edges grow in pairs in the lower parts of the plant and then singly along the stem towards the top. When the leaves or stems are crushed, they exude a gel-like liquid. Dew and raindrops form diamond-like droplets on the leaves, hence the common name, jewelweed. Both species are used interchangeably.

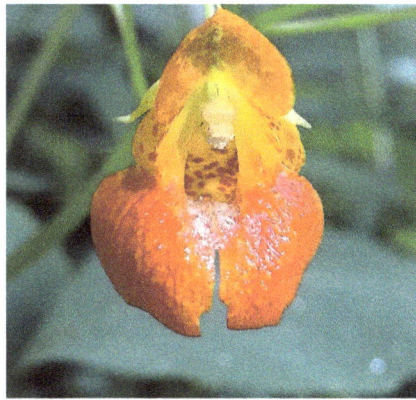

Flowers hang like pendants on short arched stems beneath the leaves. They are irregular, with five petals, the upper two united, the lower three separate, and a long spur at the back. *I. capensis* has orange flowers with tiny red dots, while *I. pallida* have yellow flowers and a shorter spur. Jewelweed is called "touch-me-not" because the ripe seed pods explode when touched, flinging the seeds a distance from the plant.

HABITAT: Abundant in cool, wet places throughout the region. According to folklore, jewelweed always grows near poison ivy, which is fortunate as it relieves the rashes they cause.

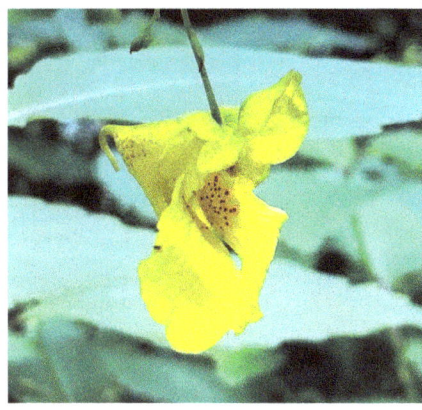

KEY ACTIONS: Astringent, anti-inflammatory, emollient

PART USED: Aerial parts

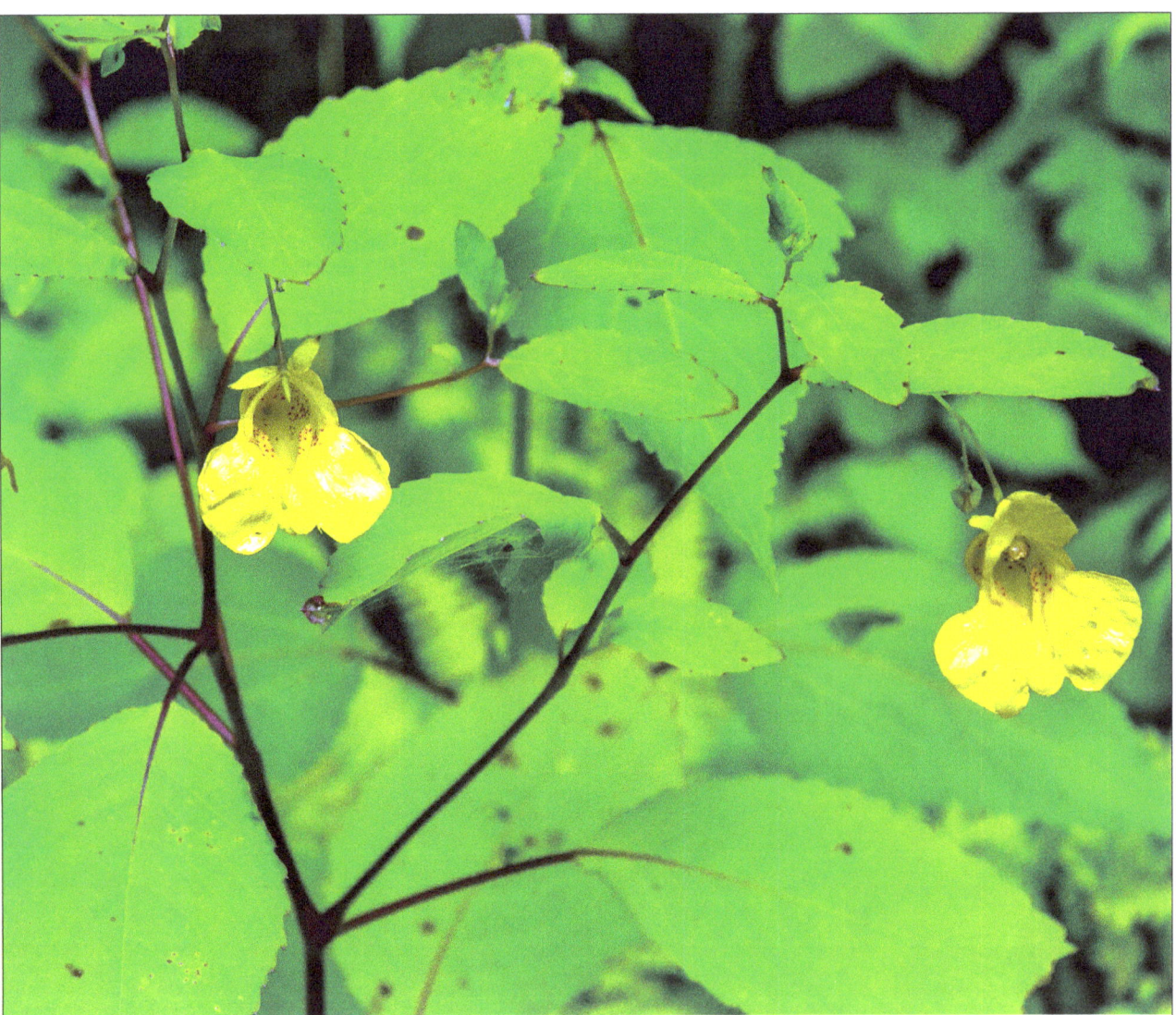

TRADITIONAL USES: The Cherokee used jewelweed juice to soothe poison ivy rash. The crushed leaves were rubbed on children's bellies to relieve a sour stomach. An infusion was used in a bath for women about to go into labor. The plant was also used ceremonially.

CURRENT USES: Jewelweed is one of the best remedies for poison ivy rash and is used for insect bites, abrasions, and other skin irritations. Some believe it can also prevent poison ivy rash if rubbed on the skin before exposure, but that may be wishful thinking. Young plants are cooked as a potherb in the early spring.

CAUTIONS: None known.

PREPARATIONS

Jewelweed is used externally to treat skin inflammation and irritation.

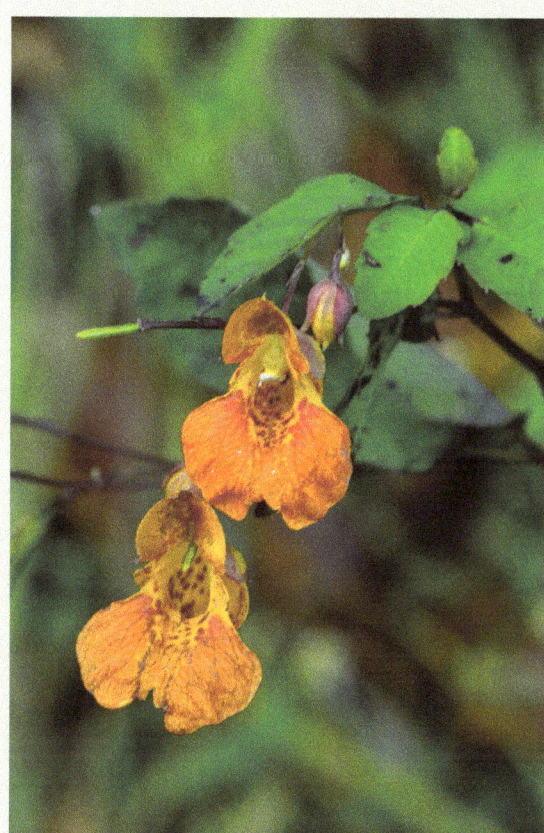

INFUSION: Fill a quart-sized canning jar with jewelweed leaves, stems, and flowers until half full. Use a wooden spoon to crush the plants and release their juices. Add boiling water to fill the jar, cover and steep it for six hours or overnight. The infusion will turn orange. Strain out and discard the spent jewelweed. Use the infusion as a skin wash, add to a bath, or pour into an ice cube tray and freeze for later use. Rub jewelweed ice cubes on poison ivy rash or other skin inflammation.

POULTICE: Put five or six fresh plants in a blender with a fourth to half a cup of aloe vera gel and eight to ten drops of lavender essential oil. Blend well. Use immediately or store in a wide-mouthed jar in the refrigerator for up to a week. Apply liberally to poison ivy rash or other inflamed, itchy skin conditions as needed.

SALVE: Allow fresh jewelweed to wilt for several hours or overnight before making a standard infused oil to be used as is or made into a salve.

DOSAGES

Use all jewelweed preparations described here as often as needed to relieve itching and inflammation of the skin.

HARVESTING

Gather jewelweed anytime during the growing season. However, like many plants, it loses vigor after it blooms, and as summer wanes, so harvest jewelweed in June or July. Jewelweed grows in large masses, making it easy to harvest many plants with little effort. Cut the plant near the roots or pull the entire plant, roots and all, out of the ground. Discard the roots. Once harvested, jewelweed wilts, so harvest twice as much as you think you need.

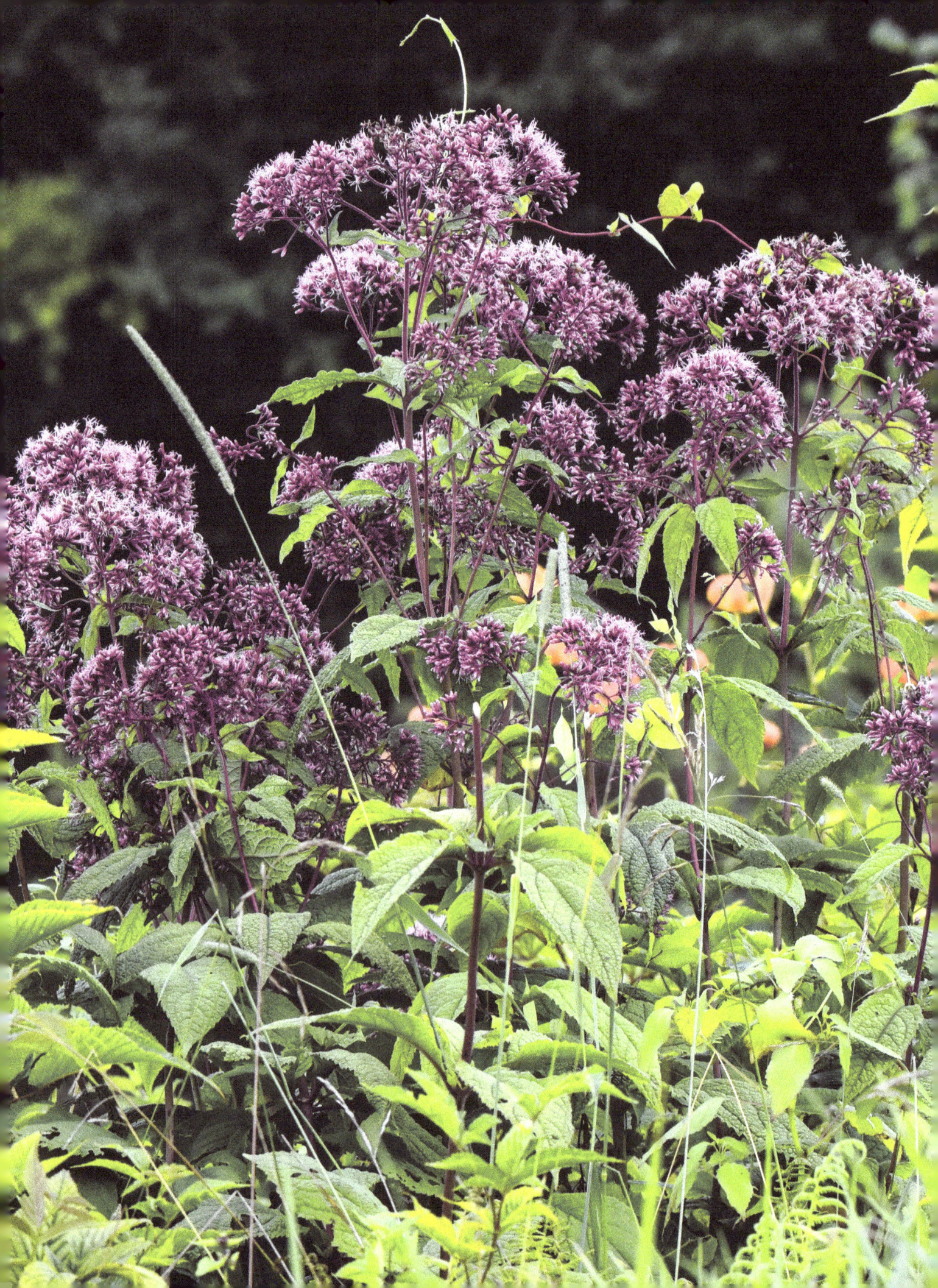

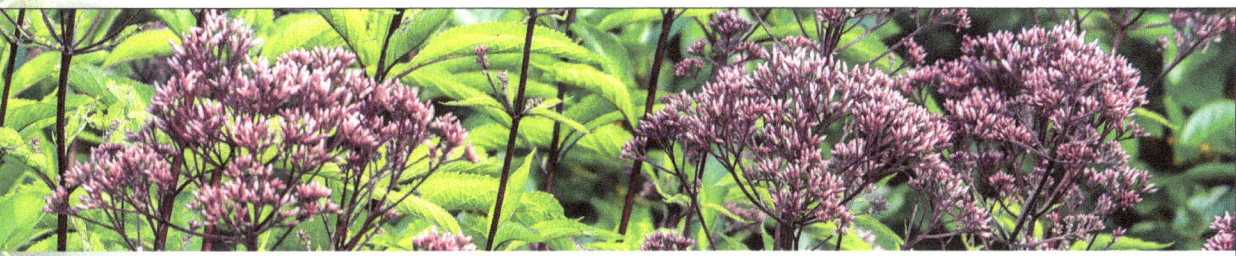

Joe Pye Weed

COMMON NAME: Joe Pye Weed

BOTANICAL NAME: *Eutrochium purpureum*

FAMILY: *Asteraceae* (Aster)

OTHER NAMES: Gravel Root, Queen of the Meadow, Sweet Joe Pye Weed, Purple Boneset

RELATED SPECIES: *Eutrochium maculatum* (Spotted Joe Pye Weed), *E. fistulosum, E. serotinum*

DESCRIPTION: Joe Pye weed is a dramatic plant that grows on a single stalk, sometimes reaching heights of ten to fourteen feet, and is topped with a regal plume of purple flowers arranged in a cluster. Lance-shaped leaves with serrated edges and a rough surface texture grow in whorls of four or six. Blooms late summer until the first frost.

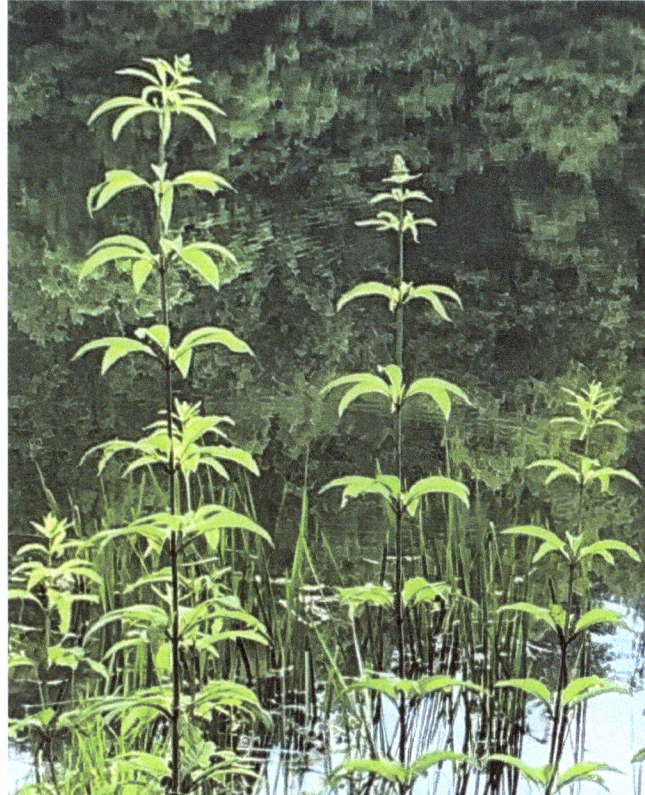

To differentiate between the two most common species found in the region, note that the flowers of *E. purpureum* form a mounded tuft; the leaves are aromatic, with dark purple marks appearing at the leaf nodes. Conversely, the flowers of *E. maculatum* form a flat-topped cluster with purple spots along the solid stem, and it is only three to four feet in height.

HABITAT: Joe Pye weed likes full sun and wet feet. It is found in sunny open areas, often at the edges of ditches, ponds and lakes. Common companion plants growing near Joe Pye weed include boneset, jewelweed and elder.

KEY ACTIONS: Diuretic, anti-lithic, anti-inflammatory, astringent, anti-rheumatic

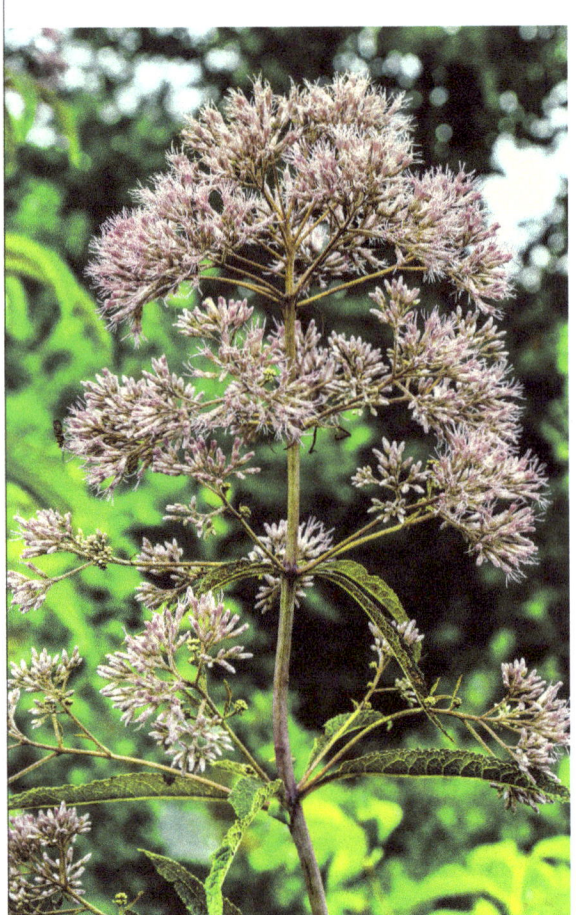

PART USED: Root

TRADITIONAL USES: The name "Joe Pye" is said to be in honor of an "Indian theme promoter" who recommended the herb to promote sweating in treating typhoid fever.[1] Another source claims the name derives from "jopi" the word for typhoid fever in an American Indian language.

The Cherokee considered Joe Pye weed leaves an important fever remedy. The hollow tubes of the stem were used to "bubble" or blow air into herbal medicines to activate them and increase their potency. They were also used to spray herbal preparations on the back of the throat.

In the nineteenth century, physicians used it to dissolve kidney stones, to soothe irritated tissues in the urinary tract, and as a general urinary system tonic. It was also used to relieve edema and treat stress incontinence.

Herbalist Tommie Bass used the root to treat kidney and bladder disease, prostate problems and kidney stones. He claimed that the root balanced blood sugar levels and used it to treat diabetes. Bass also recommended it for the relief of rheumatic pain.[2]

CURRENT USES: The roots of Joe Pye weed are a restorative tonic for the urinary tract. As a tonic, it prevents the formation of kidney stones. As an acute remedy, it helps dissolve kidney stones and soothe irritated tissues. It is a specific remedy for the treatment of prostate inflammation and swelling, cystitis, urinary tract infections, urgent or frequent urination, and vaginal discharge (leucorrhea) as a douche. The diuretic action of the root helps eliminate uric acid from the joints to relieve joint pain and inflammation.

CAUTIONS: Joe Pye weed is contraindicated during pregnancy and while nursing.

---

[1] Foster and Duke, *A Field Guide to Medicinal Plants and Herbs of North America*, 164
[2] Crellin and Philpott, *A Reference Guide to Medicinal Plants*, 274–277

PREPARATIONS

DECOCTION: For each cup of water, use two teaspoons fresh or one teaspoon dry root. Bring to a boil, reduce heat, cover and simmer for ten minutes. Strain.

TINCTURE: Fresh root – 1:2, 95%. Dried root – 1:5, 50%.

DOSAGES

DECOCTION: Drink one-half cup of cool or slightly warm decoction every half-hour to relieve acute urinary tract symptoms. As a tonic for chronic kidney problems, drink one cup of warm decoction daily for three to six months. Use as a vaginal douche as needed.

TINCTURE: Take one-half teaspoon of tincture in water every half hour for acute symptoms. For chronic kidney problems, take one-half teaspoon of tincture twice daily in water for three to six months.

HARVESTING

Joe Pye weed roots should be harvested in late summer or early fall as the flowers fade or around the first frost. Roots radiate out in all directions, so clear a wide area around the plant and loosen the soil to locate the root before digging.

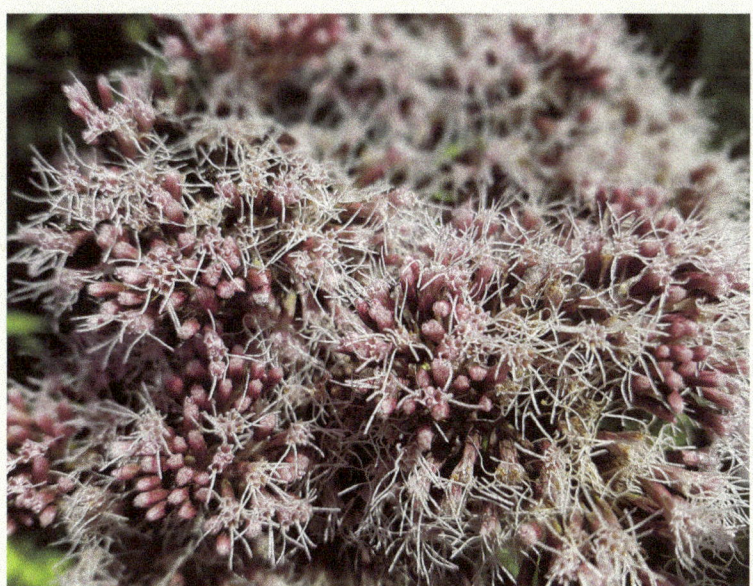

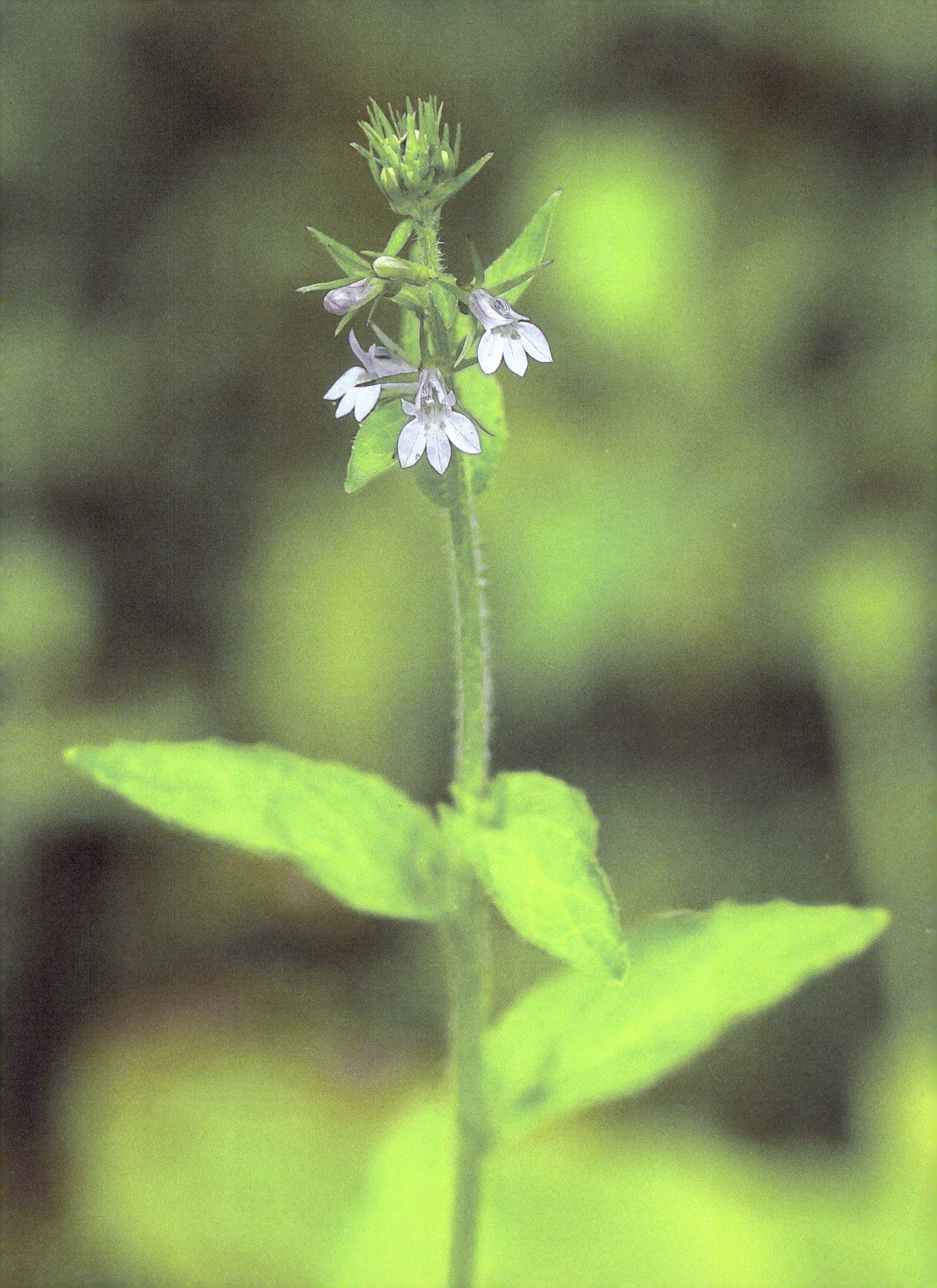

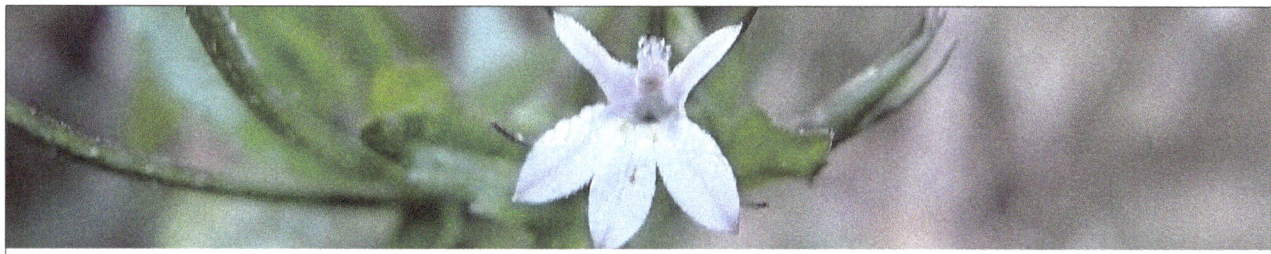

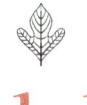

Lobelia

COMMON NAME: Lobelia

BOTANICAL NAME: *Lobelia inflata*

FAMILY: *Campanulaceae* (Bellflower)

OTHER NAMES: Indian Tobacco, Puke Weed, Asthma Weed

RELATED SPECIES: Spike Lobelia, *L. spicata var. scapose;* Greater Lobelia, *L. siphilitica;* Cardinal Flower, *L. cardinalis.*

DESCRIPTION: Lobelia is an erect annual, one to two feet tall. The alternate leaves, one to three inches long, are smooth and deep green. Tiny pale blue flowers, one-fourth inch in size, emerge at the leaf axils. Lobelia blooms appear from July to September. The plant derives its species name from the appearance of the seed-pods that swell up, or "inflate," and turn yellow when ripe.

HABITAT: Lobelia grows in partial shade along roadways and the edges of fields. It is an inconspicuous plant that is easy to overlook.

KEY ACTIONS: Antispasmodic, expectorant, emetic

PART USED: Aerial parts (leaf, flower and ripe seed pods)

TRADITIONAL USES: The Cherokee used lobelia infusions in large doses to induce vomiting and in small doses to reduce spasms in cases of colic and croup. They also used it topically to relax muscle spasms and relieve body aches. Lobelia contains lobeline, an alkaloid that generates a physiological response like that of nicotine; the dried plant was used in smoking blends as a tobacco substitute.[1]

Writing in the mid-1800s, Dr. Frances P. Porcher notes that lobelia is "one of the most valuable of our indigenous plants."[2] He

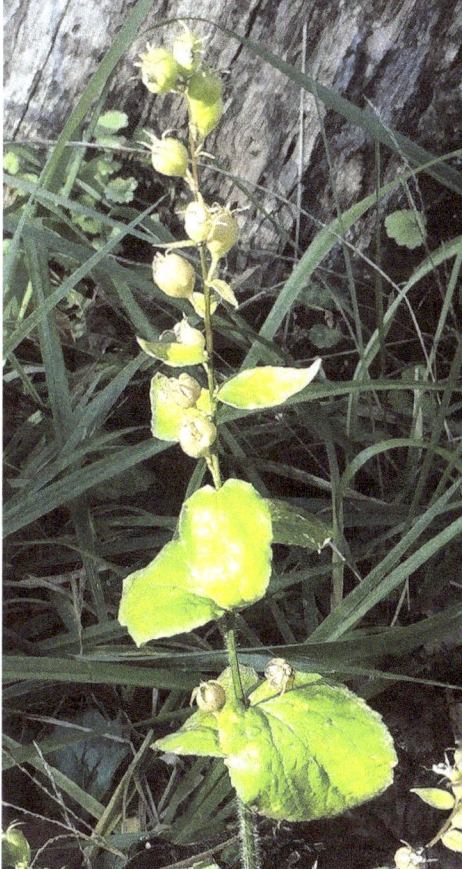

---

[1] Moerman, *Native American Ethnobotany,* 311–312

[2] Porcher, *Resources of the Southern Fields and Forests,* 401

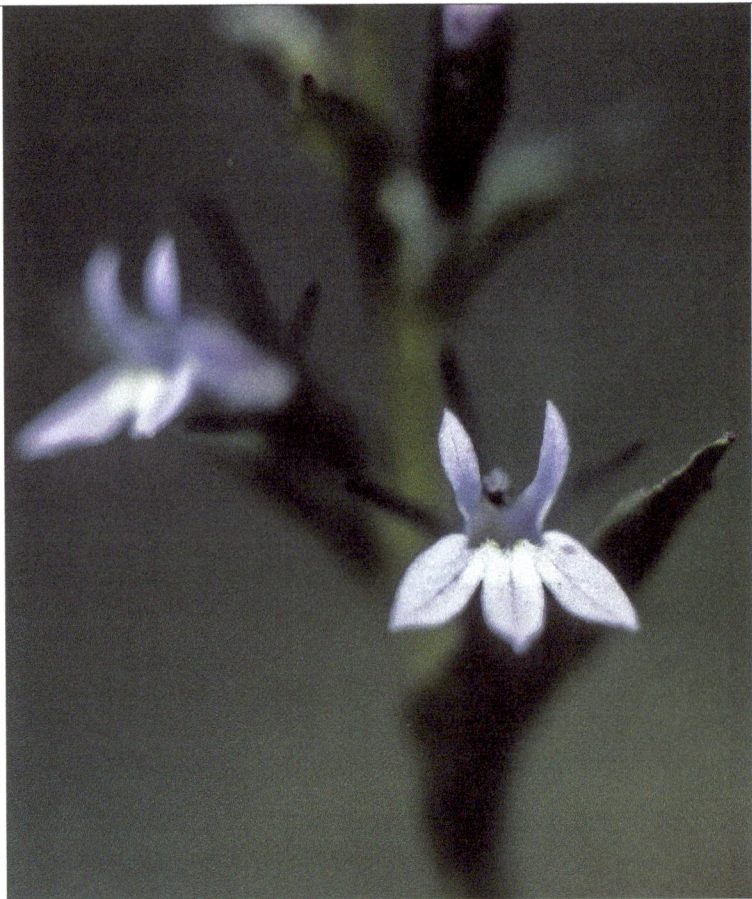

recommended using small doses of the infusion to relieve convulsions and heart palpitations, to induce sweating, and to prevent colic and croup in infants.

Although lobelia was used in both Native American and European herbal traditions, its reputation was tarnished when it was implicated in a much-publicized murder trial in 1807. A naturopathic physician, Samuel Thomson, was accused and later acquitted of killing a patient with an overdose of lobelia. Even though there is no evidence in the past two hundred years' medical literature of the plant's ever having caused any adverse effect more severe than vomiting and increased heart rate, lobelia's reputation as a poison persisted, and it fell from common usage. That said, this herb must be used with caution and strict attention to dosage recommendations.[3]

CURRENT USES: Lobelia effectively relieves acute respiratory symptoms as a bronchial dilator in proper doses. It is used for spasmodic coughs, asthmatic wheezing, and allergy-induced breathing difficulties. Lobelia tincture, used internally in small, frequent doses, relieves muscle cramps, spasms, and body aches. Lobelia tincture or liniment applied on the skin also relieves these same symptoms.

---

[3] Bergner, "Is Lobelia Toxic?" *Medical Herbalism*, Volume 10, No. 1 & 2, 1, 15–17

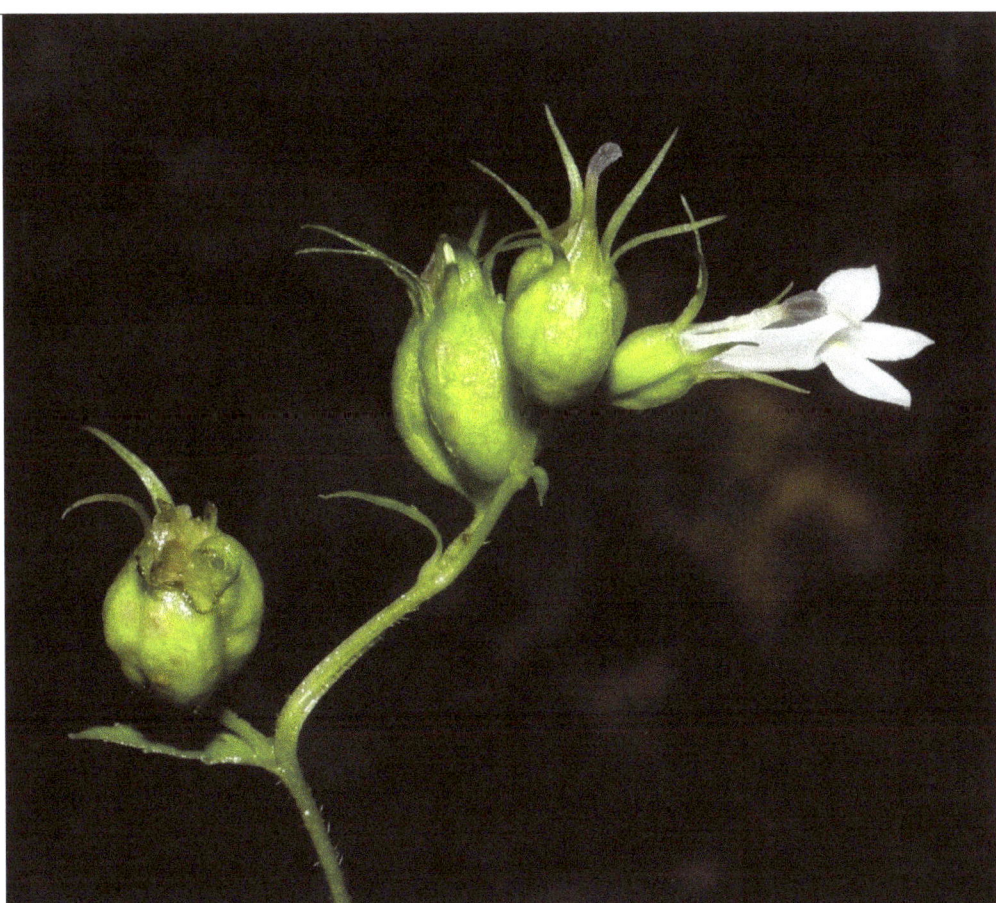

A blog post about recent research on lobelia by esteemed herbalist Jillian Stansbury explains its biphasic effect on the respiratory system.[4] Initially, lobelia acts as a respiratory stimulant; reactions include cough, excessive saliva, burning in the throat, and increased heart rate. However, this reaction lasts for only a few minutes. After this, the alkaloids in lobelia relax the respiratory system to relieve coughs, labored breathing and wheezing. This reminds us that dosage is crucial in using lobelia safely.

The herb is also used in smoking mixtures to relieve asthmatic symptoms and may ease nicotine withdrawal.

CAUTIONS: Safe use of lobelia requires careful attention to dosage. Compared to other medicinal herbs, it is used in very small amounts, usually ten drops of tincture. Because lobelia is an emetic, it will cause vomiting in large doses. However, nausea and increased heart rate are the most common side effects of taking too much lobelia, so it is obvious if you are using too much. Lobelia is contraindicated during pregnancy, while nursing or for those with heart problems.

---

[4] https://battlegroundhealingarts.com/blog/f/lobelia---newer-applications-of-a-folkloric-medicine

PREPARATIONS

Lobelia tincture is made using the standard weight-to-volume method. A second traditional method of making a simple tincture is also included below.

TINCTURE: Fresh – 1:2, 95%. Dry – 1:5, 60% plus 5% apple cider vinegar. Lobelia can also be prepared using only undiluted apple cider vinegar.

TRADITIONAL TINCTURE METHOD: Gather lobelia plants with many ripe (inflated, yellow) seed pods. Crush the fresh herb using a mortar and pestle, and slowly add some alcohol (I use brandy). Continue to add alcohol and blend with the lobelia until you have a watery mixture. Pour the mixture through a colander lined with unbleached muslin. Gather the edges of the cloth into a pouch and squeeze out every drop of liquid. Store in a brown bottle.[5]

HERBAL SMOKES: Combine dried lobelia with other herbs known to soothe the respiratory system. See the Smoky Mountain Smokes recipe on page 134.

DOSAGES

Small amounts are needed to relieve spasms, cramps, and breathing difficulties effectively. Large doses can cause nausea and even vomiting.

TINCTURE: Take ten drops in a small amount of water or tea every thirty minutes until symptoms are relieved.

SMOKE INHALATION: Take small inhalations of smoke into the lungs, hold for a few seconds and exhale. Repeat two or three times or until breathing eases. Use smoke inhalations sparingly to relieve acute symptoms because smoke is very drying to the lungs.

HARVESTING

Collect the aerial parts of lobelia when most of the seeds have ripened. Look for mature seedpods that resemble small, pale yellow balloons inflated with air. Once all the seeds ripen, the plant fades. Fresh lobelia should be tinctured or made into a liniment. Dried lobelia can be added to smoking mixtures.

Related species are often used. Spike Lobelia *(L. spicata var. scapose)* is used interchangeably with *L. inflata*. The other two species found in the region, Greater Lobelia *(L. siphilitica)* and Cardinal Flower *(L. cardinalis)*, have milder antispasmodic activity.

---

[5] Bergner and Treasure, "The Lost Forms of Lobelia," *Medical Herbalism*, Vol. 10, No. 1 & 2, 33–34

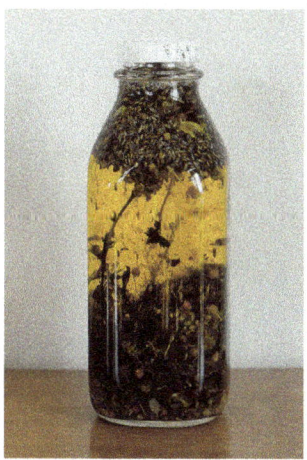

LOBELIA LINIMENT

This recipe is inspired by one shared by Canadian herbalist Chanchal Cabrera. I modified it to use our local mints, bee balm or mountain mint instead of juniper berry *(Juniperus spp.)*. It is for external use only.

INGREDIENTS

4 ounces (120 ml) lobelia tincture
4 ounces (120 ml) black haw tincture (or crampbark, *Viburnum opulus*)
4 ounces (120 ml) infused oil of poke root
4 ounces (120 ml) infused oil of mountain mint or bee balm (or any combination of the two)
¼ teaspoon (1 ml) each of any two of these essential oils: rosemary, black pepper, wintergreen or marjoram

To make the liniment, combine tinctures, infused oils and essential oils in a glass jar or bottle and shake well. Clearly label the bottle "For External Use Only" and keep it out of reach of children.

Apply the liniment with cotton to unbroken skin on tight or inflamed muscles or joints. Repeat every 30 minutes or as needed to relieve pain. Store the liniment in a cool, dark place. If stored properly, it remains potent for several years.

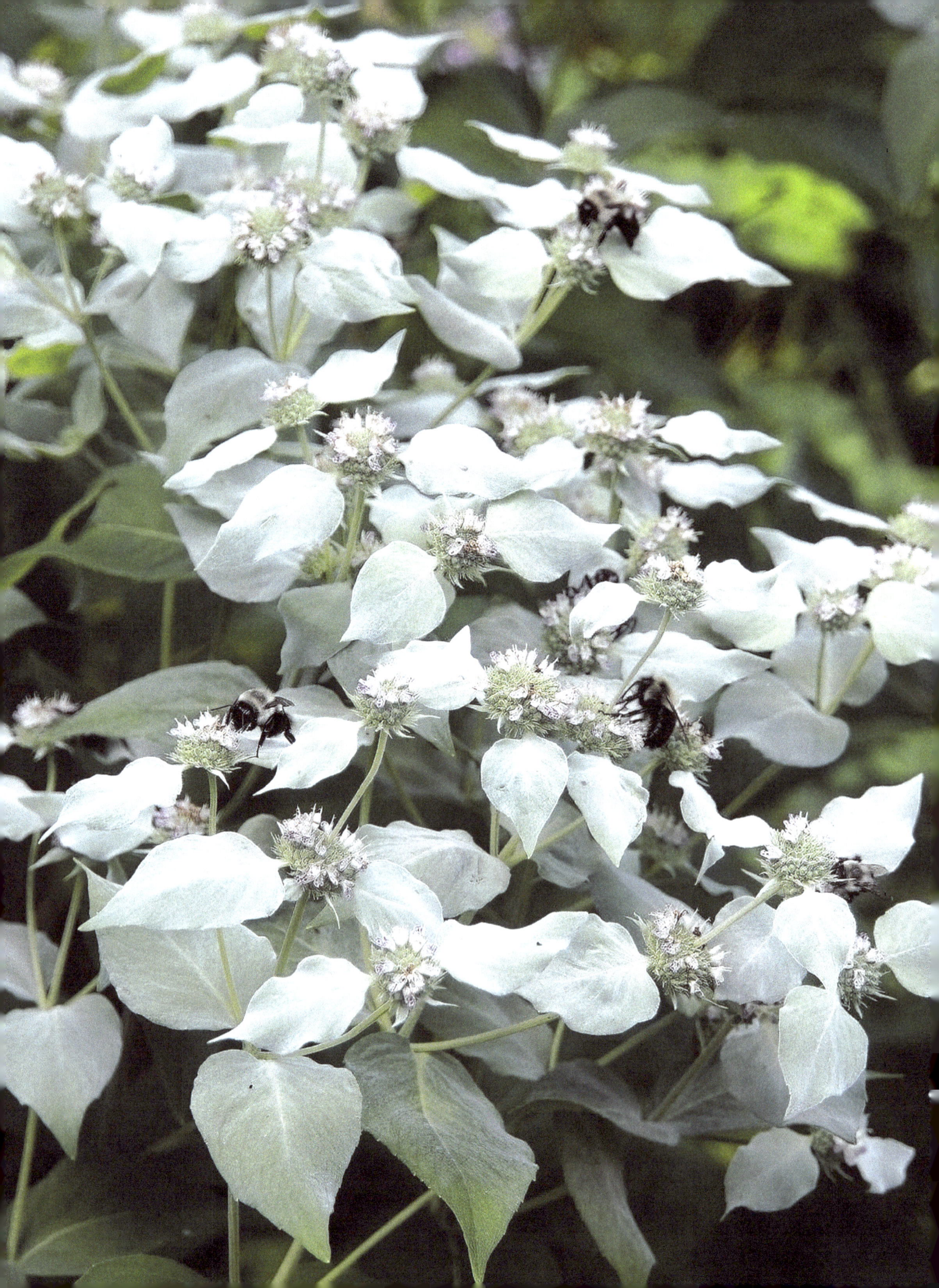

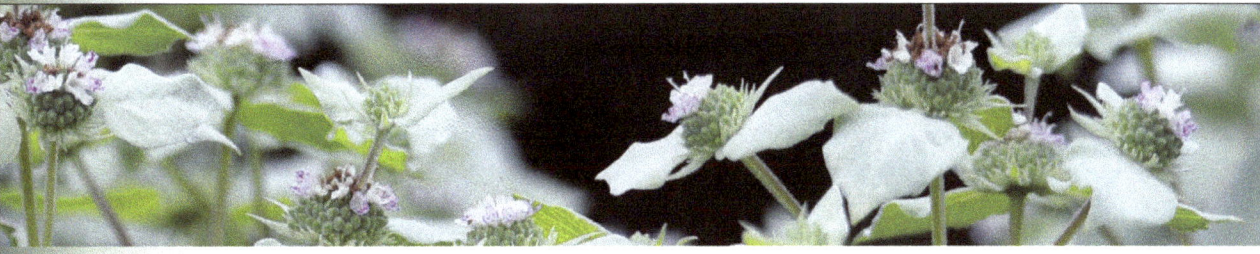

Mountain Mint

COMMON NAME: Mountain Mint

BOTANICAL NAME: *Pycnanthemum incanum*

FAMILY: *Lamiaceae* (Mint)

OTHER NAMES: Hoary Mountain Mint, Horsemint, Wild Basil

RELATED SPECIES: Beadle's Mountain Mint *(P. beadlei)*, Appalachian Mountain Mint *(P. montanum)*

DESCRIPTION: Mountain mint is a two to five feet tall perennial. Like most mints, it is very aromatic, with square stems and opposite leaves. The small, pale lavender flowers bloom in whorls in the leaf axils and at the terminal end on the branching upper stalks in midsummer. Leaves are oval, with bluntly serrated edges and pointed tips; the underside of the lower leaves are white, and the leaves of young plants are tinged with red. At midsummer, the upper leaves appear to be dusted with white powder that resembles hoar frost, hence the common name Hoary Mountain Mint.

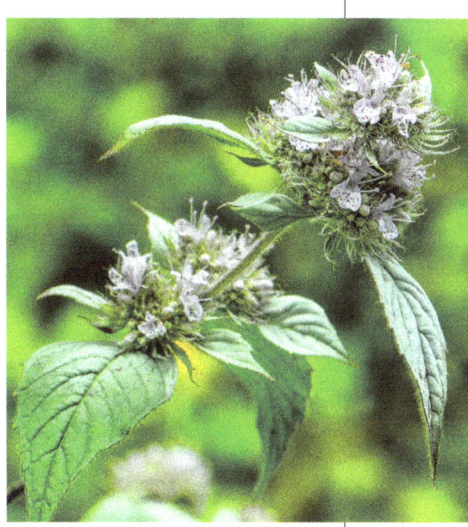

HABITAT: Sunny, open areas and along waterways or ditches.

KEY ACTIONS: Carminative, diaphoretic, antispasmodic, anti-inflammatory

PART USED: Aerial (in flower)

TRADITIONAL USES: The Cherokee used infusions of mountain mint to treat cold symptoms, reduce fevers, relieve nausea, and as an anti-inflammatory penis wash. A poultice of fresh leaves was applied to the head to relieve headaches.[1] Mountain mint has a long history of use as a folk remedy. The infusion was used for indigestion, to reduce fevers, and as an inhalation for sinus and lung congestion. It was a common home remedy used to bring on delayed menses.[2]

---

[1] Moerman, *Native American Ethnobotany*, 456

[2] Crellin and Philpott, *A Reference Guide to Medicinal Plants*, 412–413

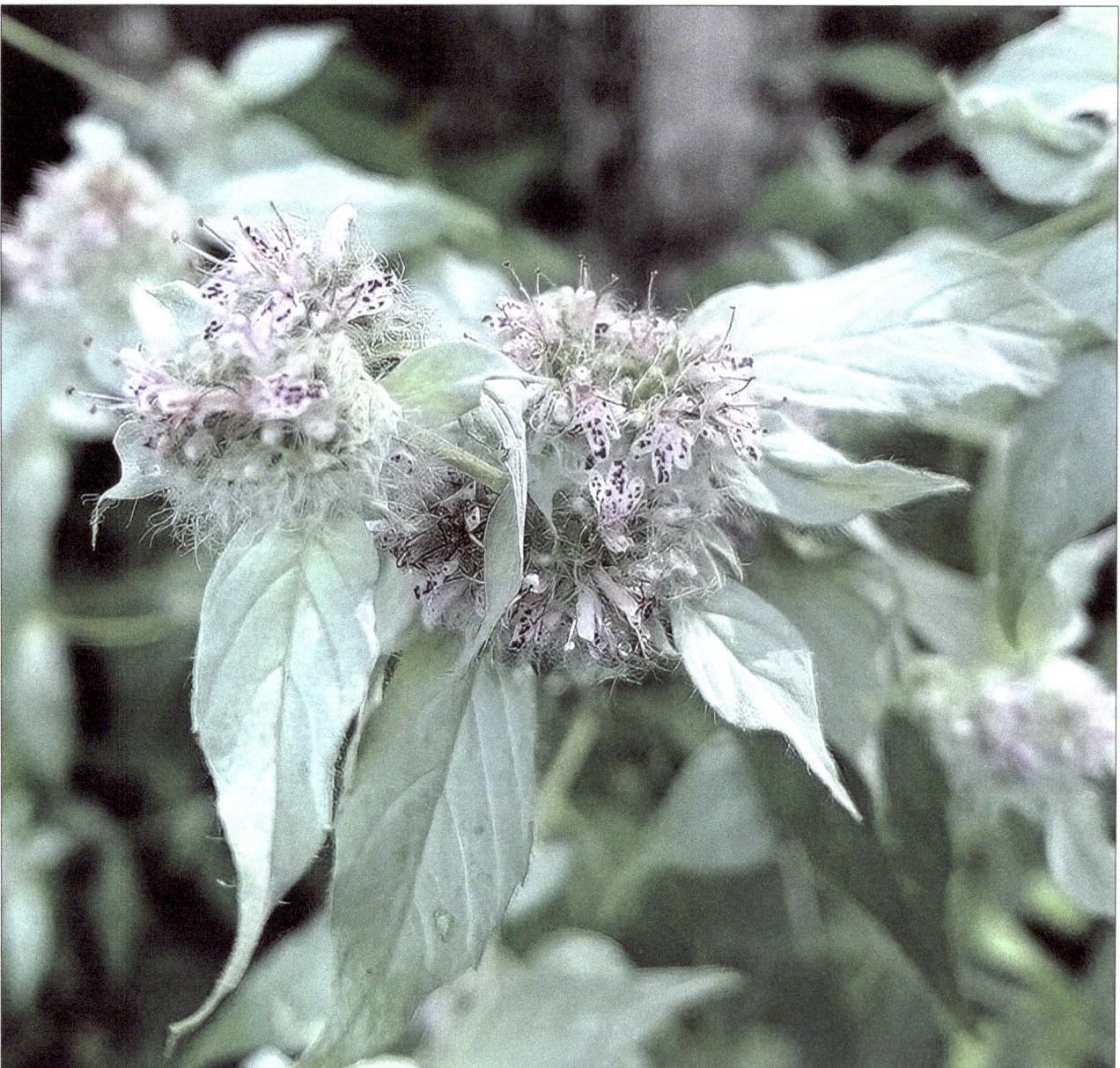

CURRENT USES: Mountain mint is a reliable remedy for indigestion, nausea, stomach cramps, and headaches caused by overeating and too much rich food. Hot infusions reduce fevers, and the vapors of hot infusions can be inhaled to relieve sinus and lung congestion.

Because it has a much stronger flavor, use mountain mint in smaller amounts than you would other members of the Mint family, such as peppermint *(Mentha piperata),* spearmint *(Mentha spicata),* or bee balm. I like to add small amounts to tea blends that include herbs with harsh or bitter flavors.

CAUTIONS: None known.

PREPARATIONS

The best way to enjoy the fragrant volatile oils of mountain mint is to prepare it as a cold infusion, as hot infusions have a harsher menthol flavor. This preserves the more delicate volatile oils. If using it as a diaphoretic to induce sweating and reduce fever, heat the cold infusion and drink as hot as possible. While mountain mint can be tinctured, I prefer to use it as tea.

INFUSION: Add one tablespoon of dried or two tablespoons of fresh herb to eight ounces of cool or room-temperature water. Cover and steep for one hour. Strain. Reheat if needed. Infusions can also be added to a foot or regular bath to relieve fevers, congestion and nausea.

INHALATION: Bring a quart of water to a boil in a pot. Remove from heat and add two big handfuls of fresh or dried mountain mint. Put the pot on a table and drape a bath towel over your head to make a tent. Breathe deeply to inhale the steam which contains the volatile oils being released by the heat. Have a good supply of tissues nearby and repeat as needed to relieve lung and sinus congestion.

DOSAGES

INFUSION: Drink eight ounces of infusion every hour or as needed until symptoms improve. For a cooling summer beverage, drink cold mountain mint infusion with a few slices of lemon.

INHALATION: Repeat every few hours or as often as needed to relieve congestion.

HARVESTING

Collect on cool summer mornings before direct sunlight and heat dissipate the essential oils. Cut the stem just above any bug-eaten leaves. Tie four or five plant stems together, put them in a paper bag and hang them in a cool, dry place until completely dry. Or strip the leaves and flowers from the stalks and dry them on a screen or in a dehydrator.

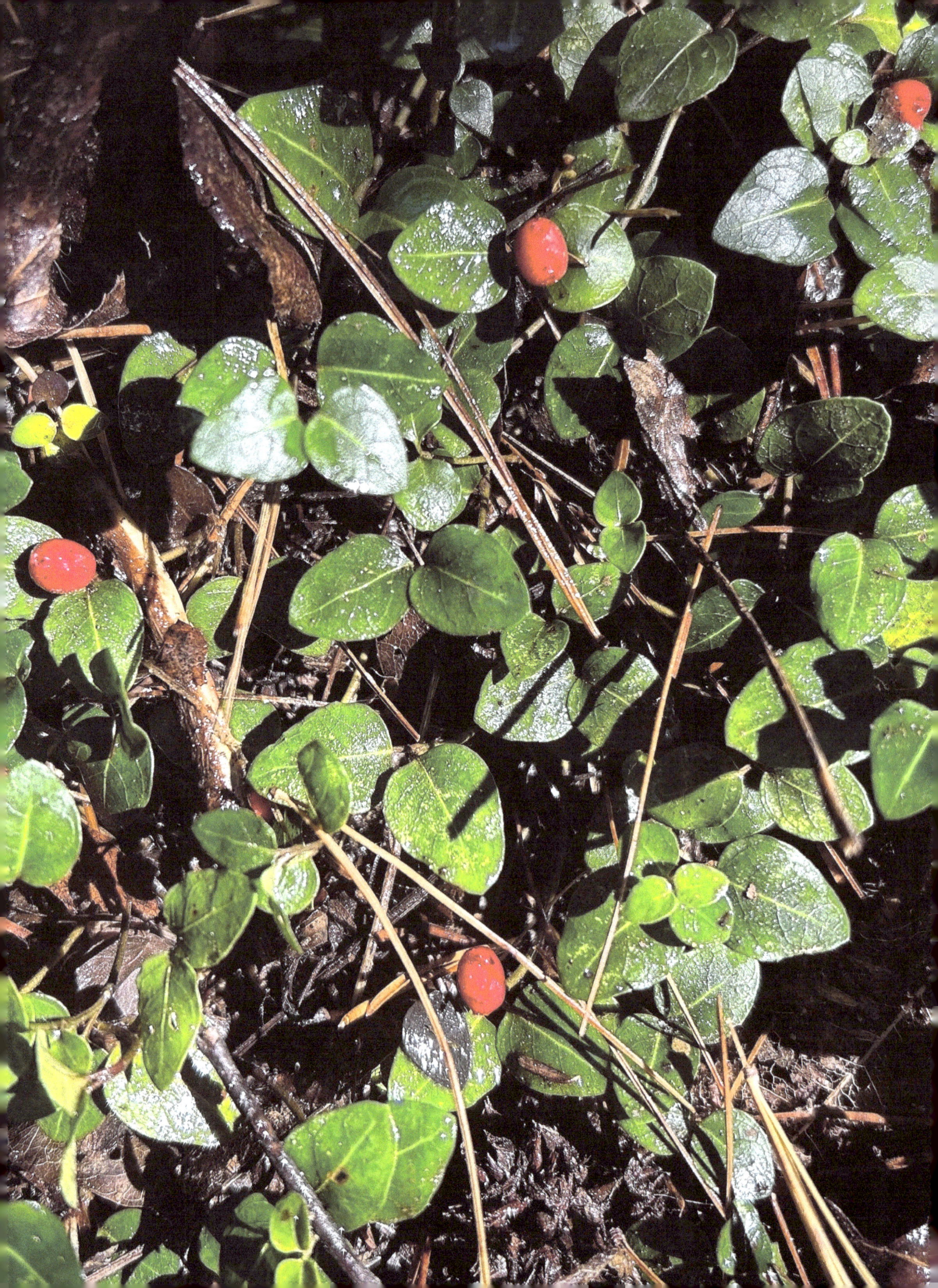

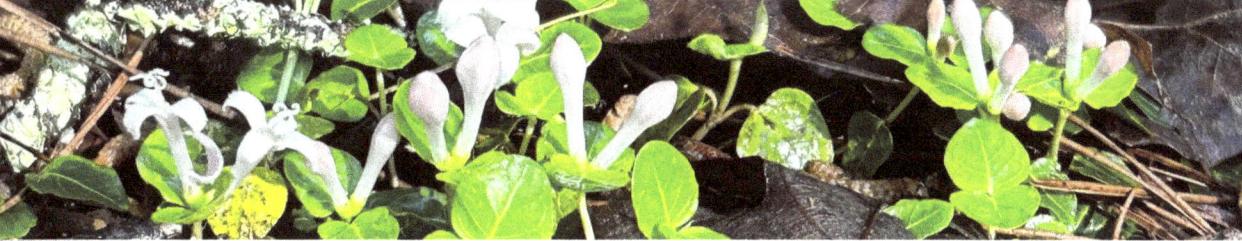

Partridgeberry

COMMON NAME: Partridgeberry

BOTANICAL NAME: *Mitchella repens*

FAMILY: *Rubiaceae* (Madder)

OTHER NAMES: Squawvine, Checkerberry

DESCRIPTION: Partridgeberry is a small, perennial evergreen vine with rounded, opposite leaves that have a shiny, leathery appearance. The top of each leaf is neatly divided in half by a white vein. The entire plant is less than three inches tall and forms lush mats on the ground. Tiny white flowers in pairs have four parts and a subtle fragrance if you can get close enough to smell them. Blooms appear in June and July. Later in the summer, flavorless, mealy berries appear and turn red when ripe. The berries persist through winter.

HABITAT: Partridgeberry grows in the deep shade of moist forests, usually on slopes or embankments.

KEY ACTIONS: Uterine tonic, astringent

PART USED: Aerial

TRADITIONAL USES: Among American Indians, partridge berry was used to remedy various female generative system symptoms, including menstrual cramps, delayed or irregular menses, heavy menstrual flow, labor difficulties, and infertility. Leaf infusions and poultices were used to soothe sore nipples, hemorrhoids, and wounds.[1]

Folk uses of partridgeberry include herbal steams to relieve rheumatic pain and a decoction of the berries in milk to stop diarrhea and treat dysentery. In the 19th and 20th centuries, partridgeberry was a popular remedy for women.[2] Though they have little flavor, the berries were also eaten.

---

[1] Moerman, *Native American Ethnobotany*, 345

[2] Crellin and Philpott, *A Reference Guide to Medicinal Plants*, 412–413

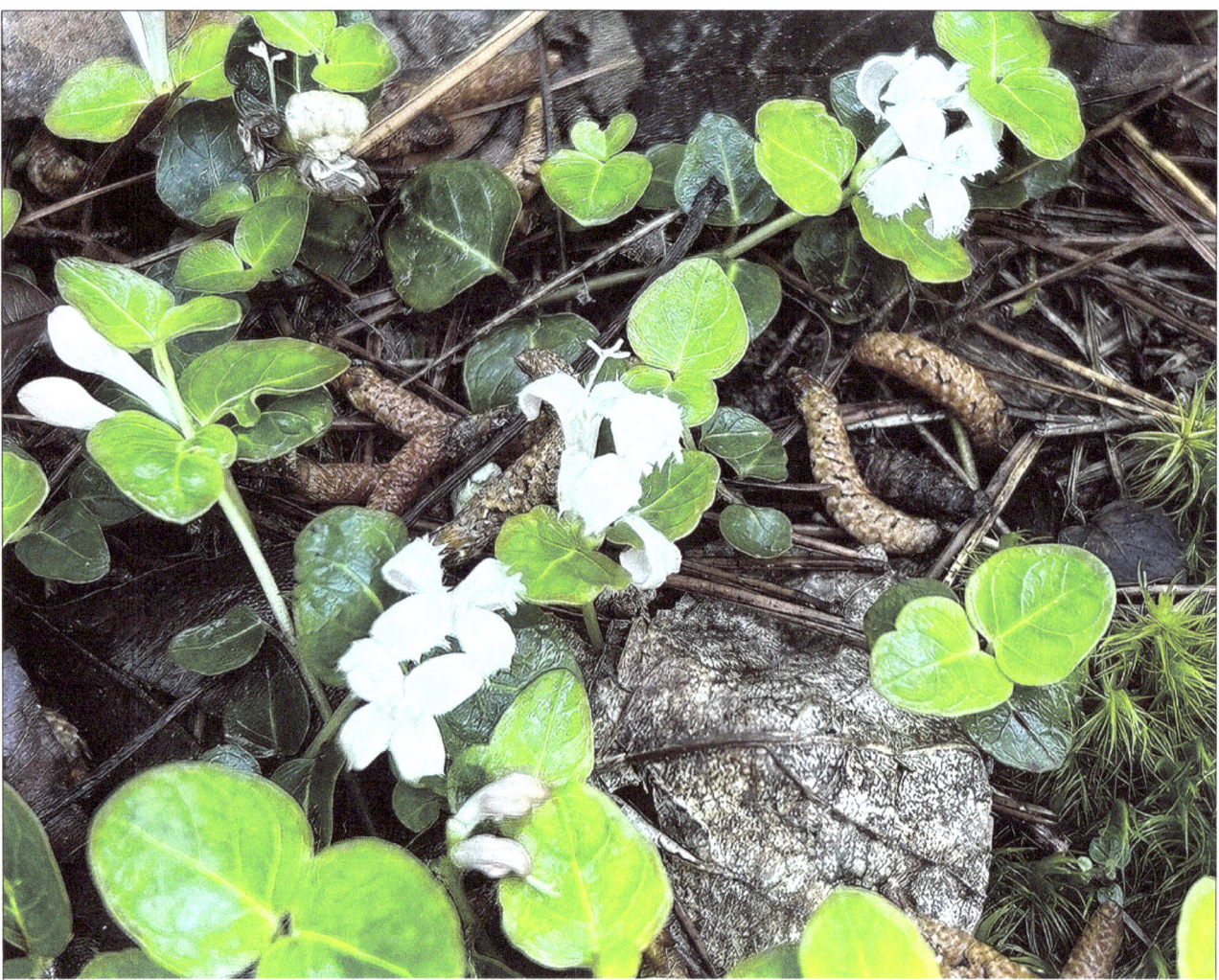

CURRENT USES: Partridgeberry is an important gynecological remedy in modern herbal practice. It is considered a reliable tonic to treat symptoms of deficiency such as infertility, lack of menses (amenorrhea), menstrual cramps (dysmenorrhea), and threatened miscarriage. It is also an effective remedy for reducing excessively heavy menstrual flow and relieving persistent vaginal discharge. Partridgeberry is also used as a uterine or labor tonic during the final trimester of pregnancy.

CAUTIONS: None known. Partridgeberry or other herbs that impact the reproductive organs should be used cautiously during pregnancy.

PREPARATIONS

Because partridgeberry leaves are leathery and dry, even when fresh, process fresh or dried leaves the same way. Although both tinctures and infusions are beneficial because partridgeberry is a tonic that should be used for several months, tincture often results in better outcomes as it is easier to use long term.

DECOCTION: Use one teaspoon of dried or two teaspoons of fresh herb for each eight ounces of water. Bring water to a boil in a pot; cover and simmer for twenty minutes. Strain.

TINCTURE: Fresh or dried – 1:5, 50%.

DOSAGES

Partridgeberry is a tonic herb that requires three to six months of daily use for best results.

DECOCTION: Drink eight ounces twice a day.

TINCTURE: Take one teaspoon in a small amount of water twice daily.

HARVESTING

Plants may be harvested at any time of the year. Cut individual vines close to the ground, careful not to damage or dislodge the roots. Because partridgeberry is a tiny plant, many are needed to make a significant amount of medicine.

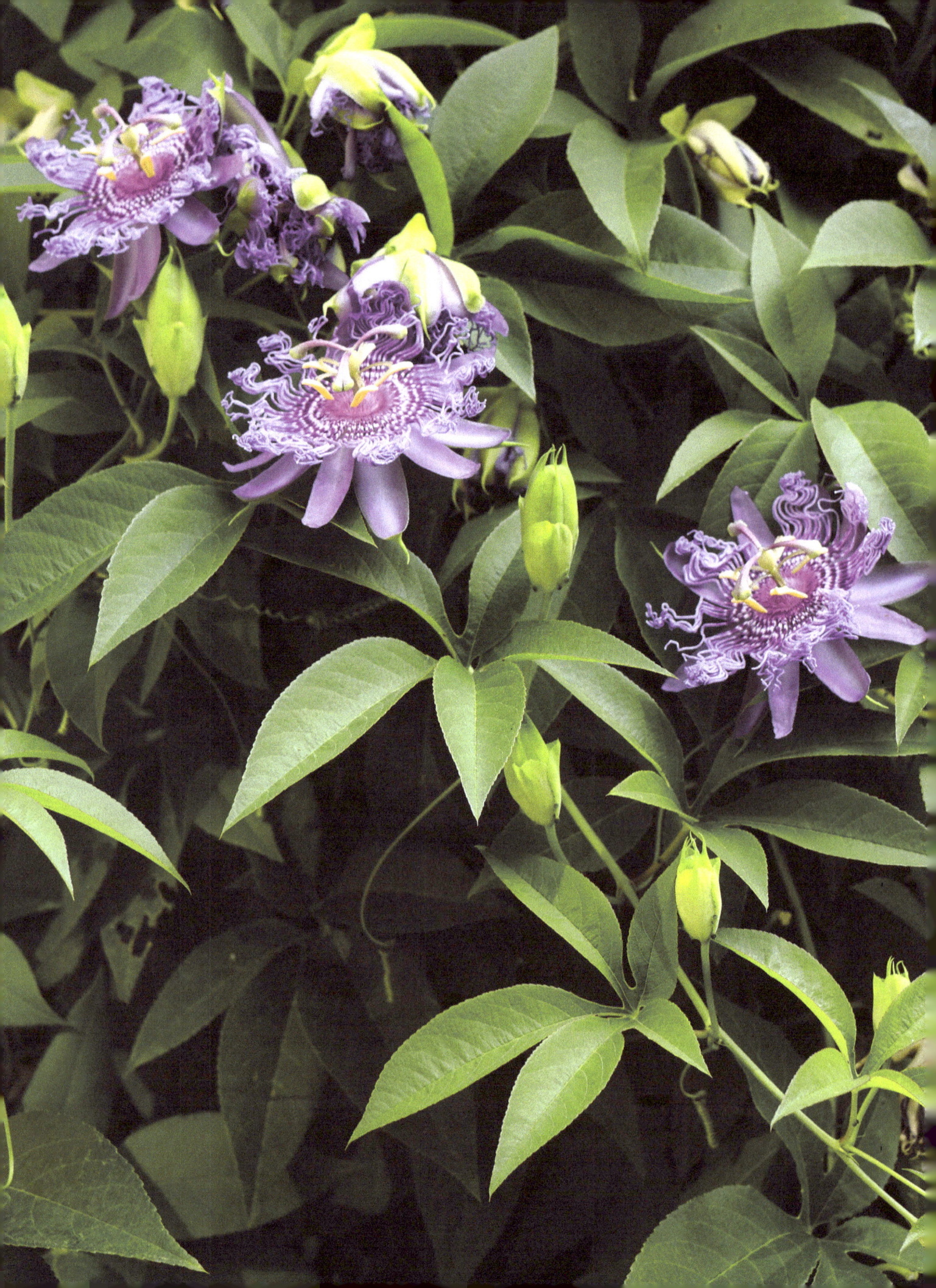

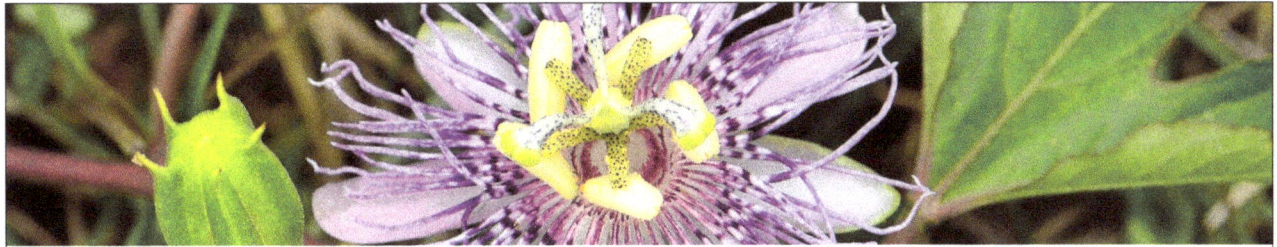

Passionflower

COMMON NAME: Passionflower

BOTANICAL NAME: *Passiflora incarnata*

FAMILY: *Passifloraceae* (Passionflower)

OTHER NAMES: Maypop

RELATED SPECIES: Yellow Passionflower *(P. lutea)*

DESCRIPTION: Passionflower is a vigorous perennial vine that grows up to twenty feet long. Leaves are deeply lobed and alternate. Dramatic, ornate purple flowers, two to three inches wide, grow singly or in pairs, blooming mid-summer. The flower has five pale purple petals and sepals, fringe-like purple and white filaments, all radiating from the five yellow anthers and upright pistil with three knobby stigmas at the center. The fruit is the size and shape of a small hen's egg; it turns from green to pale yellow when ripe. Inside the fruit, known as a maypop, are many oval black seeds in an edible gel-like pulp. A second local species, yellow passionflower *(P. lutea),* is a tiny vine with three-lobed leaves and yellow-green flowers less than one-half inch in diameter that lack the botanical complexity of *P. incarnata*.

HABITAT: Transitional zones at the edge of forests and sunny open areas. Passionflower is a common weed throughout most of the southeast.

KEY ACTIONS: Relaxing nervine, sedative, antispasmodic

PART USED: Leaf, flower, fruit (edible)

TRADITIONAL USES: Cherokees collected passionflower roots and pounded them to make a poultice or infused them for tea. The poultice was used to draw the inflammation from boils or skin infections caused by briar scratches. The infusion was used to soothe weaning babies. Drops of warm infusion were used to treat earaches. Passionflower fruits, or maypops, were crushed, and the juice was thickened with cornmeal or

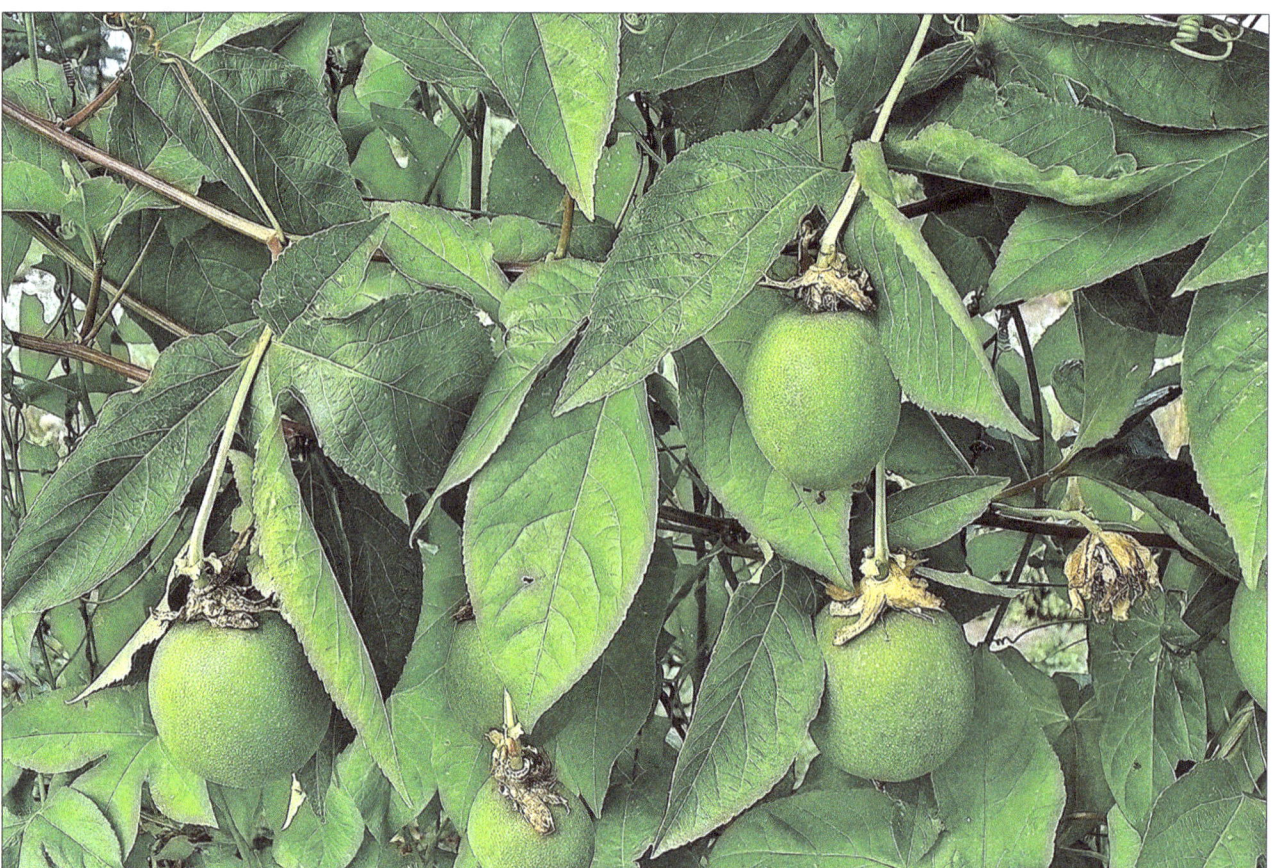

flour to make a pleasant beverage. Shoots and young leaves were cooked and eaten as a wild green.[1]

Jesuit priests who colonized South America in the early 17th century gave passionflower its common name. They believed the ornate flowers symbolized the crucifixion and passion of Jesus Christ and were a sign that they would be successful in their mission to spread Christianity.

CURRENT USES: Passionflower is a remedy that soothes the nervous system and mediates the physical symptoms caused by or made worse by stress. It can be used for tension headaches and to relax tense muscles, especially in the back, shoulders and neck. Passionflower is a specific remedy for insomnia symptoms, including difficulty falling and staying deeply asleep. When excessive tension results in shallow breathing, chest constriction, heart palpitations and the inability to relax, passionflower may effectively relax muscles and relieve the vascular constriction contributing to elevated blood pressure. The pulp collected from the ripe fruit is edible and often made into jelly or syrup.

CAUTIONS: None known.

---

[1] Moerman, *Native American Ethnobotany*, 50

PREPARATIONS

Effective as either a tincture or infusion, passionflower leaf and flower have a slightly bitter, acrid taste. Consider combining it with other aromatics like bee balm, peppermint *(Mentha piperata)* or lemon balm *(Melissa officinalis)* when making infusions.

INFUSION: Use one teaspoon dried or two teaspoons fresh leaf and flower for each eight ounces of boiling water. Cover and infuse for twenty minutes. Strain.

TINCTURE: Fresh – 1:2, 70%. Dried – 1:5, 40%.

DOSAGES

For best results, take repeated doses of passionflower until symptoms improve.

INFUSION: Drink four ounces of infusion every thirty minutes until symptoms improve or as needed.

TINCTURE: Take one-fourth to one-half teaspoon in water every thirty minutes until symptoms improve or as needed. For insomnia, take one dose an hour before bedtime, a second dose at bedtime, and if unable to sleep after about thirty minutes, take a third dose. It may take a few nights for passionflower to relax the nervous system.

HARVESTING

Collect leaves and flowers when in bloom during June and July. Gather maypop fruits after they turn pale green or yellow. Yellow passionflower is rare in the region; it should not be harvested or disturbed.

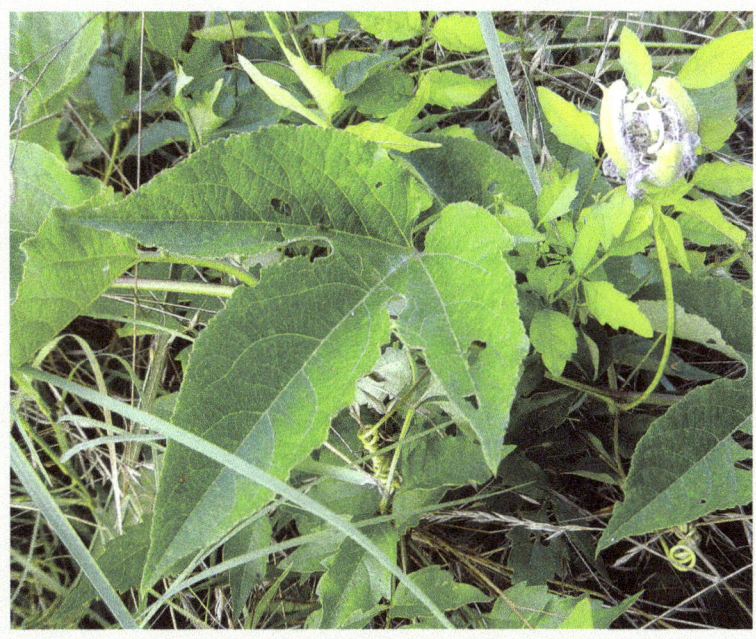

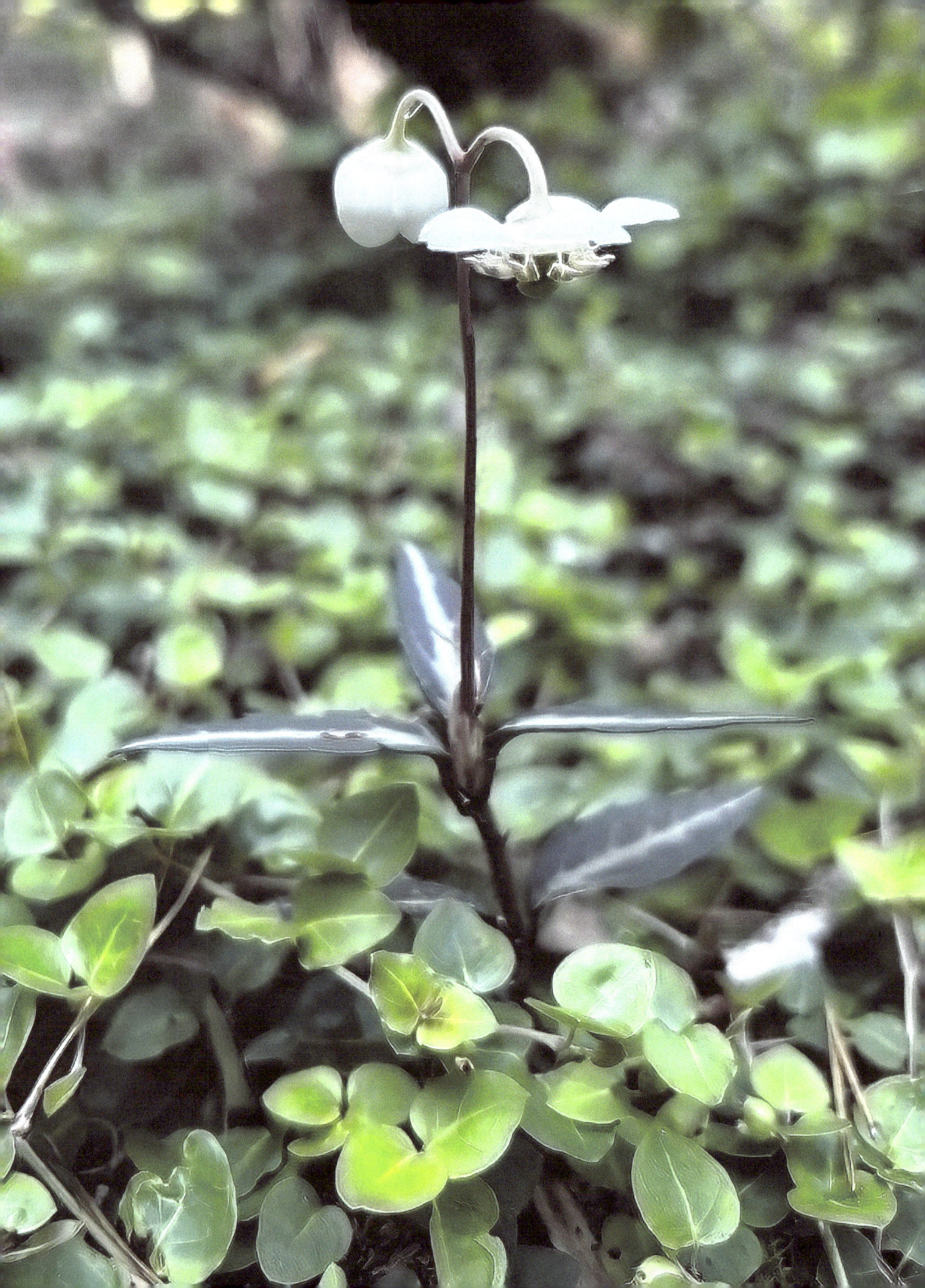

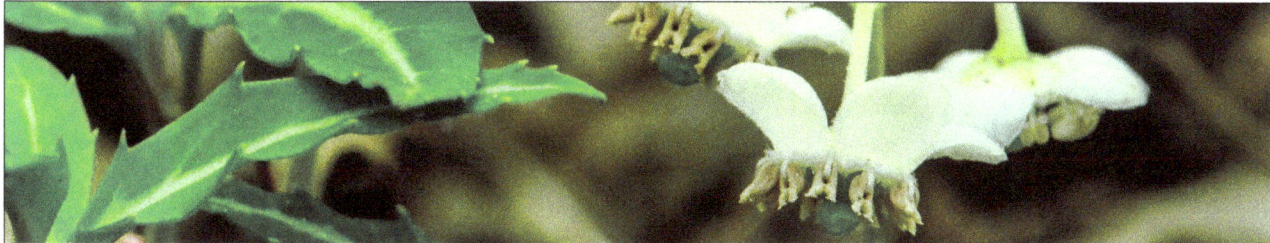

Pipsissewa

COMMON NAME: Pipsissewa

BOTANICAL NAME: *Chimaphila maculata*

FAMILY: *Ericaceae* (Heath)

OTHER NAMES: Spotted Pipsissewa, Rat's Bane, Rat's Vein

RELATED SPECIES: *C. umbellata,* also known as pipsissewa, is found farther north and west. It has similar properties, and the two can be used interchangeably.

DESCRIPTION: Pipsissewa is a four to five-inch-tall evergreen perennial with dark green, leathery leaves with a milky white strip down the center and shallowly toothed edges. The leaves are technically alternate, but they are so close together that they appear to grow in pairs or whorls. In early summer, nodding, waxy white flowers tinged with pink, a knobby green center, and a subtle fragrance (if you can get down on the ground close enough to smell them!) bloom on upright stems. The leaves of *C. umbellata* are similar but without white markings and arranged in more pronounced whorls. The whitish-pink flowers have distinctive red anthers.

HABITAT: Common in dry, deciduous forests.

KEY ACTIONS: Alterative, lymphatic, diuretic, tonic, antiseptic, vulnerary, anti-inflammatory

PART USED: Leaf

TRADITIONAL USES: The Cherokee drank pipsissewa infusions for rheumatic pain, colds, fevers, and kidney problems. Strong decoctions were used as a wash to treat ringworm and skin ulcers.[1]

During the Civil War, doctors recommended pipsissewa to treat digestive problems, kidney issues, and general debility. It was said to stimulate the appetite and revive flagging energy. Decoctions were used internally and externally to heal obstinate ulcers. A simple tincture made with

---

[1] Moerman, *Native American Ethnobotany,* 50

pipsissewa leaves steeped in whiskey was used as a remedy for rheumatism to warm joints and relieve stiffness and pain.

Folk usage of pipsissewa includes combining it with mullein leaf *(Verbascum thapsus)* to prevent children from wetting the bed and as a spring tonic to increase energy. Pipsissewa root was an ingredient in many traditional

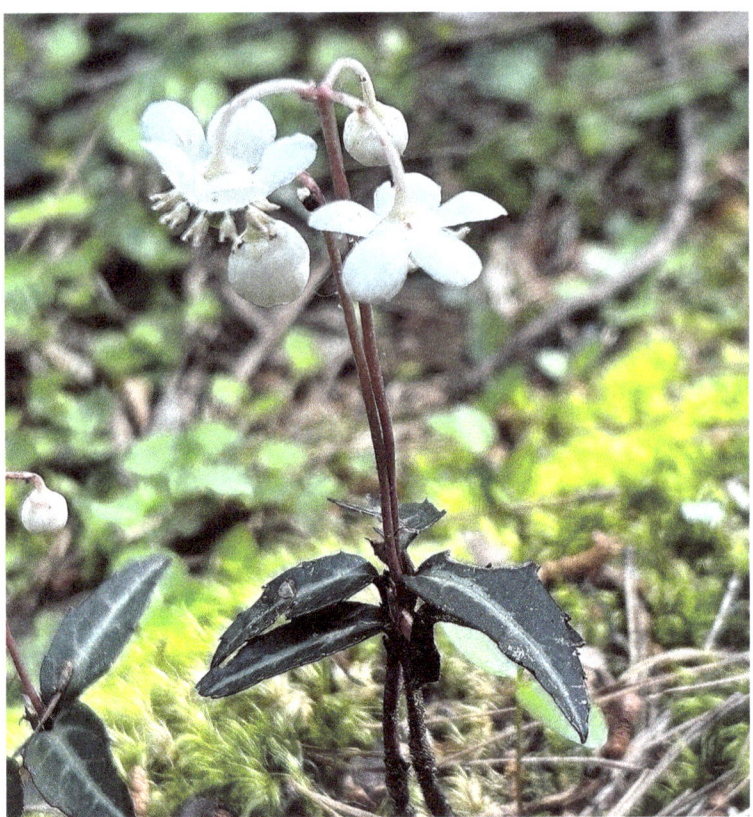

root beer recipes. According to Southern folklore, pipsissewa will repel or kill rats, hence the common name "rat's bane."

CURRENT USES: In modern herbal practice, pipsissewa is frequently used to treat acute and chronic urinary tract problems. It is a tonic for symptoms of chronic kidney issues with a pattern of frequent bladder infections, incontinence, or a history of kidney disease. Pipsissewa is also used for acute symptoms such as bladder infections, prostatitis, cystitis and urethritis, kidney stones, and painful or frequent urination. Pipsissewa is an excellent diuretic to include in general detoxifying formulas along with liver tonics (hepatics), blood cleansers (alteratives) and lymphatics. The infusion used as a douche reduces vaginal discharge (leucorrhea).

CAUTIONS: Acute kidney symptoms (listed above), when accompanied by sharp pains in the lower back and fever, may indicate a life-threatening kidney infection. If these symptoms occur, immediately seek help from a medical professional who can accurately diagnose kidney infections before using herbal remedies.

PREPARATIONS

Pipsissewa leaves are leathery, and fresh or dried leaves are processed similarly.

INFUSION: Add two tablespoons of chopped fresh or dried leaf to eight ounces of boiling water. Cover and steep for thirty minutes. Strain.

DECOCTION: Add two tablespoons of chopped fresh or dried leaf to eight ounces of cold water. Bring to a boil, then reduce heat to a simmer, cover and decoct for thirty minutes.

TINCTURE: Dried – 1:5, 50%.

DOSAGES

Although both tinctures and infusions are beneficial, when using pipsissewa as a tonic, dosing with tincture often results in better outcomes as it is easier to use long-term.

INFUSION: For acute symptoms, drink four ounces every hour. Drink four ounces twice daily for one month or longer as a tonic.

DECOCTION: Appy topically as a skin wash or use warm preparation as a vaginal douche as needed.

TINCTURE: For acute symptoms, take one-half teaspoon in a small amount of water every hour. As a tonic, take one-half teaspoon in water twice daily for a month or longer.

HARVESTING

Gather pipsissewa leaves any time of year. Cut the stem just above the ground, careful not to dislodge the roots. You can carefully strip leaves from the stem or just use all aerial parts. Rinse well before drying or processing fresh. Because pipsissewa is so tiny, many leaves are needed, so be sure you are harvesting from a large, healthy population.

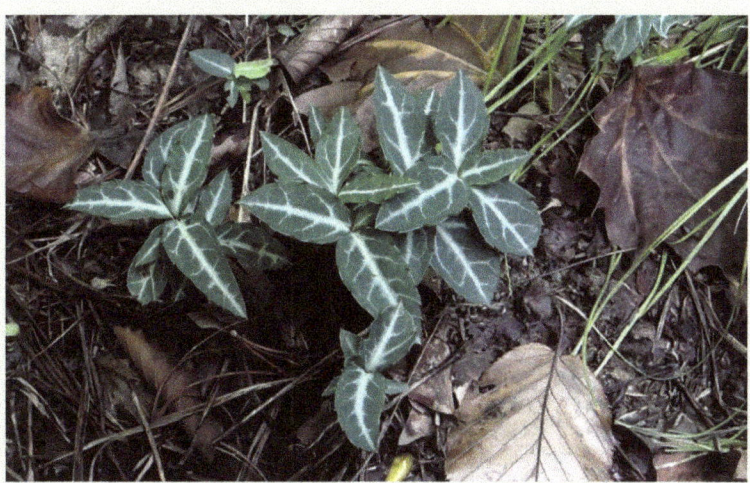

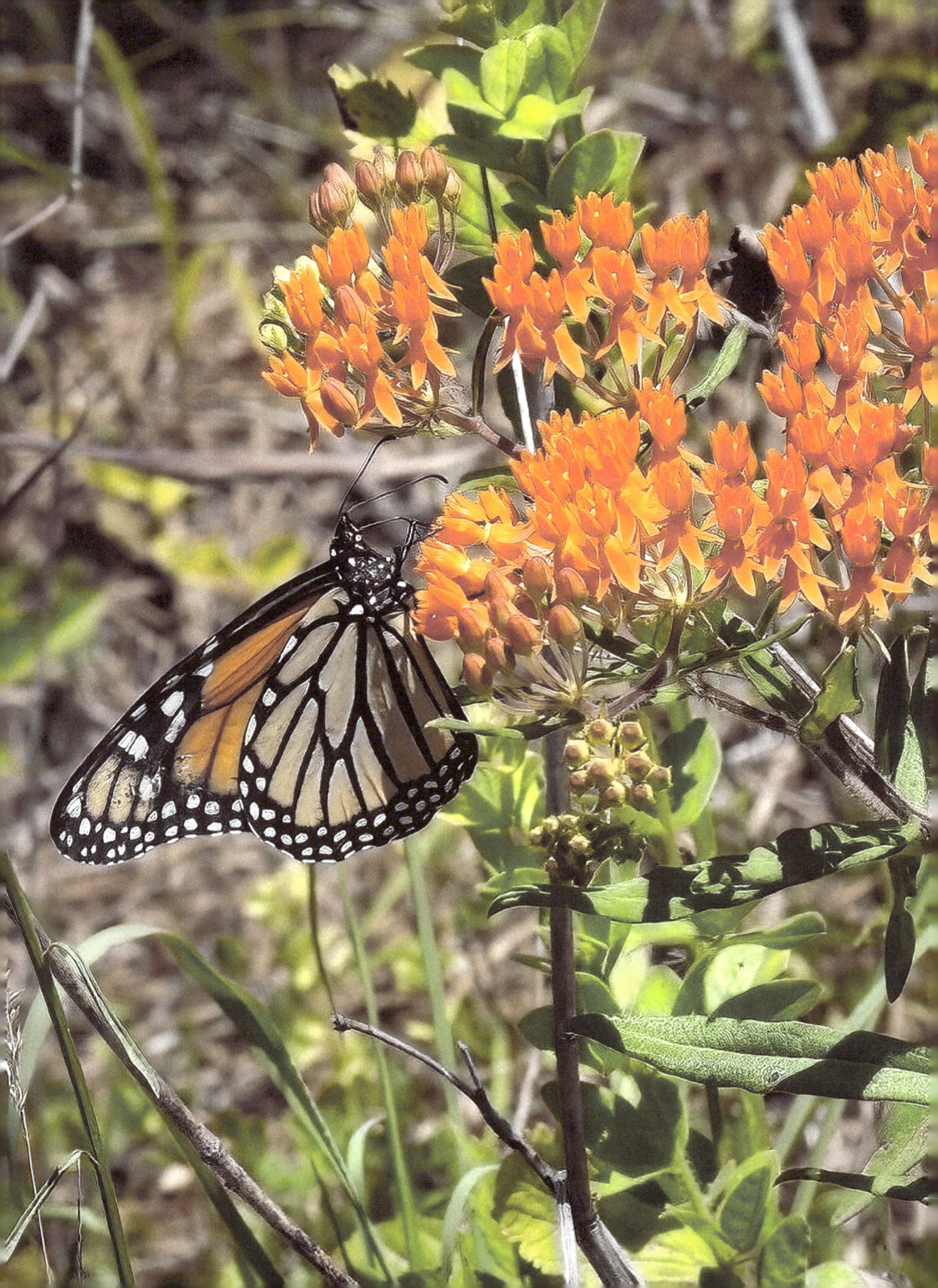

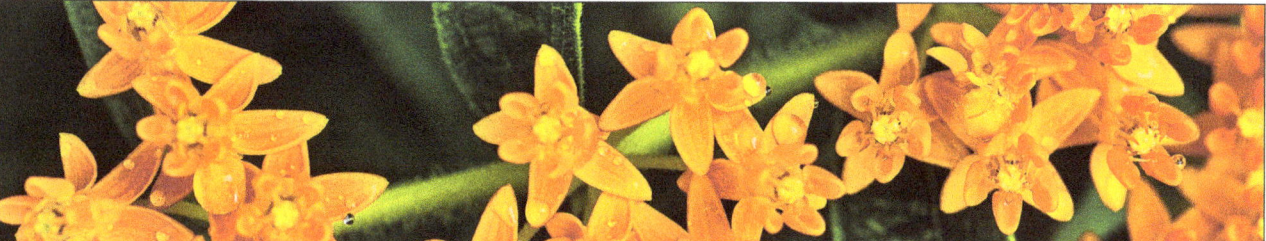

Pleurisy Root

COMMON NAME: Pleurisy Root

BOTANICAL NAME: *Asclepias tuberosa*

FAMILY: *Asclepiadaceae* (Milkweed)

OTHER NAMES: Butterfly Weed, Colic Root

DESCRIPTION: Pleurisy root is a perennial, two to three feet tall, with hairy, narrow leaves with rounded tips arranged alternately along a thick, slightly hairy stem. Distinctive fluorescent orange flowers bloom in clusters from June to August. Individual flowers have five sepals, five petals (that curve sharply downward), and five coronas. The flowers are very fragrant, and their nectar is sweet. Two to four inches long seed pods have a bumpy surface. When ripe, the pod cracks open, and brown seeds, each attached to silky, down-like plumes that act like a navigational system, are dispersed by the wind. Pleurisy root is part of a large plant family of over 2,000 species, most in tropical climates.

Pleurisy root flowers are an essential food source for monarch and swallowtail butterflies and should be part of every pollinator garden. The leaves, which contain an alkaloid toxic to birds, are a larval food source for monarch butterflies. The alkaloids are stored in the caterpillar's body, and later, after they metamorphose into butterflies, if birds eat them, they become nauseous. Several other butterfly species mimic the monarch's appearance to ward off predatory birds, although they do not feed on the leaves of pleurisy root.

HABITAT: Look for neon orange pleurisy flowers in sunny, open areas and in transitional zones at the edge of forests and along roads.

KEY ACTIONS: Stimulating expectorant, bronchial dilator, anti-inflammatory, antispasmodic, anti-catarrhal, lymphatic, cardio stimulant

PART USED: Root

TRADITIONAL USES: Pleurisy root has been used in American Indian and folk medicine to treat respiratory and pulmonary symptoms. It was considered a specific remedy for coughs, lung congestion, and breathing

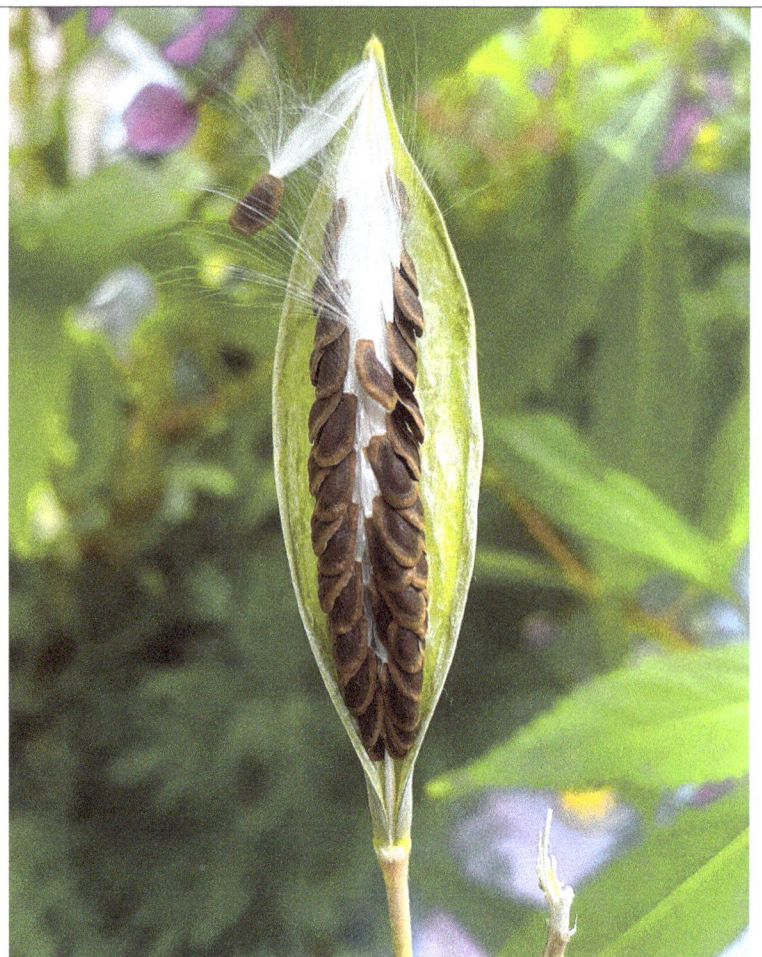

"From early days, this Asclepias has been regarded as a valuable medicinal plant. It is one of the most important indigenous American remedies, and until lately, it was official in the United States Pharmacopoeia."

Maude Grieve,
(1031)
A Modern Herbal

difficulties. Pleurisy root was also used in combination with other herbs to treat bronchitis, pleurisy, and pneumonia. It was also used to drain fluids from the chest in pulmonary edema.

CURRENT USES: Use pleurisy root for respiratory infections; however, attention to dosage is essential for safe use. As a bronchial dilator and stimulating expectorant, pleurisy root relieves breathing difficulties and effectively breaks up and eliminates lung congestion. One of its unique actions is reducing inflammation of the pleura, the fluid-filled sac that surrounds the lungs and separates them from the ribcage. This inflammation causes the painful coughs typical of respiratory infections. Pleurisy root is a specific remedy for colds, chest infections, bronchitis, pleurisy, and pneumonia, but usually in combination with other expectorants. It also improves lymphatic drainage and may help resolve mild pulmonary edema.

CAUTIONS: Pleurisy root should only be used for short periods to treat acute symptoms. Large doses may cause vomiting and nausea. Reduce the dosage or discontinue use if stomach upset occurs. Contraindicated during pregnancy, while nursing or for babies and children.

PREPARATIONS

Use dried roots only.

DECOCTION: Use one teaspoon of dried root for each eight ounces of water. Bring water to a boil in a pot; cover and simmer for ten minutes. Strain.

TINCTURE: Dried – 1:5, 50%.

DOSAGES

Precise dosing is needed to avoid nausea.

DECOCTION: Drink four ounces of decoction every few hours or at least three times a day.

TINCTURE: Take twenty drops in a small amount of water every few hours or at least three times a day.

HARVESTING

Harvest the root in the fall after the seed is ripe. Pleurisy root has a thick taproot that is notoriously hard to extract from the ground; it seems to wedge itself into the hardest earth available. Immediately after harvesting, clean and slice the root into small pieces. Dry completely.

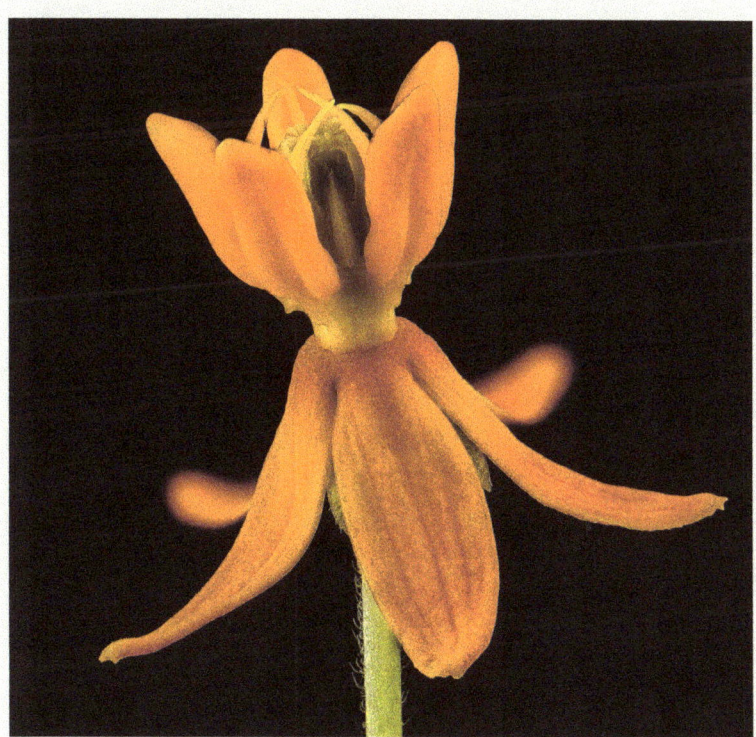

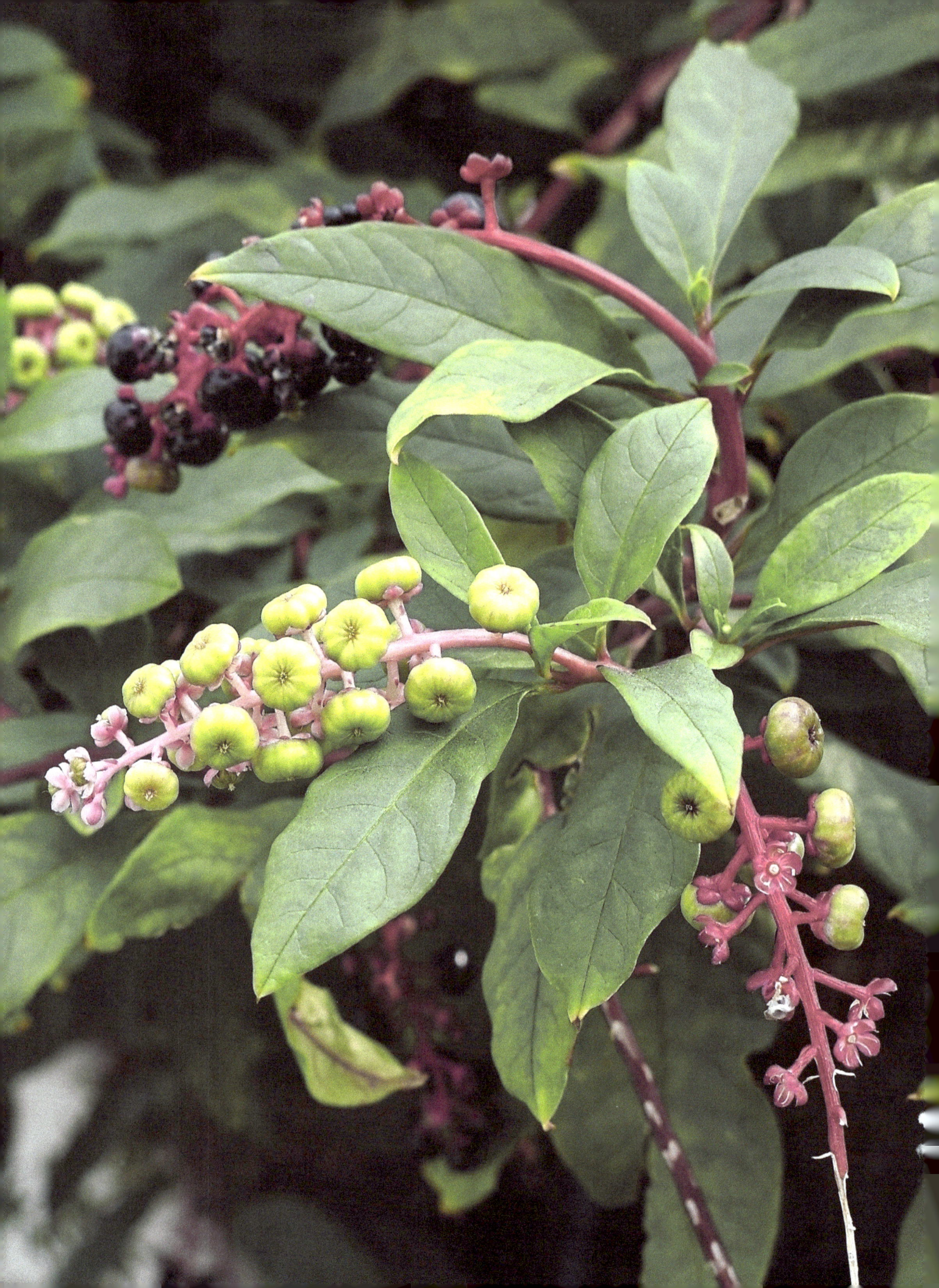

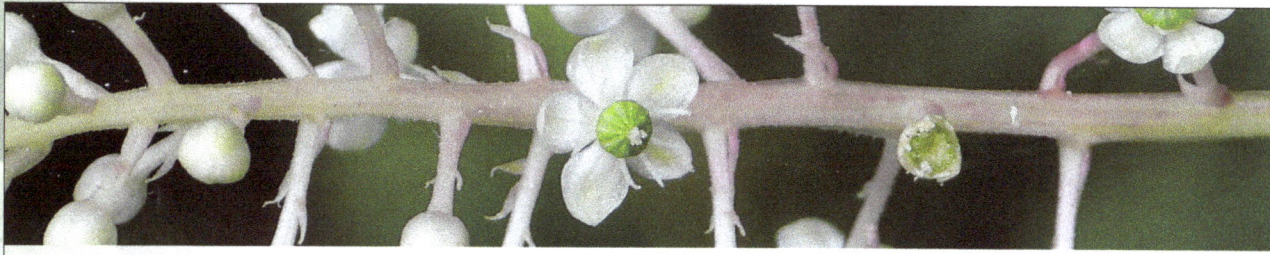

Poke Root

COMMON NAME: Poke Root

BOTANICAL NAME: *Phytolacca americana*

FAMILY: *Phytolaccaceae* (Pokeweed)

OTHER NAMES: Poke Salad, Poke Sallet

RELATED SPECIES: None

DESCRIPTION: Large perennial, four to ten feet tall, with alternate, entire leaves, three to eight inches long. If you examine the small green and white flowers arranged in racemes, you will see there are no petals, only five small white sepals. Ripe berries are dark purple with a large seed, and often, you'll find ripe berries on the same stem with flower buds and blossoms. The smooth, hollow stems are green until late summer, when they turn a brilliant magenta, making poke one of the most striking herbs of late summer. The white, fibrous tap root is enormous; a single root may weigh three to five pounds!

HABITAT: A common wayside plant found in masses in open sunny areas, transition zones at the edge of woodlands, and disturbed soil throughout Eastern North America.

KEY ACTIONS: Lymphatic, alterative, emetic, cathartic, narcotic, abortifacient

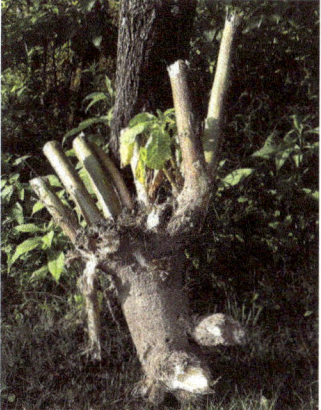

PART USED: Root, berries (leaves are edible in early spring)

TRADITIONAL USES: Poke roots, berries and leaves were all used by indigenous healers, as a folk remedy, and by 19th-century physicians. Uses vary, and there are anecdotal accounts of all parts of the plant being used internally and externally for cancerous tumors, persistent ulcerous skin conditions, scabies, eczema, inflammation of the throat and

"Dr. Moore, of South Carolina, informs me that the berries of the poke in alcohol or whiskey, a dessert spoonful, repeatedly given, has been found one of the most efficient remedies we possess in rheumatism."

Frances Peyre Porcher, (1863) Resources of the Southern Fields and Forests

mouth, hemorrhoids, lymphatic swelling, breast pain, and mastitis. The berries in brandy or other alcohol were a popular remedy for rheumatic pain and inflammation. Strong decoctions made with poke roots and leaves have also been used as a wash to treat dogs with mange. Cooked poke leaves collected early in spring are a traditional Southern delicacy known as Poke Sallet. Ink made from ripe berries was used extensively during the Civil War when standard ink was in short supply; it has a rich magenta color.

CURRENT USES: While poke root has a place in the modern herbal apothecary, it must be used with extreme caution. It is toxic if not prepared carefully and appropriately dosed. It is a powerful lymphatic used internally in low doses to reduce lymphatic swelling and resolve persistent bacterial infections. Include a small amount of poke in alterative formulas following acute infections, often combined with cleavers *(Galium aparine)*, red clover *(Trifolium pratense)*, and red root.

Because of its affinity for the lymph system, it is one of the most effective remedies for mastitis and acute symptoms of fibrocystic breast disease. In treating mastitis, use poke root tincture internally and apply the root salve topically. The salve may also be applied to persistent skin problems like eczema and slow-healing ulcers.

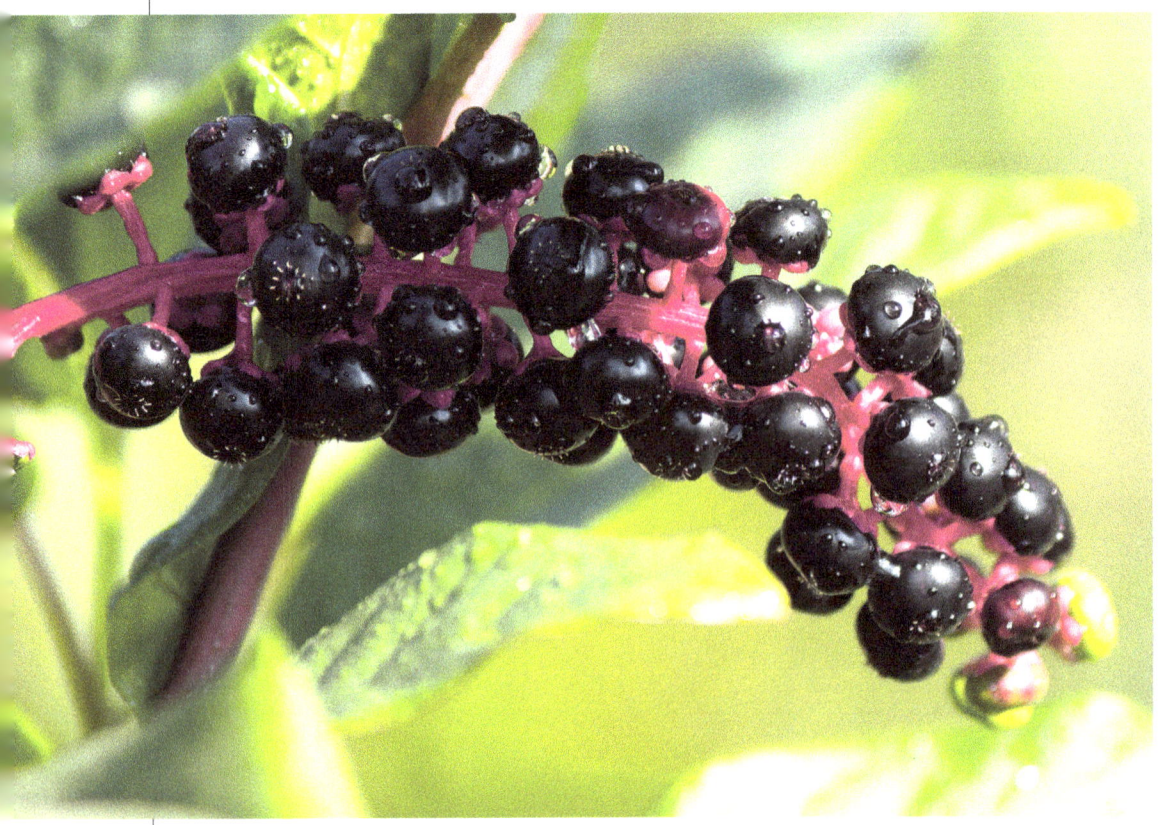

"No other remedy equals Phytolacca in acute mastitis. Sore nipples and mammary tenderness, or morbid sensitiveness of the breasts during the menstrual period, call for Phytolacca."

Harvey W. Felter and John U. Lloyd, (1898) King's American Dispensary

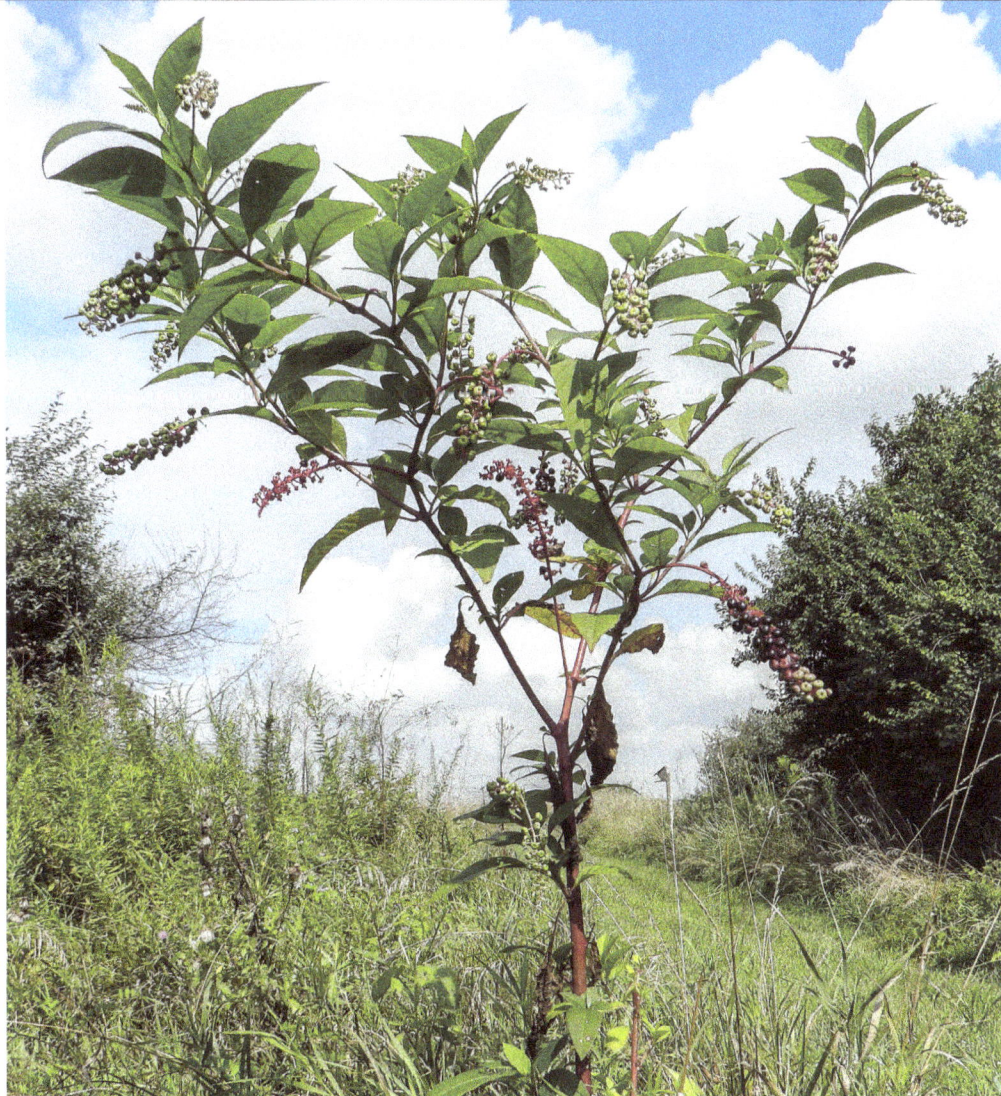

"Of late, there have been some Quacks, who pretend to cure Cancers with this herb, but I have not met with one instance of its having been serviceable in that Disorder."

Philip Miller, *(1731) The Gardener's Dictionary*

Poke berry brandy relieves arthritic and rheumatic inflammation and pain, especially if symptoms are worse in cold, damp weather. Properly cooked poke leaves, gathered in the early spring, are a delicious wild food with a flavor reminiscent of asparagus.

CAUTIONS: All parts of the poke plant contain compounds that may cause nausea, vomiting, diarrhea, headache, sweating, blurred vision, and low blood pressure. The onset of these reactions may be delayed by several hours, making it possible to take a toxic dose without realizing it. If any of these symptoms occur, discontinue use immediately. Contact with fresh leaves, roots, and berries can irritate the skin and mucus membranes; always wear gloves when handling poke. Poke is strictly contraindicated for internal use in pregnancy, for children and for anyone with kidney disease. Despite these cautions, don't be afraid of poke! I have used poke root tincture and salve with excellent results, but I always follow the guidelines under Preparations and Dosages.

PREPARATIONS

TINCTURE: Poke root is considered a low-dose botanical. To safely use the tincture, it is prepared at a 1:10 ratio using one part root to ten parts menstruum. Root – 1:10, 50%.

INFUSED OIL AND SALVE: Prepare a standard infused oil or salve using fresh root at a ratio of two parts finely chopped fresh root to five parts oil. If you only have dry root, use one part ground herb to five parts oil.

DOSAGES

Poke root tincture should not be used daily for over one or two weeks to relieve acute symptoms, and you must pay close attention to dosage. Small doses of poke root brandy used to relieve rheumatic and arthritic symptoms are safe for longer-term use.

TINCTURE: Take three to five drops in water every two to three hours until symptoms improve. Be sure to drink plenty of water or herbal teas when taking poke root tincture.

INFUSED OIL AND SALVE: Apply topically to swollen glands and inflamed, painful breasts. Repeat three to four times daily until symptoms improve. Use poke root tincture internally and poke oil or salve externally for mastitis symptoms.

HARVESTING

Wear gloves when harvesting or processing poke roots, berries or leaves. In the spring, collect poke leaves just as they emerge from the ground and before they unfurl. Never collect leaves from a plant over ten to twelve inches tall. Collect berries when they are a deep purple color, midsummer.

Harvest poke root in the fall before the leaves begin to fade. Poke root is large and tuberous, so be prepared to dig! Clean the root and cut it into slices. Since only small doses are required for tincture, you only need a few ounces of the root and have enough to last for years.

POKE SALLET

Collect young poke leaves before they unfurl entirely, usually when the plant is less than ten to twelve inches tall. Bring a pot of water to a boil, add the leaves, bring to a boil and cook for five minutes. Drain the leaves in a colander. Refill the pot with fresh water, add the same poke leaves, boil them for five minutes and drain. When cooled slightly, taste a small portion of the leaves; if they're still bitter, repeat the boiling process. Refill the pot with fresh water a third time and bring it to a boil. This time, add the poke leaves and simmer for twenty minutes. Drain the leaves well. Heat a frying pan over medium heat, add some olive oil, or go traditional, using bacon drippings or other animal fat. Add the poke leaves, some salt and pepper, and toss to coat the poke with the oil (or fat) for five to ten minutes. Serve hot, sprinkled with vinegar or lemon juice.

POKE BERRY BRANDY

Crush one cup of fresh poke berries in a wire mesh strainer to separate the seeds from the fruit. Discard the seeds. Put the berry pulp in a quart canning jar and fill the jar with good brandy. Shake well, steep for two weeks, and continue to shake the jar daily. Strain the berries and discard them. Pour the brandy into a clean bottle and label it.

Take one tablespoon of brandy twice a day. It can be added to tea or coffee.

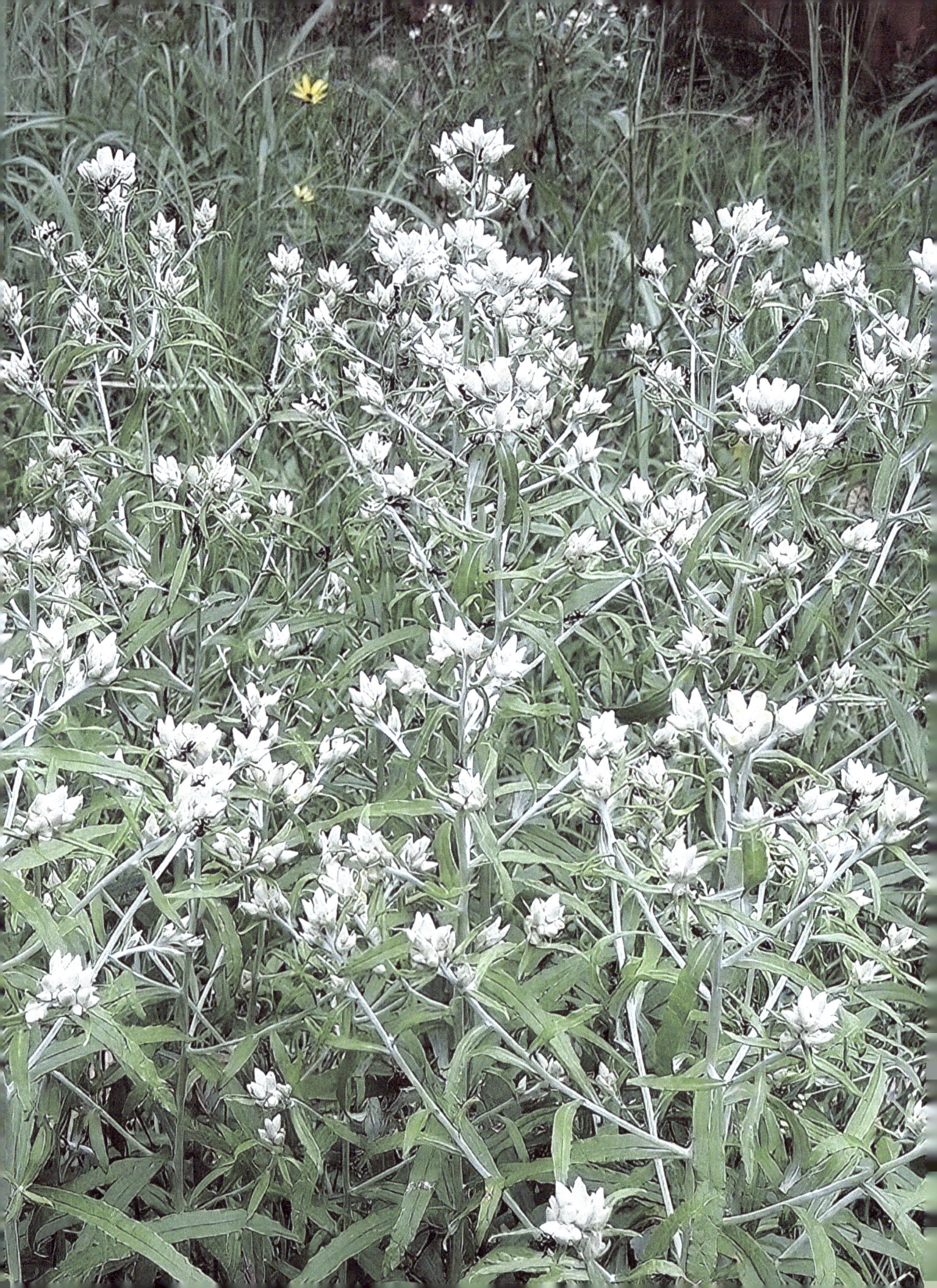

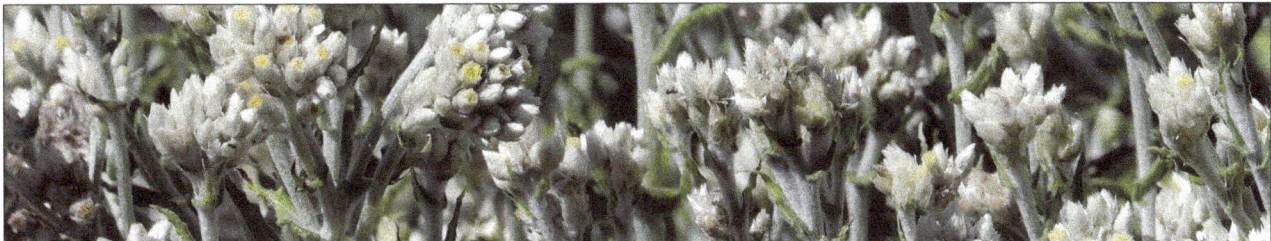

Rabbit Tobacco

COMMON NAME: Rabbit Tobacco

BOTANICAL NAME: *Gnaphalium obstusifolium*
(also known as *Pseudognaphalium obtusifolium*)

FAMILY: *Asteraceae* (Aster)

OTHER NAMES: Sweet Everlasting, Life Everlasting, Cudweed

DESCRIPTION: Rabbit tobacco is an upright biennial herb, one to three feet tall, with tiny white flowers in branching terminal clusters. The leaves are alternate, lance-shaped and without stalks. Foliage is silver-gray, with a dry, wooly appearance and a pleasant aroma.

HABITAT: Found in dry, open areas. Common throughout the region.

KEY ACTIONS: Decongestant, relaxing expectorant, antispasmodic, astringent, mild sedative

PART USED: Aerial (in flower)

TRADITIONAL USES: Rabbit tobacco was used extensively for respiratory symptoms, including colds, coughs, sinus congestion, and sore throats. Tommie Bass used it in cough syrups and tea to relieve migraine headaches and lung and sinus congestion. He recommended adding the dried herb to boiling water, covering the head with a towel and inhaling the vapors.[1] The dried herb was smoked to relieve asthmatic symptoms and sinus congestion. The Cherokee used rabbit tobacco as a ceremonial smudge and a wash to treat persons bothered by ghosts or those who "wanted to run away."[2] In the South, teenagers often smoke rabbit tobacco in hand-rolled cigarettes.

CURRENT USES: Although rabbit tobacco has a long history of use as a folk remedy, it has only mild therapeutic properties. Drink hot infusions to relieve chest pain, lung and sinus congestion, and spasmodic coughs. Rabbit tobacco may also be used in inhalations (as described below) or

> *"It's awful simple, but it's one of the most valuable plants for making cough syrup and a cold remedy."*
>
> Tommie Bass, (1988)
> *A Reference Guide to Medicinal Plants*

---

[1] Crellin and Philpott, *A Reference Guide to Medicinal Plants*, 157–158

[2] Moerman, *North American Ethnobotany*, 250

smoked to relieve wheezing caused by asthma, lung congestion, and chest pain. Its soothing antispasmodic and mild sedative properties make it a valuable addition to cough syrups.

CAUTIONS: None known.

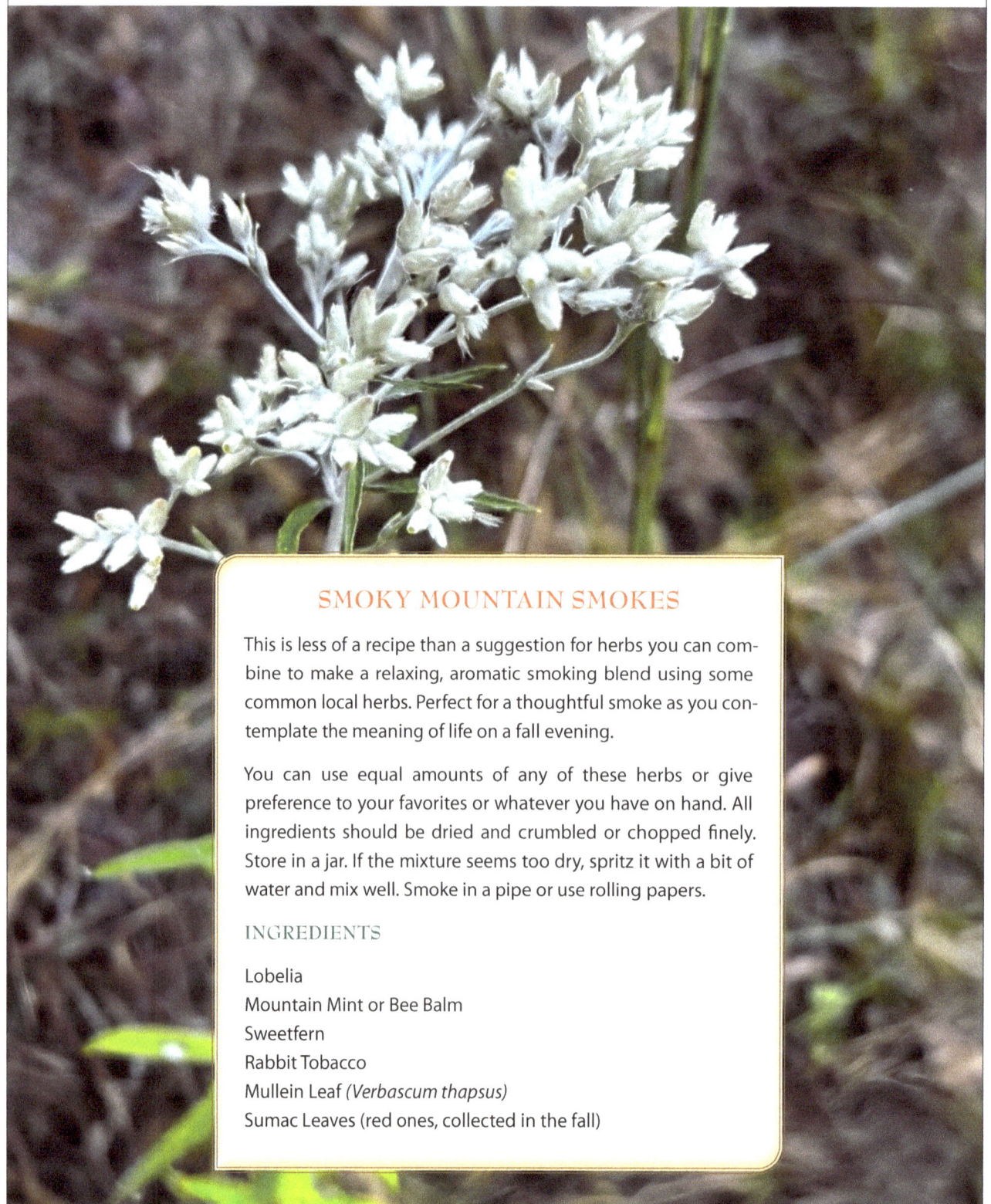

SMOKY MOUNTAIN SMOKES

This is less of a recipe than a suggestion for herbs you can combine to make a relaxing, aromatic smoking blend using some common local herbs. Perfect for a thoughtful smoke as you contemplate the meaning of life on a fall evening.

You can use equal amounts of any of these herbs or give preference to your favorites or whatever you have on hand. All ingredients should be dried and crumbled or chopped finely. Store in a jar. If the mixture seems too dry, spritz it with a bit of water and mix well. Smoke in a pipe or use rolling papers.

INGREDIENTS

Lobelia
Mountain Mint or Bee Balm
Sweetfern
Rabbit Tobacco
Mullein Leaf *(Verbascum thapsus)*
Sumac Leaves (red ones, collected in the fall)

PREPARATIONS

INFUSION: Use two tablespoons of fresh or dried rabbit tobacco for each eight ounces of water. Cover and steep for twenty minutes. Strain and sweeten. This infusion is most effective if you drink it hot. Use cold infusion as a wash or compress for inflamed skin conditions.

INHALATION: Prepare a simple infusion by steeping a generous handful of dried or fresh rabbit tobacco and two pints of freshly boiled water in a wide ceramic bowl. Make a tent by draping a bath towel over your head and the bowl while inhaling the steam for ten minutes. Add more hot water if needed to produce more steam.

HERBAL SMOKE: Grind or crush dried leaves and flowers as finely as possible. Fill a pipe or use rolling papers to make a cigarette. Inhale the smoke deeply, hold it for a few seconds, and then exhale through the nose. Repeat several times or as needed to relieve sinus congestion and wheezing.

DOSAGES

INFUSION: Drink three to four cups of tea daily until symptoms improve. A cold infusion is a soothing wash for poison ivy or other skin rashes, combined with fresh jewelweed leaves *(Impatiens capensis)*, if available, to increase anti-inflammatory actions.

INHALATION: Use an inhalation every two to three hours until symptoms improve.

HERBAL SMOKE: Use as needed to relieve lung or sinus congestion, asthmatic wheezing and as a gentle sedative. Don't overuse rabbit tobacco smoke, as it can dry the lungs.

HARVESTING

Collect the entire plant when in bloom. Bundle stems and hang to dry, though rabbit tobacco is a fairly dry herb and, as Tommie Bass put it, "It looks the same dead or alive…gather it before frost, but it can be gathered in winter. It keeps about as good in the field as it does stored inside."[3] When dried leaves crumble to the touch, strip the leaves and flowers from the stem and store them in a jar.

---

[3] Crellin and Philpott, *A Reference Guide to Medicinal Plants*, 365

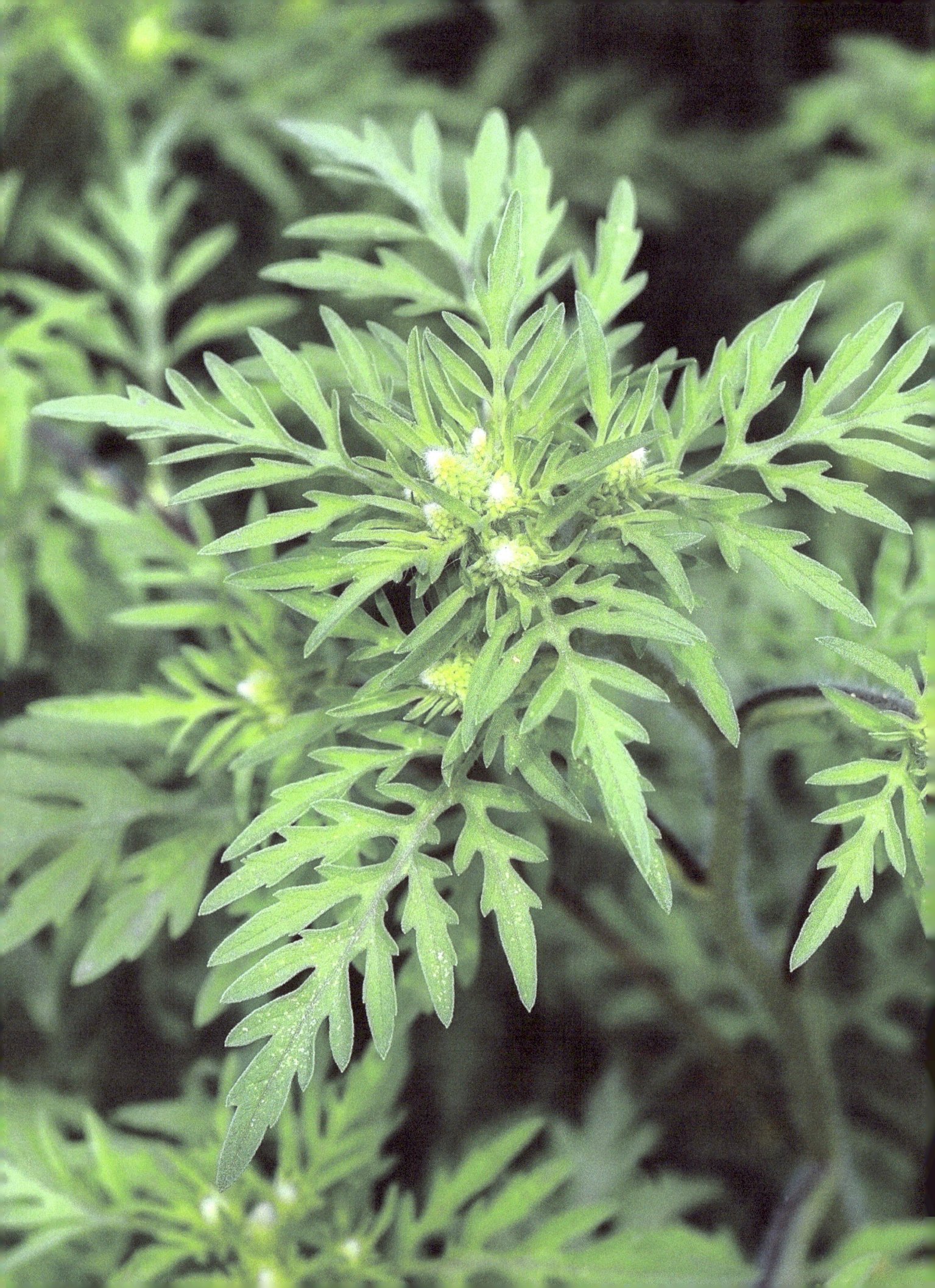

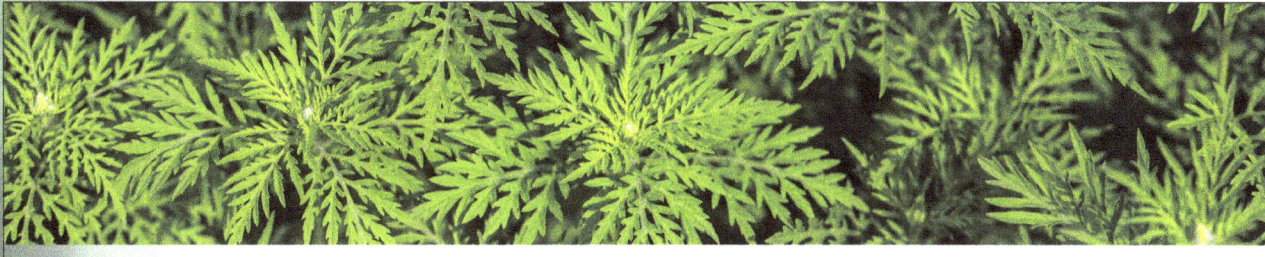

Ragweed

COMMON NAME: Ragweed

BOTANICAL NAME: *Ambrosia artemesiifolia*

FAMILY: *Asteraceae* (Aster)

OTHER NAMES: Bitter Weed, Hayfever Weed, Wild Wormwood

RELATED SPECIES: Greater Ragweed *(A. trifida),* Lanceleaf Ragweed *(A. bidentata)*

DESCRIPTION: Common annual, one to four feet tall, with deeply dissected leaves, opposite on the lower stem and becoming alternate towards the top. The inconspicuous green flowers are tiny, less than half an inch wide, and arranged in terminal racemes.

HABITAT: Common in sunny, open areas and transition zones in sun or part shade.

KEY ACTIONS: Astringent, decongestant, antihistamine

PART USED: Aerial parts (in flower).

TRADITIONAL USES: The Cherokee used ragweed as a topical astringent, rubbing the fresh leaves on bug bites and using the infusion as a wash for hives.[1] It was also used internally as an astringent tea to control diarrhea.

CURRENT USES: Ragweed is used as an herbal antihistamine for seasonal allergies. Oddly enough, its wind-pollinated flowers contribute to fall allergy symptoms, while the entire plant relieves them. Ragweed relieves a stuffy, runny nose, itchy eyes, and scratchy throat. It won't prevent allergy symptoms but relieves them for several hours. Add ragweed to skin salves as an astringent, or use the infusion as a wash for rashes, hives and insect bites.

CAUTIONS: None known.

---

[1] Moerman, *Native American Ethnobotany,* 66

PREPARATIONS

Use fresh plants to make tincture if possible.

INFUSION: Use one cup of dried leaves and flowers or two cups of fresh leaves and flowers per quart of boiled water. Cover and steep for twenty minutes. Strain.

TINCTURE: Fresh – 1:2. Dried – 1:5, 40%.

SALVE: Prepare a standard salve using infused oil made with fresh or dried ragweed.

DOSAGES

Ragweed is a mild but effective remedy for acute allergy symptoms. Repeat dosing as needed to relieve symptoms. Combine with goldenrod *(Solidago spp.)* for an even more effective allergy remedy.

INFUSION: Drink one cup every hour until symptoms improve. Use the cool infusion as a wash for inflamed, irritated skin and bug bites.

TINCTURE: Take half to one teaspoon of tincture every thirty minutes until symptoms improve.

SALVE: Apply as needed to soothe inflamed, irritated skin.

HARVESTING

Collect the ariel parts in flower, strip leaves and flowers from the stem, and discard the stem. Use fresh or dry for future use.

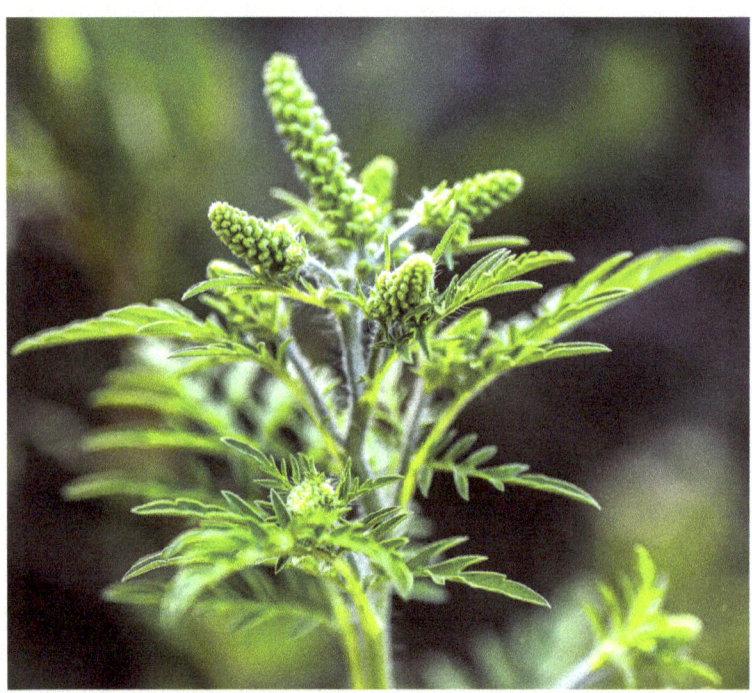

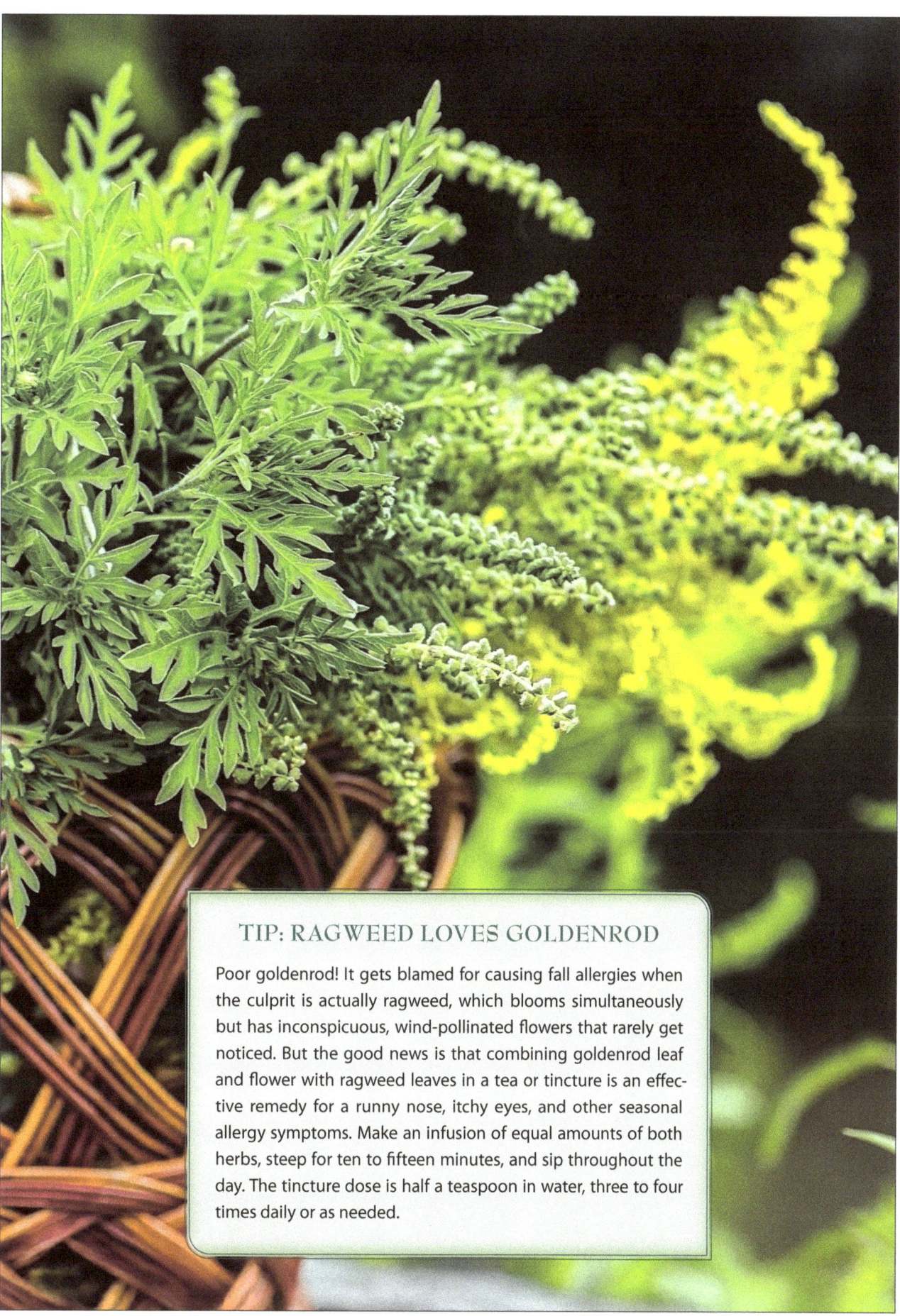

TIP: RAGWEED LOVES GOLDENROD

Poor goldenrod! It gets blamed for causing fall allergies when the culprit is actually ragweed, which blooms simultaneously but has inconspicuous, wind-pollinated flowers that rarely get noticed. But the good news is that combining goldenrod leaf and flower with ragweed leaves in a tea or tincture is an effective remedy for a runny nose, itchy eyes, and other seasonal allergy symptoms. Make an infusion of equal amounts of both herbs, steep for ten to fifteen minutes, and sip throughout the day. The tincture dose is half a teaspoon in water, three to four times daily or as needed.

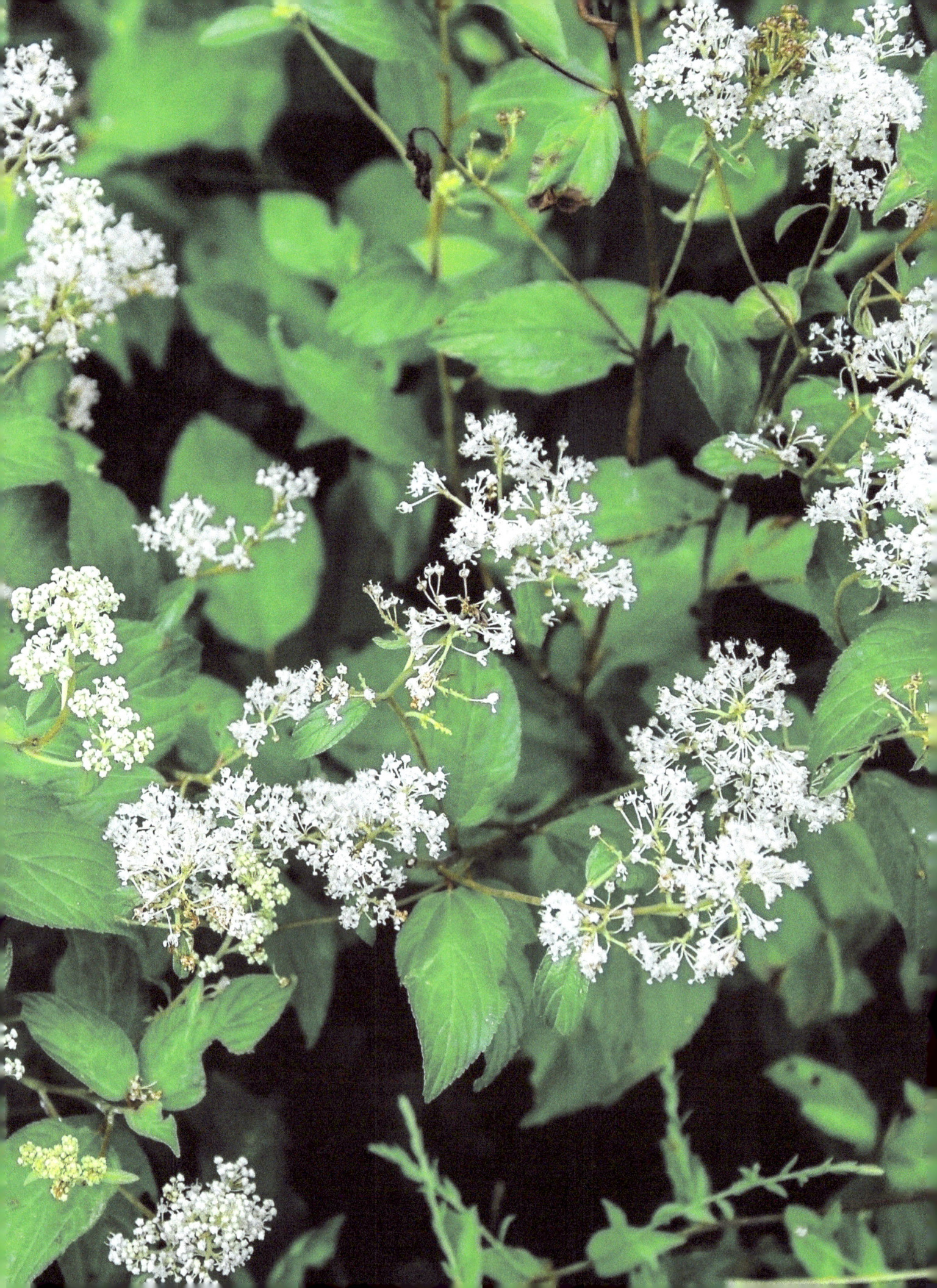

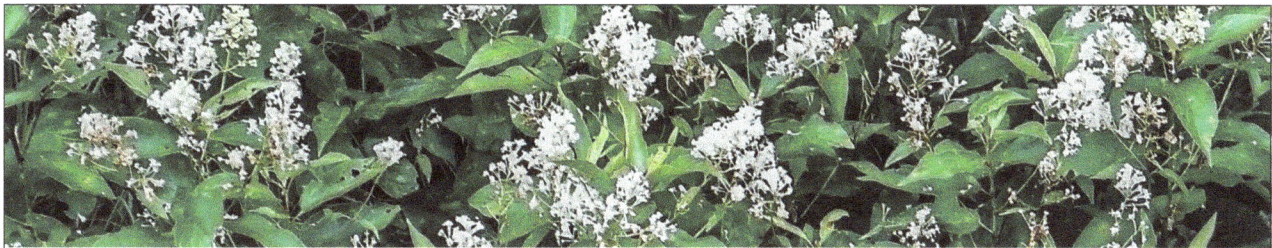

Red Root

COMMON NAME: Red Root

BOTANICAL NAME: *Ceanothus americanus*

FAMILY: *Rhamnaceae* (Buckthorn)

OTHER NAMES: New Jersey Tea, Redshank

DESCRIPTION: Red root is a shrub that is two to four feet tall, with alternate, oval leaves one to three inches long, finely serrated and rounded at the base. A distinctive feature of the leaves is the three prominent veins that run from the base to the outer margin and are most visible on the underside. Clusters of tiny white flowers with five petals on long stalks bloom from May to September. The root has a reddish bark.

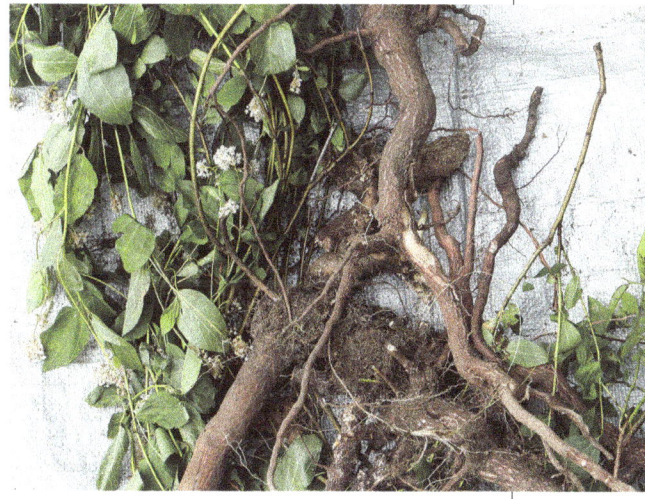

HABITAT: Common throughout the region, it thrives on dry, rocky soil in sunny open areas and transition zones.

KEY ACTIONS: Lymphatic, alterative, astringent

PART USED: Root, leaf

TRADITIONAL USES: Red root was used extensively to treat syphilis and gonorrhea, though it was ineffective.[1] *The Complete Herbalist*, published in 1872, recommended red root for asthma, chronic bronchitis, whooping cough, and consumption. Tommie Bass used decoctions of the root as a gargle for sore throats, thrush and inflammation in the mouth, and internally for prostate inflammation, psoriasis, and swollen glands.[2] Leaves were used for tea during the Revolutionary War when imported tea from China was unavailable.[3]

---

[1] Porcher, *Resources of the Southern Fields and Forests*, 109

[2] Crellin and Philpott, *A Reference Guide to Medicinal Plants*, 370

[3] Porcher, *Resources of the Southern Fields and Forests*, 110

CURRENT USES: Red root relieves lymphatic congestion and supports immune response. It stimulates lymphatic drainage to reduce swollen lymph glands and relieve symptoms of fibrocystic breast disease. A specific treatment (internally) for congestion and inflammation in tissues and organs in the pelvis. Red root astringes vaginal discharge (leucorrhea) and reduces prostate gland inflammation. Red root works slowly and deeply, so it should be used daily for a month or longer for best results.

The astringent properties of the leaf infusion or root decoction can be used as a wash or compress for eruptive, weeping skin conditions, as a vaginal douche, and as a first aid treatment for burns. Internally, the decoction's astringency helps control diarrhea.

CAUTIONS: None known.

TIP: LYMPHATIC HERBS

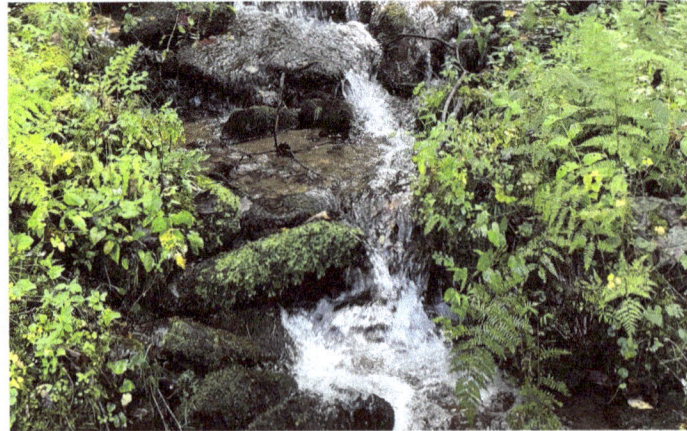

Lymphatic herbs stimulate and support the function of the lymphatic and immune systems. In the folk tradition, lymphatic herbs are said to "clean the blood," though this isn't accurate. Instead, it would make more sense to say that they increase the ability of the immune system to respond to and eliminate infections. Swollen glands are the most common indication that your immune system is working to fight an infection. This is when herbs like red root, poke root, and immune-stimulating herbs like echinacea *(Echinacea spp.)* and garlic *(Allium sativa)* should be used to fight infections.

PREPARATIONS

Fresh and dried roots are used interchangeably.

INFUSION: Make a standard infusion using about two tablespoons of fresh or dried leaves in eight ounces of water. Infuse for fifteen minutes or to taste.

DECOCTION: Make a standard decoction using one tablespoon of fresh or dried root in eight ounces of water. Decoct for 20 minutes. Strain.

TINCTURE: Fresh or dried root – 1:5, 50% alcohol.

DOSAGES

Red root is most effective in small, regular doses taken over several weeks or months to address chronic conditions such as fibrocystic breast disease or prostatitis. For acute symptoms, use larger doses until symptoms improve and then smaller doses for an extended period.

INFUSION: Infused leaves as tea or externally as a skin wash.

DECOCTION: Drink one to two cups of root decoction daily for several weeks or months. Use the decoction externally as an astringent skin wash, vaginal douche, or gargle.

TINCTURE: Take one-half teaspoon three times daily for chronic symptoms and up to one tablespoon three times daily to relieve acute symptoms. Drink plenty of water while taking red root to support lymphatic drainage.

HARVESTING

Harvest the root in late summer after the flowers have faded or in winter (if you can accurately identify it). The roots are tough, even when freshly dug, so cut them up immediately after harvesting. You will need serious clippers, loppers, or possibly a small hatchet. Collect and dry leaves anytime during the growing season.

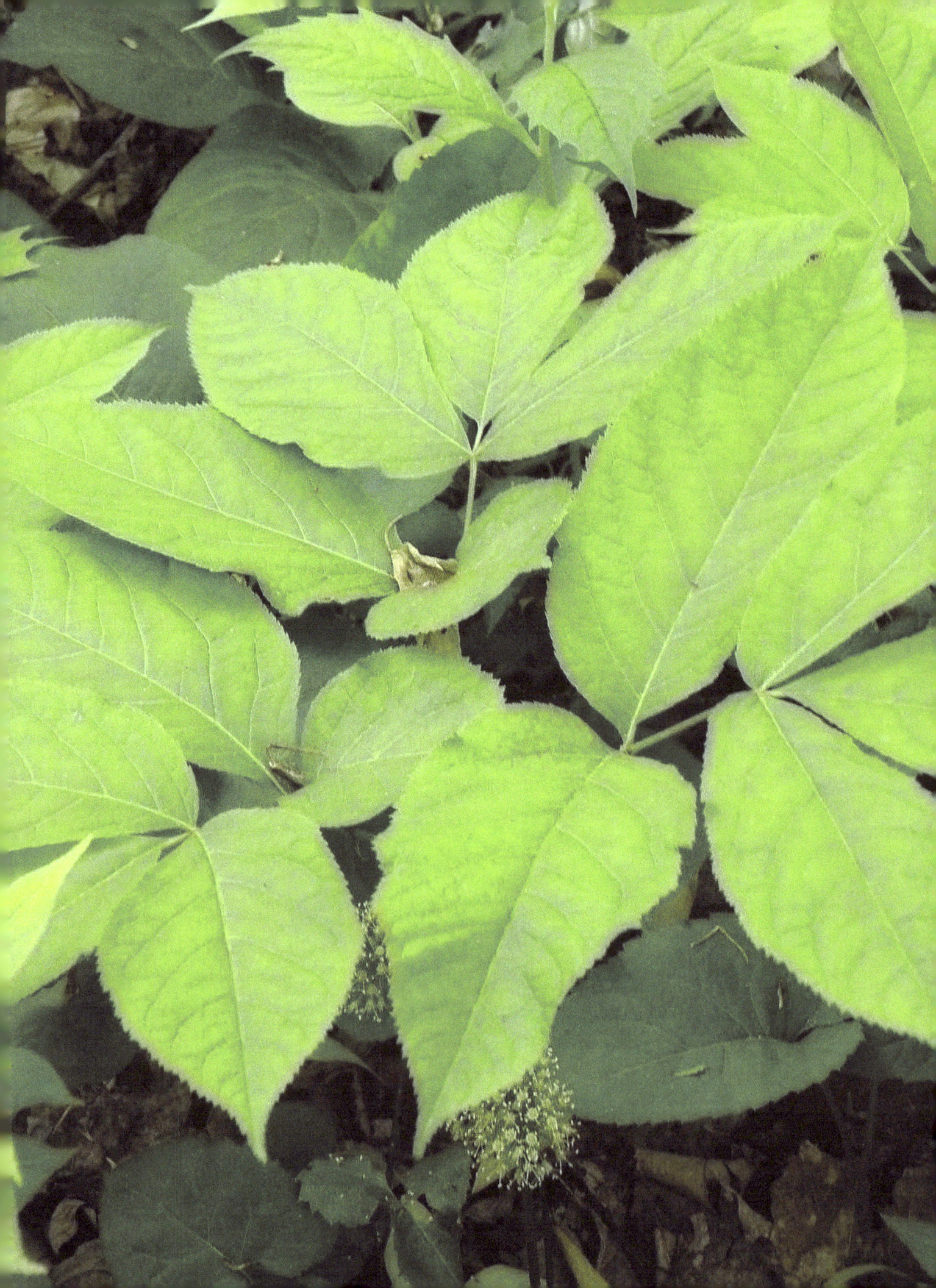

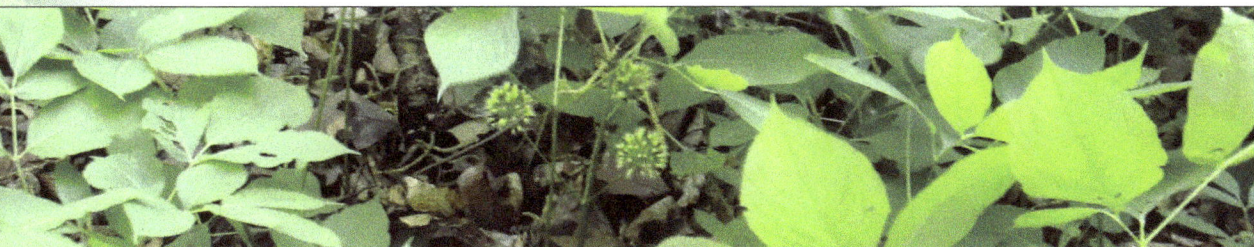

Sarsaparilla

COMMON NAME: Sarsaparilla

BOTANICAL NAME: *Aralia nudicaulis*

FAMILY: *Araliaceae* (Ginseng)

OTHER NAMES: American Sarsaparilla, Wild Sarsaparilla, False Sarsaparilla, Spignet, Spikenard

RELATED SPECIES: Two other plants found throughout the region, *Smilax glauca* and *S. rotundifolia,* are also known by the common name sarsaparilla, though they have entirely different properties.

DESCRIPTION: Sarsaparilla is a perennial about two feet tall, with pinnately compound leaves on long stems and three to five leaflets on each stem. Small white flowers in round umbels on separate stems bloom from June to August. In late summer, sarsaparilla has wine-colored, slightly translucent berries that are edible with a spicy, tart taste. Its thick and fleshy roots grow horizontally.

HABITAT: Common in dense woods in deep shade, sarsaparilla is often surrounded by black cohosh *(Actaea racemosa)* and blue cohosh *(Caulophyllum thalictroides).*

KEY ACTIONS: Alterative, lung tonic, general tonic

PART USED: Root, berries (edible)

TRADITIONAL USES: In North America, the Cherokee and other American Indians considered sarsaparilla a panacea and used it alone or combined with other herbs to treat physical weakness. Sarsaparilla root decoction was given to children to treat pneumonia, teething sickness, and kidney weakness. It was also used as a restorative blood tonic for various chronic diseases and externally to treat skin and mouth infections.[1]

---

[1] Moerman, *Native American Ethnobotany,* 181–182

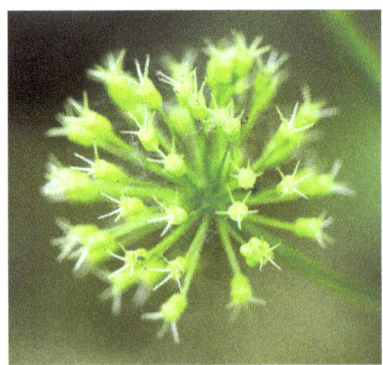

During the 16th century, sarsaparilla was one of the many New World remedies that caused a sensation in Europe, where it was used as a remedy for syphilis symptoms. The aromatic root was a traditional ingredient in root beer recipes. It was also used as a warming tonic to relieve rheumatic pain and stiff joints.

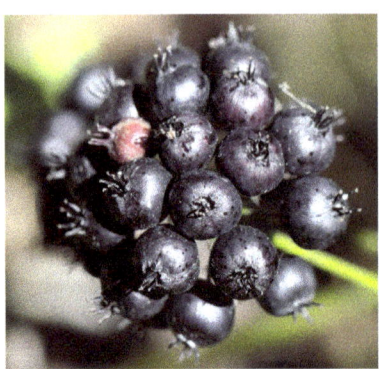

CURRENT USES: Despite its rarity in modern herbal practice and on the commercial herb market, sarsaparilla, a member of the Ginseng family, has its own unique mild tonic properties. It may not be as potent as American ginseng *(Panax quinquefolius),* but its gentle nature makes it a perfect remedy for fatigue, especially after long periods of stress, overwork, or when recovering from severe respiratory infections. It is usually combined with other lung herbs as a specific remedy for lingering dry coughs following bronchitis and other respiratory illnesses. When brewed into a tea, its roots offer a pleasant-tasting, mild tonic that can be enjoyed daily.

CAUTION: While no studies have been done to establish the safety of sarsaparilla in pregnancy or while nursing, it has a long history of traditional use with no reported side effects or cautions.

TIP: THE PROBLEM WITH COMMON NAMES

Always pay careful attention to the scientific name of plants for proper identification and because common names vary from place to place. In the case of sarsaparilla, my survey of the historical uses of sarsaparilla reveals just how confusing a common name can be. Sarsaparilla is the common name used for another member of the *Araliaceae* family, *A. racemosa*, several local *Smilax* vines, and a tropical *Smilax* known as Jamaican Sarsaparilla. To complicate the issue even more, all of these roots were used in traditional root beer recipes, making it almost impossible to recreate them without knowing the scientific names of the plants they used.

PREPARATIONS

Prepare a tincture from freshly harvested root whenever possible.

DECOCTION: Use one tablespoon of dried root or two tablespoons of finely chopped fresh root for each eight ounces of water. Bring to a boil; cover tightly and simmer for twenty minutes. Strain.

TINCTURE: Fresh – 1:2. Dried – 1:5, 50%.

DOSAGES

Use sarsaparilla daily for a month or longer as a tonic. For acute symptoms, combine with mullein *(Verbascum thapsus)*, elecampane *(Inula helenium)*, rabbit tobacco *(Gnaphalium obtusifolium)* or wild cherry bark *(Prunus serotina)* in tincture formulas or cough syrups.

DECOCTION: As a general tonic, drink two to three cups of decoction daily for one month or longer. Decoct sarsaparilla alone or with other expectorant herbs for coughs and other respiratory symptoms.

TINCTURE: As a general tonic, take a half teaspoon in a small amount of water two to three times a day for one month or longer. Combine with other lung herbs for coughs and other respiratory symptoms. The tincture can also be added to throat-soothing teas.

HARVESTING

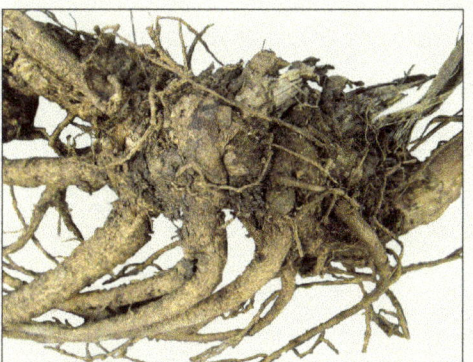

Harvest roots in late summer or after the berries ripen but before the foliage fades. Thick, fleshy sarsaparilla roots grow horizontally just below the ground. Before digging the root, clear away dirt and leaves from around the base of the main stem; then, dig carefully into the soil, using your hands as needed, to determine which direction the root is growing. Remove soil from either side of the root, following its shape until you can lift it from the ground. Wash and slice the fresh root immediately after harvest.

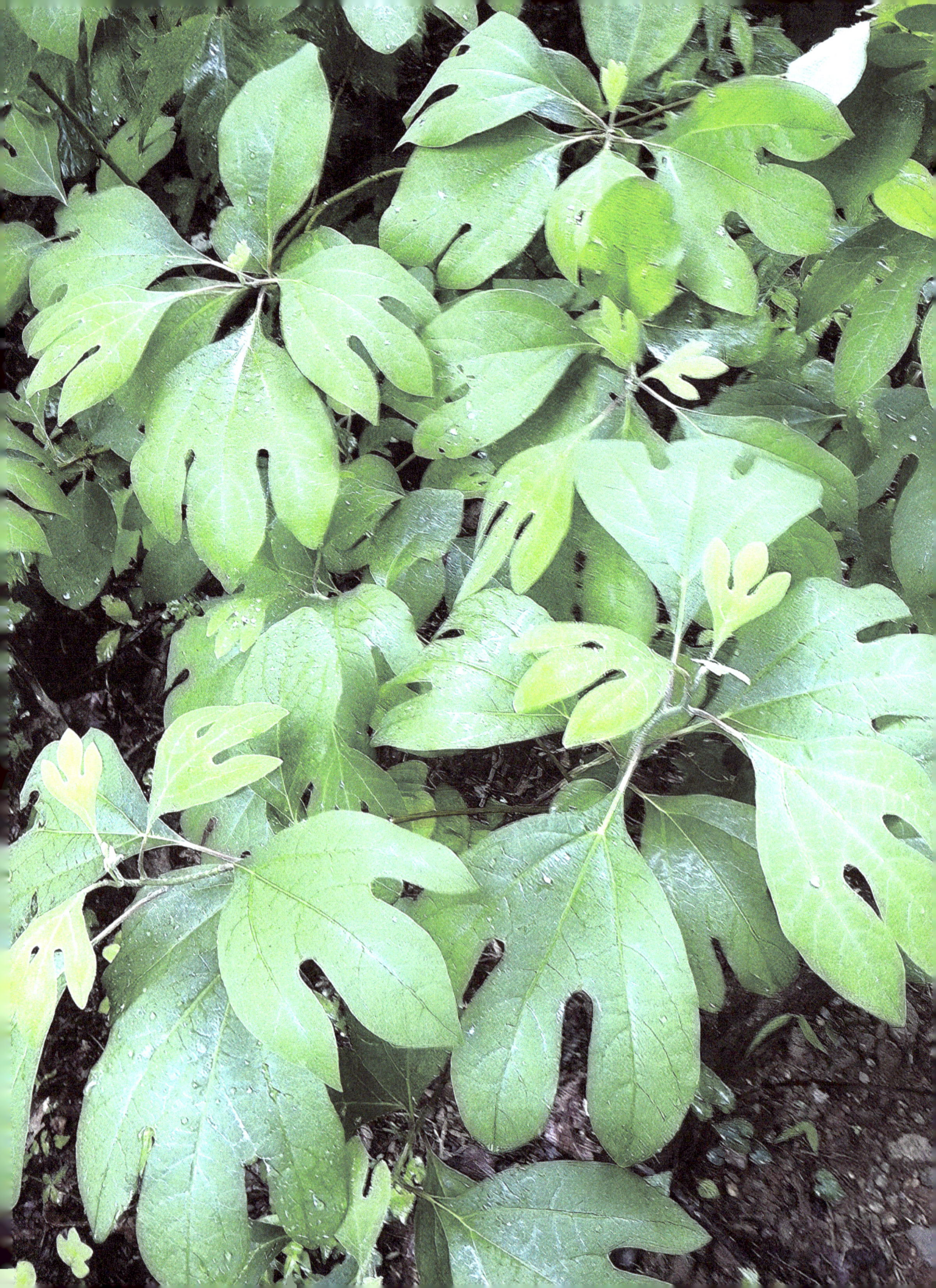

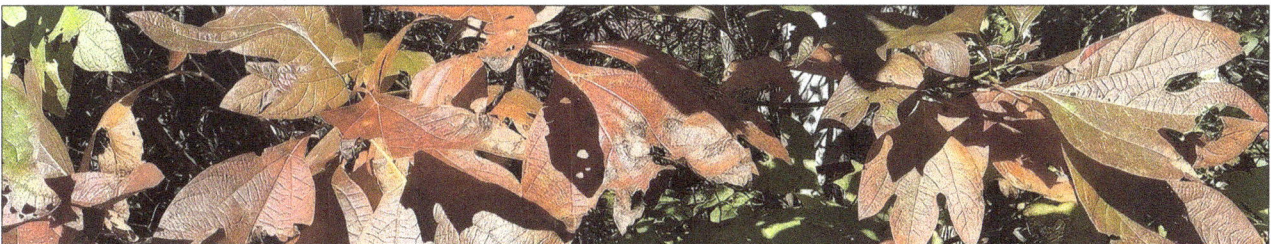

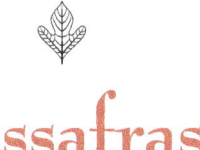

Sassafras

COMMON NAME: Sassafras

BOTANICAL NAME: *Sassafras albidum*

FAMILY: *Lauraceae* (Laurel)

OTHER NAMES: Cinnamon Wood, Ague Tree

DESCRIPTION: Sassafras is a distinctive tree with bark furrowed in horizontal ridges. Alternate, entire leaves are lobed and found in three unique shapes that resemble footballs (no lobes), mittens (two lobes), and ghosts (three lobes). Tiny clusters of stemless yellow flowers bloom along the branches in April and May, followed in late summer by small, blue, egg-shaped fruits containing one seed each. Roots grow horizontally away from the trunk just below the ground. All parts of the sassafras are aromatic; when crushed or bruised, they release a pleasant cinnamon-like fragrance.

HABITAT: Common understory tree throughout deciduous forests and open areas of eastern North America. Mature trees are often surrounded by saplings of various sizes that rarely reach maturity in dense forest shade.

KEY ACTIONS: Carminative, alterative, demulcent, diaphoretic

PART USED: Root, bark, leaf and pith

TRADITIONAL USES: Sassafras has a long history of use particularly among American Indians who used it as a beverage, cooking spice, and medicine. It was considered a blood tonic and used for many conditions believed to be caused by toxins or heat in the blood, such as rheumatism, hives, measles, skin eruptions, and rashes. Infusions of the bark were also used to treat diarrhea, worms, and parasites.

Sassafras leaf was and is a popular spice; the dried leaves were powdered and used to spice meats and as a thickening agent for soups and stews. In Louisiana, French Creole settlers, influenced by African and Native American culinary traditions, used the dried, powdered leaves to thicken and flavor a classic Creole and Cajun dish known as "Filé Gumbo."

Sassafras is a traditional folk remedy in the southern Appalachians, where it is still used as a tonic to clean and thin the blood in the spring. The pith, or spongy inner layer of the outermost branches, was dissolved in water to make a soothing wash for sore eyes and as a demulcent tea for the stomach and intestines. Hot sassafras root tea is used to relieve fevers. Until recently, sassafras extract was used as a flavoring agent in commercial root beer.

CURRENT USES: While sassafras is rarely used in modern herbal practice due to safety concerns, it is a gentle and effective alterative. As a carminative, sip small amounts of sassafras root or leaf tea to ease nausea, indigestion, and gas. It may also be helpful for soothing acute symptoms of irritable bowel syndrome. As an ingredient in alterative or hepatic formulas, aromatic sassafras roots cover the taste of bitter herbs. Sassafras root decoction is an effective tea that is drunk hot to reduce fevers and is used as a wash to relieve poison ivy rash. The pith, or spongy inner part of young sassafras branches, can be collected and steeped in warm water to make a mucilaginous infusion that soothes irritation in the upper respiratory system and digestive tract and externally as a wash for the eyes.

"[The pith] of young branches is advantageously given as a demulcent drink in disorders of the respiratory organs, bowels, and bladder… and as an application to inflamed eyes."

Frances Peyre Porcher, (1863) Resources of the Southern Fields and Forests

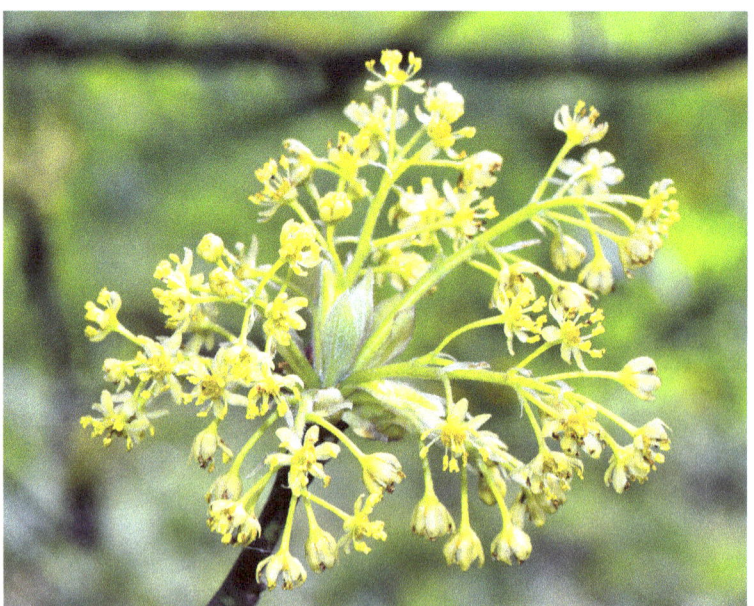

CAUTIONS: In the United States, sassafras was banned from sale in commercial preparations in the 1960s. This was due to safety concerns related to safrole, a compound in sassafras. Safrole was classified as a carcinogen by the Food and Drug Administration after an animal study in which rats that were fed purified safrole over two years later developed liver cancer. *The Botanical Safety Handbook* states this was "the equivalent to approximately 68 years of human exposure." No known human cases of toxicity have been documented, and the occasional use of sassafras tea is considered safe except during pregnancy. However, it is important to

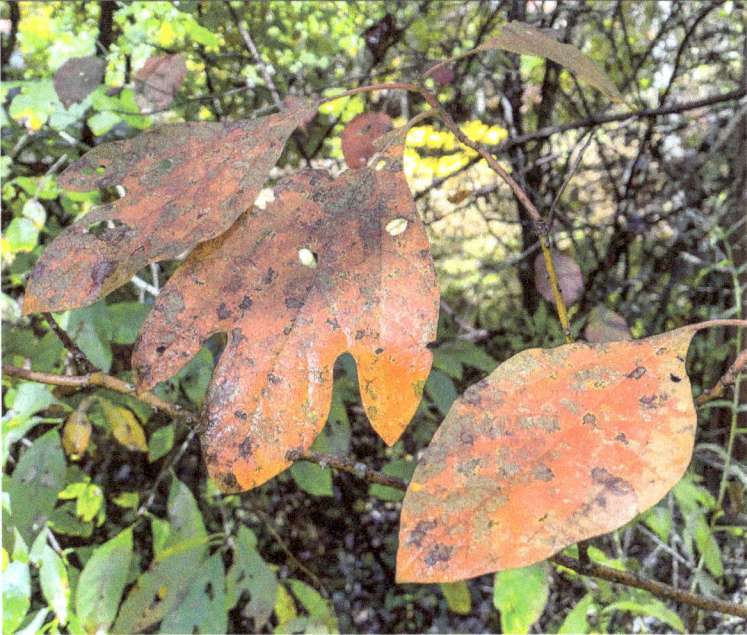

note that the safety of sassafras is still a subject of debate in the scientific community, and caution should be exercised when using it.[1]

Because safrole is not water-soluble, use only infusions and decoctions to avoid actual or speculative dangers. Do not use sassafras essential oils or alcohol tinctures. Sassafras tea should not be consumed daily for over three weeks. Additionally, it should not be used during pregnancy or with children under seven. If you follow these precautions, water-based extracts of sassafras should be a safe addition to your apothecary.

---

[1] Gardner and McGuffin, *AHPA's Botanical Safety Handbook, Second Edition*, 787–778

PREPARATIONS

I like to add a small amount of sassafras leaf or root to help reduce the taste of strong or bitter herbs in tea formulas.

INFUSION: Leaf—Use two tablespoons of dried leaves or a handful of coarsely chopped fresh leaves for each eight ounces of water. Cover and steep for thirty minutes. Strain and sweeten if desired.

INFUSION: Pith—Using cold water, infuse one-fourth cup of sassafras pith for each eight ounces of water. Cover and steep overnight. Strain. See directions below for collecting pith.

DECOCTION: Root and Bark—Use two teaspoons of root or bark, finely chopped, for every eight ounces of water. Bring roots to a boil; cover tightly and simmer for ten to fifteen minutes. Strain and sweeten if desired.

DOSAGES

Review the Cautions on page 150 for using sassafras safely.

DECOCTION/INFUSION: Drink one to two cups of leaf infusion or root decoction daily for a week or as needed. Drink one cup of infused pith every thirty minutes or as needed to relieve gastric discomfort. Apply the cooled, strained pith infusion to wash irritated eyes as needed.

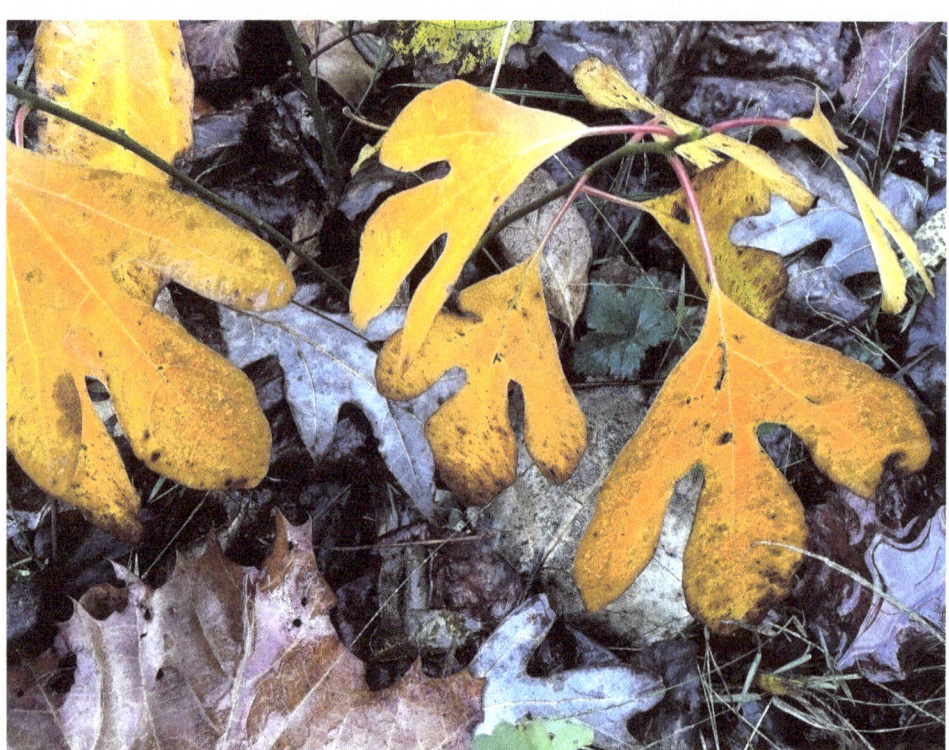

HARVESTING

Look for the seedlings that have sprouted up around mature sassafras trees. You will usually find many small saplings, two to four feet tall, within a thirty-foot radius of older trees; their stick-like roots are thin and easy to dig.

Traditionally, sassafras root and bark are harvested from January through March — they can also be collected throughout the spring and summer though the flavor is not as strong. Harvest leaves in spring and early summer. To harvest sassafras roots in late winter or early spring, mark sassafras saplings with colored yarn in the fall to correctly identify them in the winter.

The root bark of mature trees is sometimes harvested by digging the surface roots that lie just below the drip line (just below the tips of the branches that extend farthest from the trunk). Because of the riot of interwoven roots found just beneath the soil's surface in the forest, learn to recognize the roots by their appearance, but verify it by scraping the bark to see if it has the characteristic sassafras aroma.

Sassafras roots grow horizontally from the base of the main trunk. Before digging, determine which direction the root extends from the trunk. Once the soil is loosened around the base of the sapling and along the root, it can usually be pulled out of the ground with a firm tug. If the root is thicker than one inch in diameter, use a knife to remove the outer bark from the root; if it is smaller in circumference, cut the roots into thin slices without removing the bark. Dry the outer root bark or sliced root. Roots turn rich reddish brown when dry. Collect bark from the saplings in early spring just as leaves appear. Do not collect bark from mature trees, as it makes them vulnerable to disease and will often kill them. Gather green leaves as soon as they emerge through June. As the summer progresses, the leaves are less succulent and less potent.

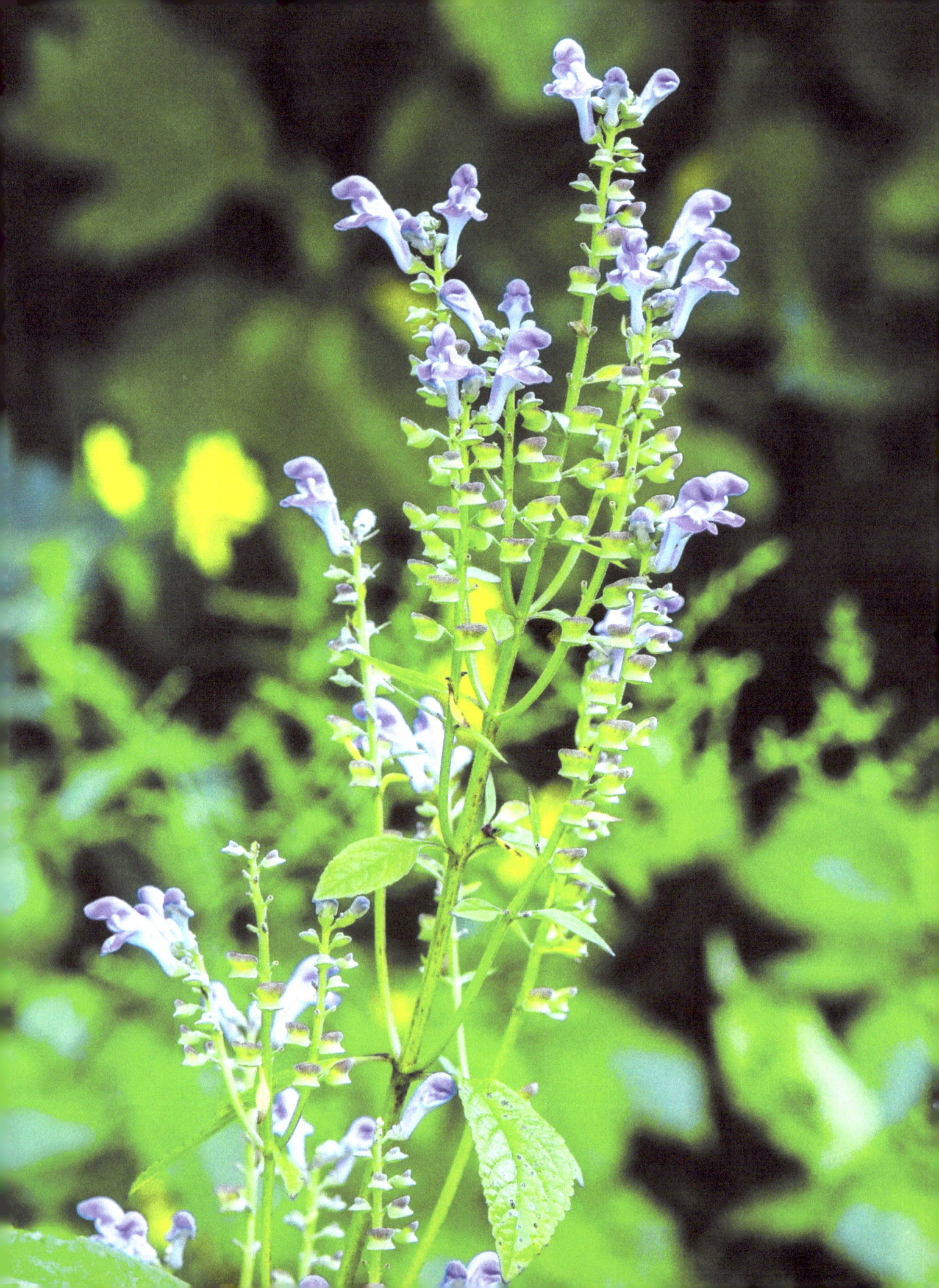

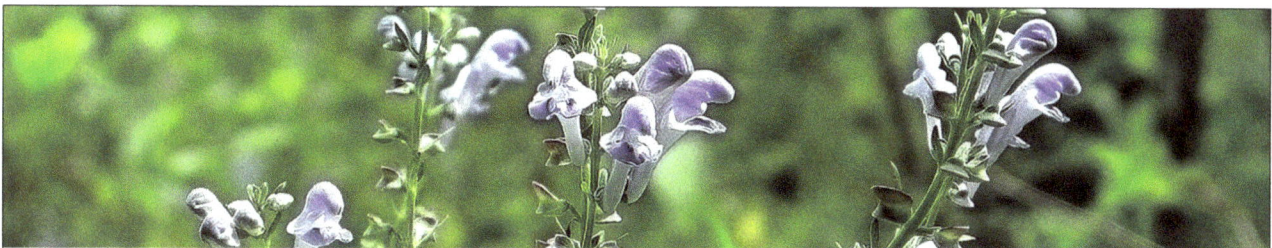

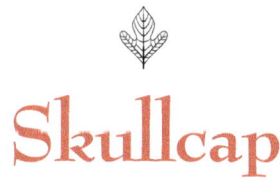

Skullcap

COMMON NAME: Skullcap

BOTANICAL NAME: *Scutellaria incana, S. lateriflora*

FAMILY: *Lamiaceae* (Mint)

OTHER NAMES: Hoary Skullcap *(S. incana),* Mad Dog Skullcap *(S. lateriflora)*

DESCRIPTION: Both regional species of skullcap are upright perennials, one to two feet tall. Like other Mint family herbs, they have square stems and opposite leaves that are oval with slightly toothed edges and a round base. The pale blue or sometimes lavender flowers are two-lipped on racemes, but *S. lateriflora* flowers are only on one side of the flower stalk and emerge from the leaf axils, while *S. incana* flowers are on branching stems at the top of the plant. Blooms from late June to August. Noted botanist Alan Weakley points out that all *Scutellaria* species are "recognizable by the "tractor seat-shaped" protuberance on the upper calyx."[1] Despite being in the Mint family, skullcap lacks the characteristic spicy aroma and has a bitter flavor.

HABITAT: Common in sunny, open fields or partial shade.

KEY ACTIONS: Nervine relaxant, antispasmodic, nerve tonic, bitter, emmenagogue

PART USED: Aerial (in flower)

TRADITIONAL USES: The Cherokee used skullcap to relieve menstrual cramping, bring on delayed menses, and ease breast tenderness. Strong tea was given to women immediately after labor to induce vomiting to help expel the afterbirth.[2]

Skullcap was a folk remedy to relieve symptoms of hydrophobia caused by dog bites, hence the common name Mad Dog Skullcap. It was also used as

---

[1] Weakley, *Plants of the Southern and Mid Atlantic States* (Print Version, March 2010), 760

[2] Moerman, *Native American Ethnobotany,* 524

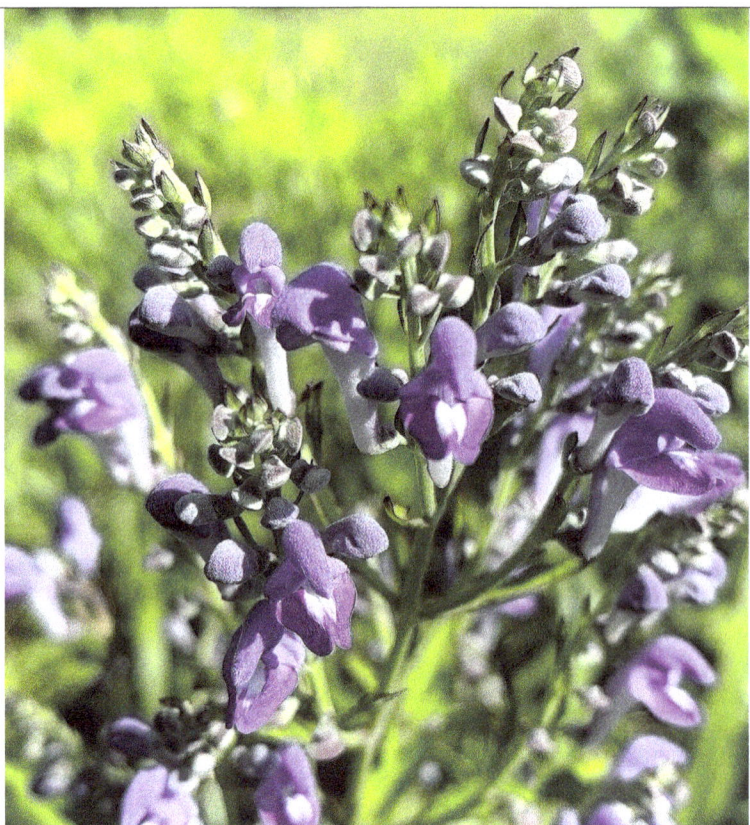

a restorative remedy for the nervous system to address nervous exhaustion accompanied by insomnia, depression, anxiety, and muscle tremors or spasms.

CURRENT USES: Skullcap, a versatile nervine, soothes and restores the nervous system. It relieves acute symptoms, while long-term use harmonizes and rejuvenates the nervous system. It is particularly effective for combating mental fatigue and nervous exhaustion induced by over-stimulation, overwork, and prolonged stress. A reliable remedy for insomnia with difficulty falling asleep, stress-aggravated migraine headaches, and general feelings of anxiety. As an antispasmodic, it relieves menstrual cramping, general muscle tension, sciatic or back pain, and tight neck and shoulders. Skullcap also plays a crucial role in easing the symptoms associated with drug and alcohol withdrawal.

CAUTIONS: Skullcap is generally considered safe during pregnancy and nursing. There have been some reports of liver toxicity caused by skullcap; however, it is widely believed that these reports are due to adulteration with Germander *(Teucrium canadense),* another regional herb that closely resembles skullcap.[3]

---

[3] Gardner and McGuffin, *AHPA's Botanical Safety Handbook* (Second Edition), 802

PREPARATIONS

Tincture prepared with fresh skullcap has the most potent tonic properties, while the dry herb is more sedating and better suited to treating acute symptoms.

INFUSION: Use two teaspoons of dried or three teaspoons of fresh herb for eight ounces of water. Cover and steep for 15 minutes. Strain.

TINCTURE: Fresh – 1:2, 95%. Dried – 1:5, 50%.

DOSAGES

Skullcap quickly relieves acute symptoms but acts as a tonic for the nervous system when used daily for extended periods. Due to its bitter taste, I often combine it with more aromatic herbs like bee balm *(Monarda spp.)* and mountain mint *(Pycnanthemum incanum)*.

INFUSION: For acute conditions, drink one cup every thirty minutes or as needed to relieve symptoms. As a nerve tonic, drink two cups daily for a month or longer.

TINCTURE: Take half to one teaspoon every thirty to sixty minutes or as needed for acute conditions. Take a half teaspoon twice daily for a month or longer to use as a tonic.

HARVESTING

Collect skullcap when in full bloom in late June through August. Cut the stem just above any yellowed or bug-eaten leaves. Either prepare a tincture using fresh herbs or bundle the stems of five or six plants with a rubber band and hang them to dry. When leaves crumble to the touch, strip the leaves and flowers from the stems and store them in a glass jar.

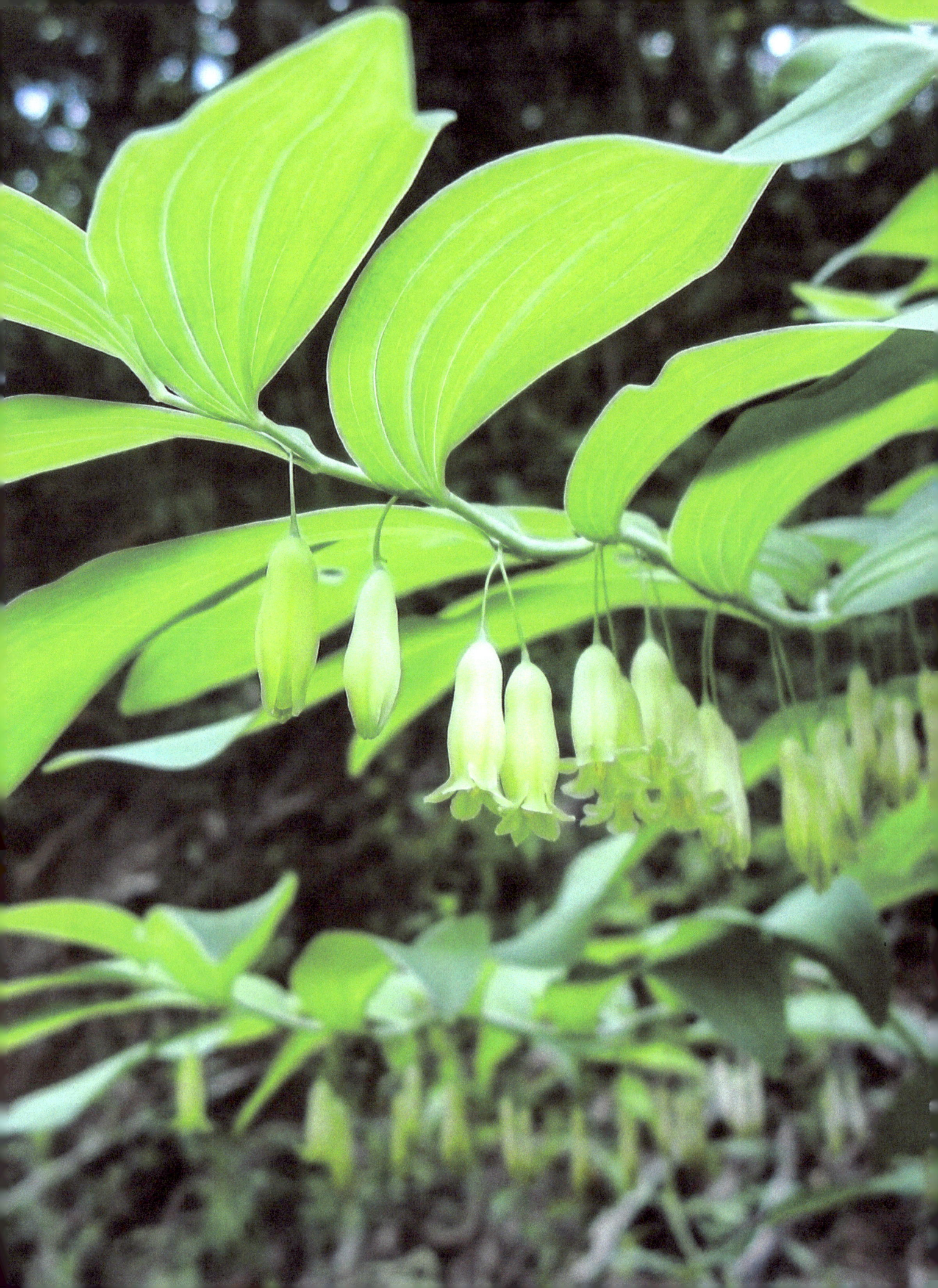

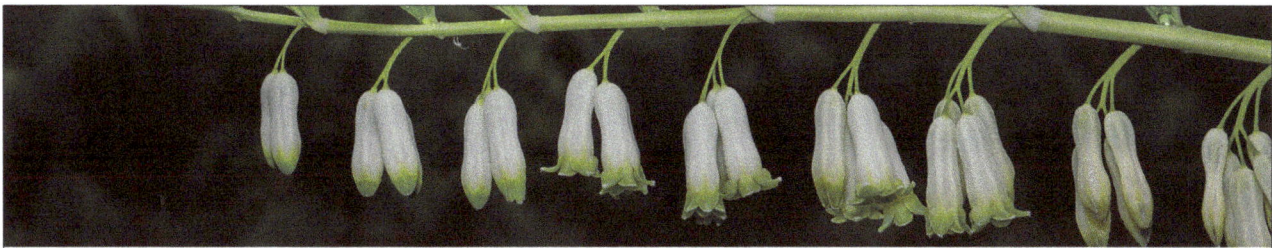

Solomon's Seal

COMMON NAME: Solomon's Seal

BOTANICAL NAME: *Polygonatum biflorum*

FAMILY: *Liliaceae* (Lily)

OTHER NAMES: True Solomon's Seal, King Solomon's Seal

RELATED SPECIES: Greater Solomon's Seal *(P. multiflorum)* and Hairy Solomon's Seal *(P. pubescens)* are used interchangeably with *P. biflorum*. Solomon's Plume or False Solomon's Seal *(Maianthemum racemosum,* formerly known as *Smilacina racemosa)* does not have the same therapeutic properties, though the root and aerial sprout are edible.

DESCRIPTION: Solomon's seal, a beautiful perennial, stands one to three feet tall, with a single graceful arching stem and narrow alternate leaves with parallel veins. Its tubular whitish-green flowers, each with six lobes, dangle in pairs from every leaf axil along the stem. It blooms from May to June, followed by bead-like berries, which change from green to dark blue in late summer. Greater Solomon's Seal is a larger variant with three or more flowers at each leaf axil. Hairy Solomon's seal *(P. pubescens)* has fine hairs along each vein on the underside of the leaf and is slightly smaller than *P. biflorum*.

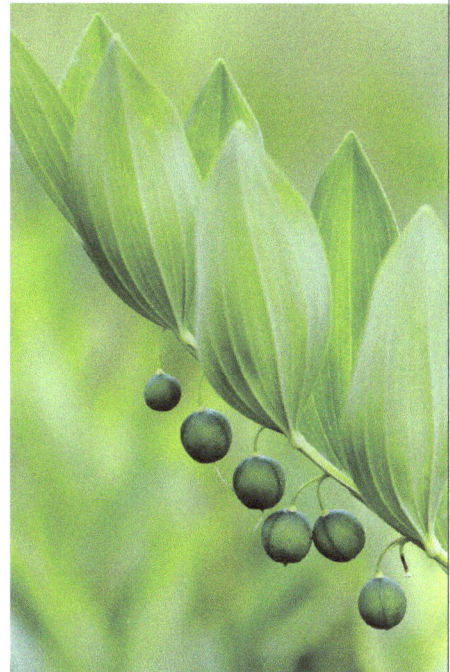

Solomon's seal takes its name from the rootstock scars, which resemble a wax seal marked with an "S." The rhizome runs horizontally just beneath the ground and is knobby, with delicate root hairs along its length. Stem scars or "seals" indicate the age of the plant, with one scar for each year of growth.

Solomon's plume or false Solomon's seal *(Maianthemum racemosum)* often grows near Solomon's seal, and the two plants are sometimes confused. However, Solomon's plume can be distinguished by its distinctive zigzag stem, small star-like flowers that bloom in a terminal cluster from May to

July, and reddish-pink berries. Solomon's plume has an edible root but no medicinal properties.

CAUTIONS: None known.

HABITAT: Deciduous forests throughout the region. Solomon's seal favors cool, moist slopes. Often found growing alongside black cohosh (*Actaea racemosa*), blue cohosh (*Caulophyllum thalictroides*), and bloodroot (*Sanguinaria canadensis*).

KEY ACTIONS: Demulcent, expectorant, lung tonic, sedative, demulcent tonic

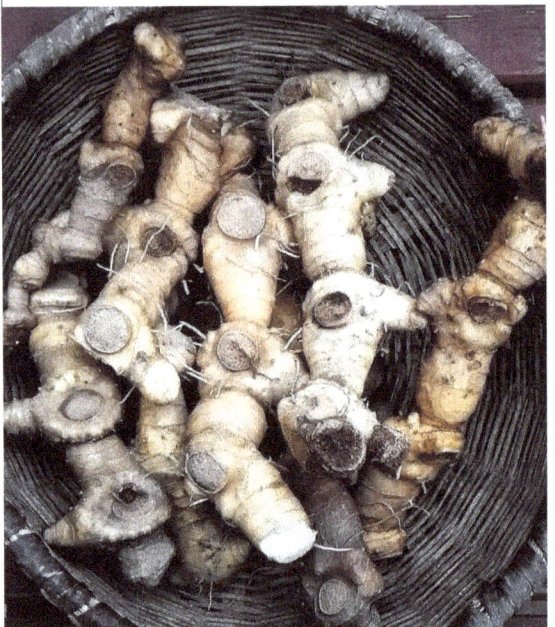

PART USED: Root, shoots (edible in the early spring)

TRADITIONAL USES: The Cherokee used Solomon's seal as food and medicine. Edible young shoots with a flavor like asparagus were collected in spring. Roasted roots were ground to make flour. Crushed, fresh roots were applied as a poultice to bruises and swellings. Strong root decoctions were used for consumption, as well as coughs, breathing difficulties, and chronic lung weakness. This same preparation was used to treat inflammation of the stomach and bowels. It was also used internally to heal broken bones, torn or strained ligaments, tendons and muscles. Solomon's seal also has a long history as an herb with magical properties. American Indians burned the root to clean sleeping quarters and guarantee restful sleep.[1]

CURRENT USES: Use Solomon's seal as a mild tonic for general debility and weakness, especially after a long illness when symptoms such as lack of appetite, a dry hacking cough and restlessness are present. As a tonic, Solomon's seal restores essential fluids throughout the body, which contributes to its reputation as a longevity tonic and strengthens respiration. Use Solomon's seal for extended periods to loosen stiff ligaments and tendons and restore essential fluids to mucus membranes, dry skin and hair. Contributes to the healing of broken bones, torn and sprained muscles, ligaments and tendons. Decoctions soothe inflammation and irritation of the lungs, stomach, and intestinal tract. For bruises, use tincture internally and apply a fresh root poultice to bruises to break up blood stagnation and move the blood.

"...the roots must be stamped, some ale or wine put thereto, strained and given to drink...to knit broken bones, against bruises, blacke or blew marks gotten by stripes, falls or the like; against inflammation...or swellings."

John Gerard, (1030) *Gerard's Herbal*

---

[1] Moerman, *Native American Ethnobotany*, 422

PREPARATIONS

DECOCTION: Use two tablespoons of dried root or one tablespoon of fresh root in eight ounces of water. Bring to a boil; cover and simmer for twenty minutes. Strain.

TINCTURE: Fresh – 1:2, 95%. Dried – 1:5, 50%.

POULTICE: Grate fresh root and use a mortar and pestle to pound into a paste. Add a little aloe vera gel to make a smooth mixture that holds together if needed. Use immediately.

DOSAGES

Internal use as a tonic often requires a month or longer of daily use.

DECOCTION: Drink one cup three or four times daily for extended periods.

TINCTURE: Take one-half teaspoon twice a day. Long-term use (three months or more) is needed to address symptoms of dryness caused by overall deficiency and aging.

POULTICE: Apply as needed to relieve pain and swelling from bruises.

HARVESTING

Dig roots mid to late summer after berries ripen. The white bud protruding from the terminal end of the rhizome and several inches of the root may be replanted to generate a new plant. After digging the root, discard leaves and berries, wash roots, slice thinly and dry till brittle, or make fresh herb tincture. Berries are toxic. Solomon's seal stems, collected before leaves are fully unfurled, are a delicious wild edible with a flavor like asparagus.

TIP: STAYING JUICY

As we age, we often notice more symptoms of dryness, like dry hair and skin, less joint flexibility, a chronic dry cough, indigestion, and constipation. Herbs like Solomon's seal are so effective at relieving these issues because they act as moistening tonics. Other moistening tonics include burdock *(Arctium lappa)* and licorice *(Glycyrrhiza glabra)*. They all help restore essential fluids in the mucosal lining of the stomach, intestines, and lungs, relieve vaginal atrophy and restore the synovial fluid in the joints, and revive dry skin and hair. Used daily for several months or longer, along with adequate hydration, these herbs can restore crucial bodily fluids and slow down symptoms associated with aging.

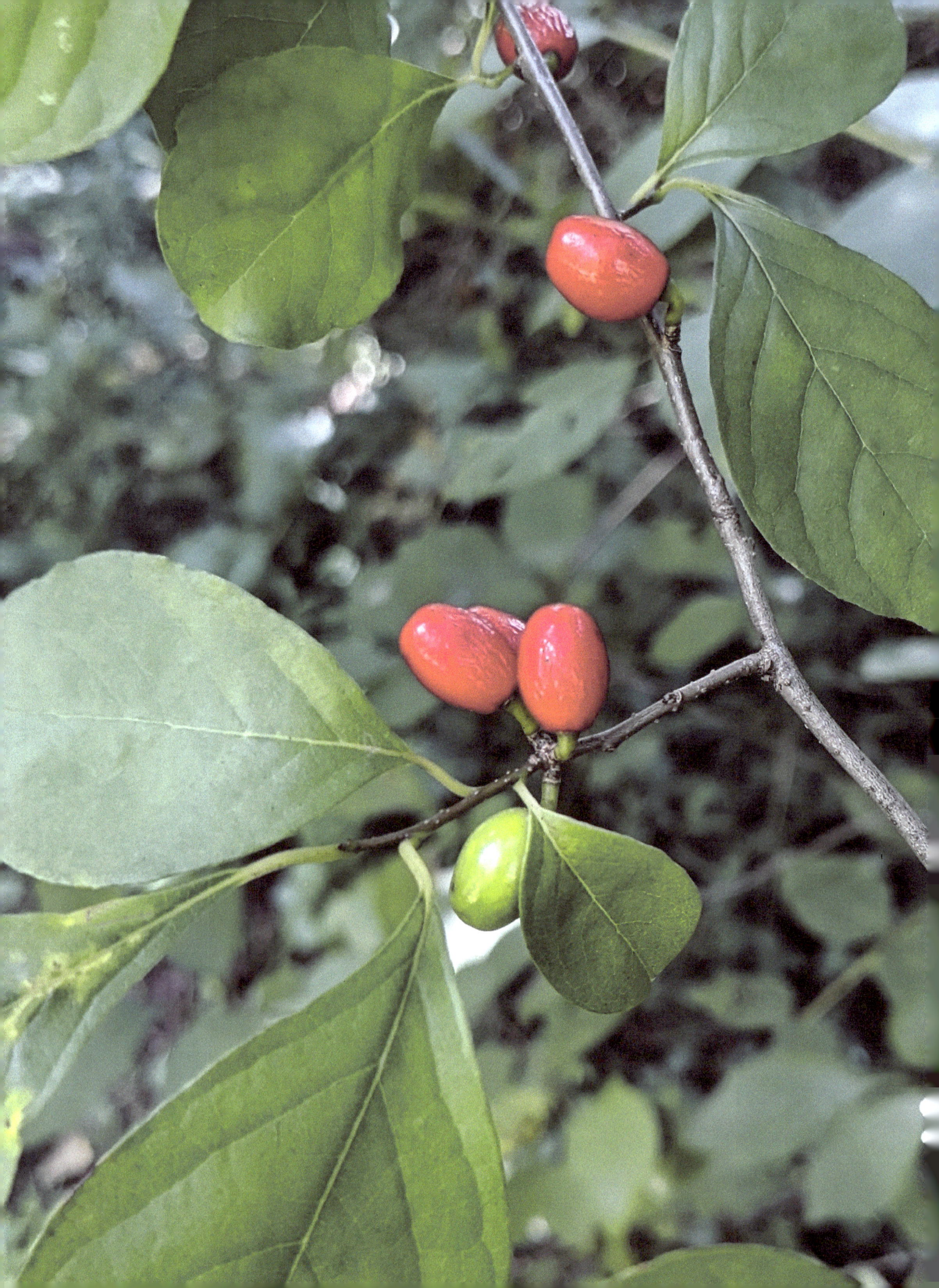

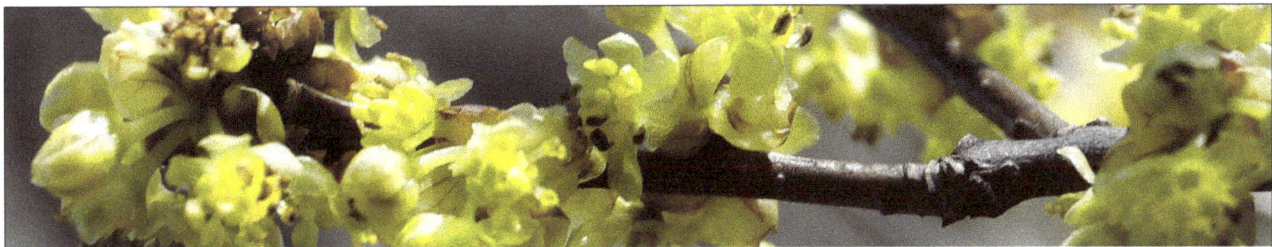

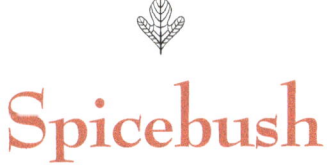

Spicebush

COMMON NAME: Spicebush

BOTANICAL NAME: *Lindera benzoin*

FAMILY: *Lauraceae* (Laurel)

OTHER NAMES: Wild Allspice, Spicewood

DESCRIPTION: Spicebush, a deciduous shrub five to fifteen feet tall, has alternate, oval leaves with smooth edges. Female plants have small clusters of yellow flowers that bloom in early spring before the leaves emerge and shiny, oblong red berries, each containing one hard seed that ripens in the late summer. The berries are spicy, and taste somewhat like allspice. All parts of the plant are aromatic.

HABITAT: Common understory plant in deciduous forests, often found growing along streams and creeks.

KEY ACTIONS: Diaphoretic, carminative, stimulant, aromatic, expectorant

PART USED: Leaf, bark, twig, berry

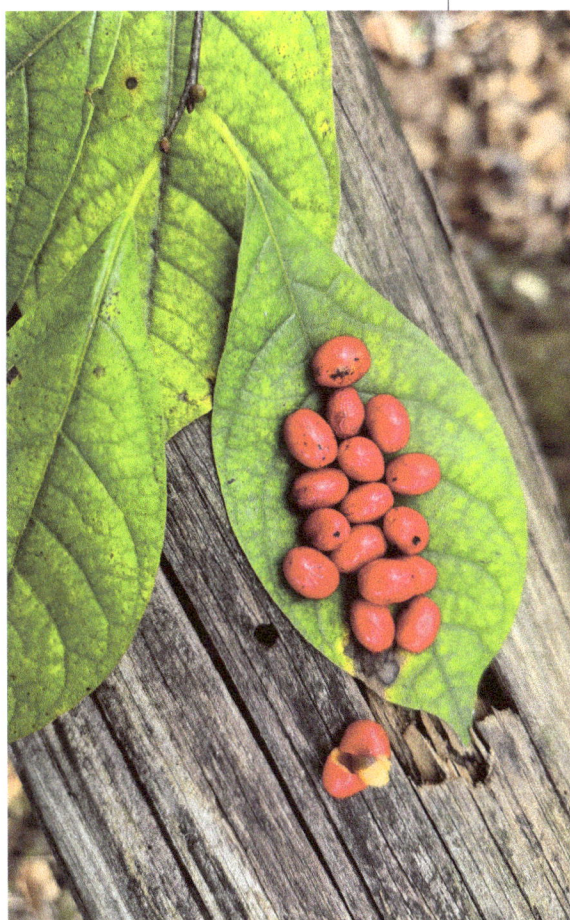

TRADITIONAL USES: American Indians made tea from all parts of the spicebush. They drank the tea as a spring tonic and to relieve coughs, reduce fevers, and treat measles. Spicebush was also used to bring on delayed menses.[1] During the Revolutionary War, spicebush berries were used as a substitute for allspice *(Pimenta dioica)*. In the Civil War, spicebush was regularly used a reliable diaphoretic remedy for intermittent fevers.[2]

---

[1] Moerman, *Native American Ethnobotany,* 308

[2] Porcher, *Resources of the Southern Fields and Forests,* 355

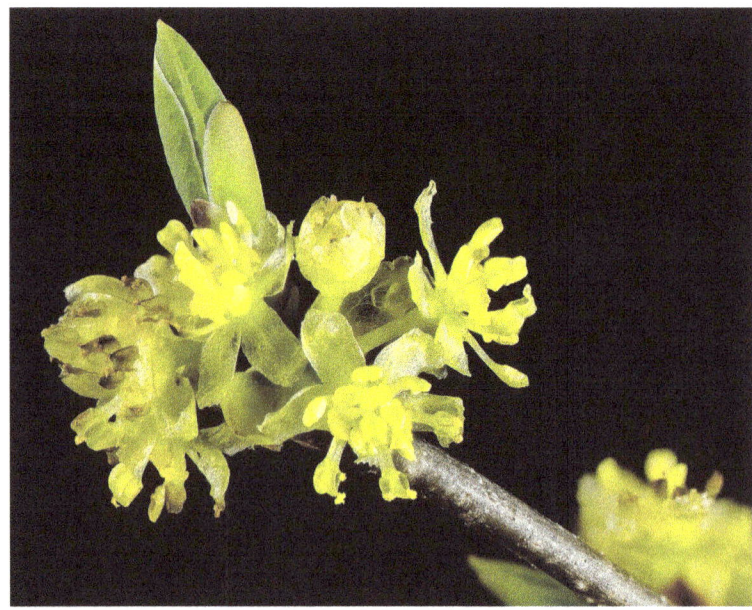

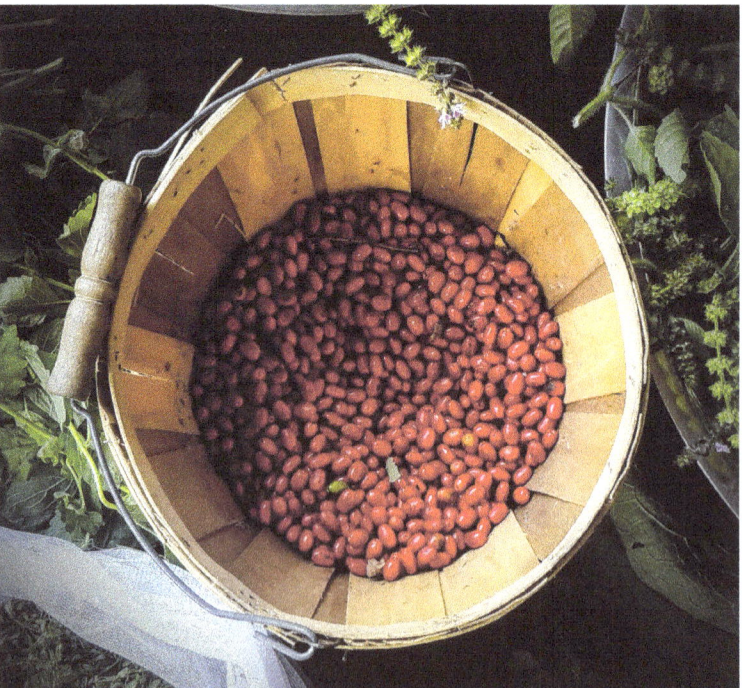

"The soldiers of the upper country of South Carolina... came into camp fully supplied with the spice bush for making a fragrant, aromatic, diaphoretic tea."

Frances Peyre Porcher, *(1863) Resources of the Southern Fields and Forests*

CURRENT USES: Spicebush is not well known in modern herbal practice. However, it is a common understory bush and a mild but effective remedy that warms the stomach to relieve indigestion with bloating, nausea and gas. Drink the warming, aromatic decoction as hot as possible to stimulate sweating, reduce fevers, ease menstrual cramps, and bring on delayed menses.

CAUTIONS: None known.

PREPARATIONS

DECOCTION: Use one-half cup dried or one cup of finely chopped fresh leaves and twigs for each eight ounces of water. Bring to a boil; cover tightly and simmer for at least twenty minutes. Strain and sweeten.

CONDIMENT: Berries are challenging to dry. The best way to preserve them is to freeze fresh berries. When ready to use, grind in a food processor or small spice grinder. Use them immediately after grinding to flavor apple, pumpkin or squash pies, applesauce, and apple cider, or add to any recipe that calls for allspice or cinnamon.

DOSAGES

A mild herbal remedy used to relieve acute symptoms.

DECOCTION: As a diaphoretic, drink eight ounces of hot decoction every few hours and stay well covered with blankets or warm clothes, as this tea causes sweating.

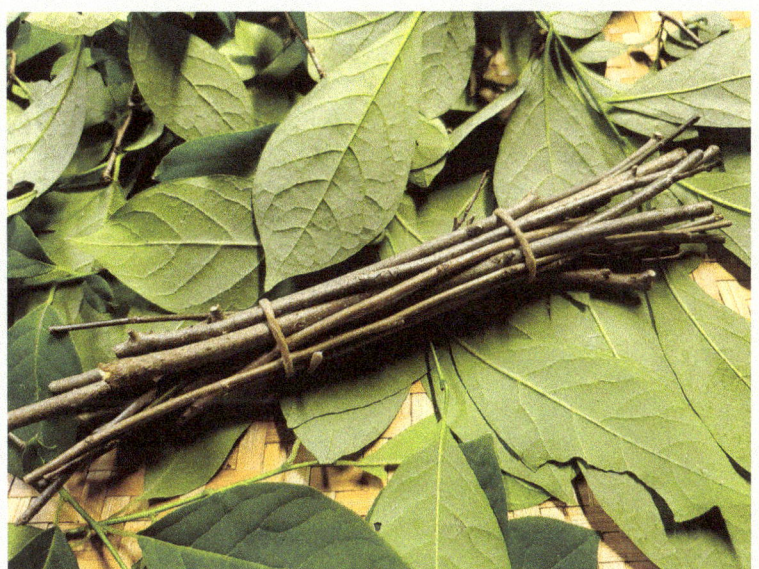

HARVESTING

Harvest leaves, bark, and twigs at any time, though they are most potent during early spring to mid-summer. Collect four or five-inch tips from the outer branches. Harvest berries when they turn a deep scarlet color in early fall. Seeds fall from the branches soon after they ripen, so keep a sharp eye out to harvest them before they drop. Prepare berries using the Condiment directions.

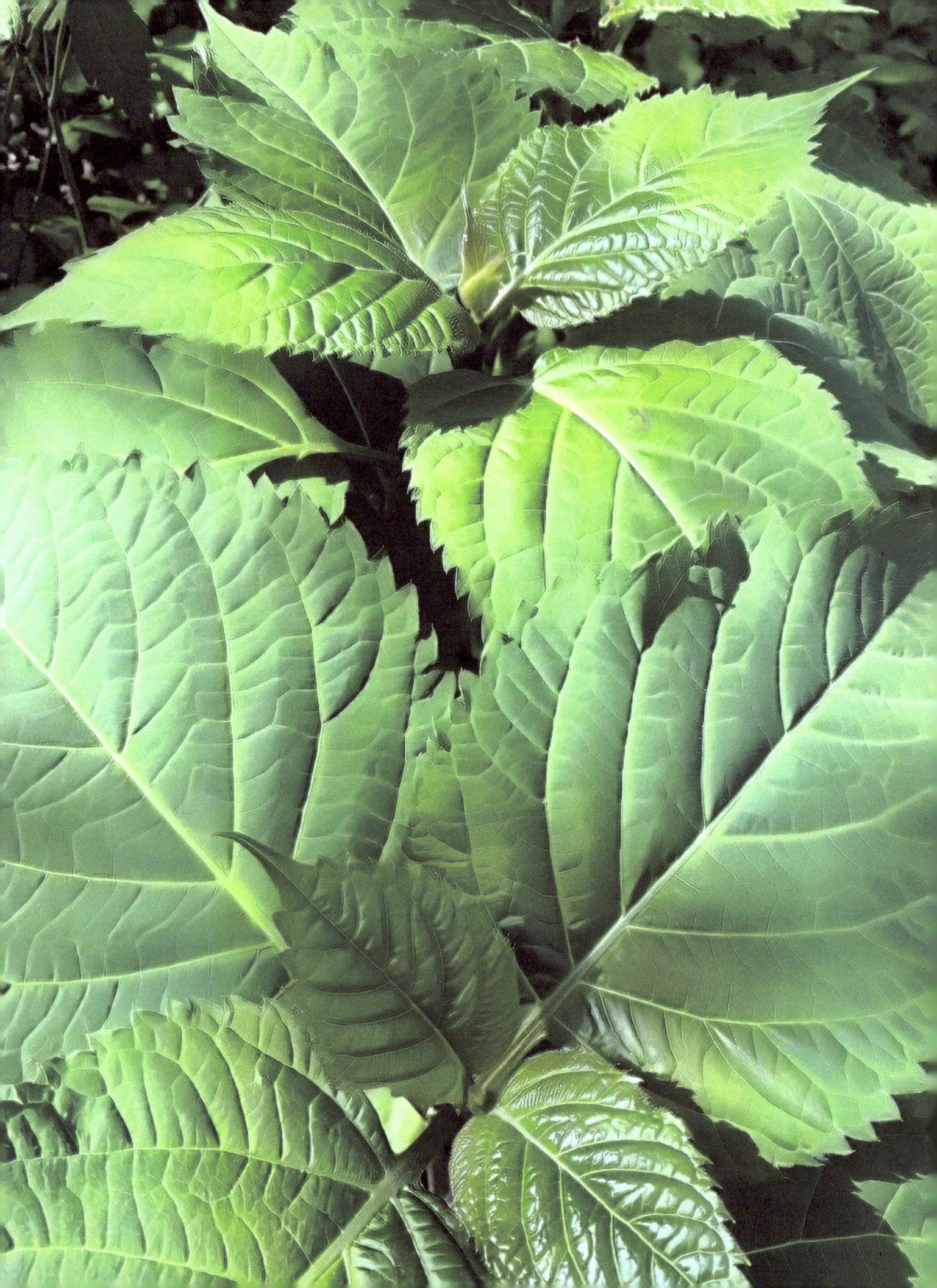

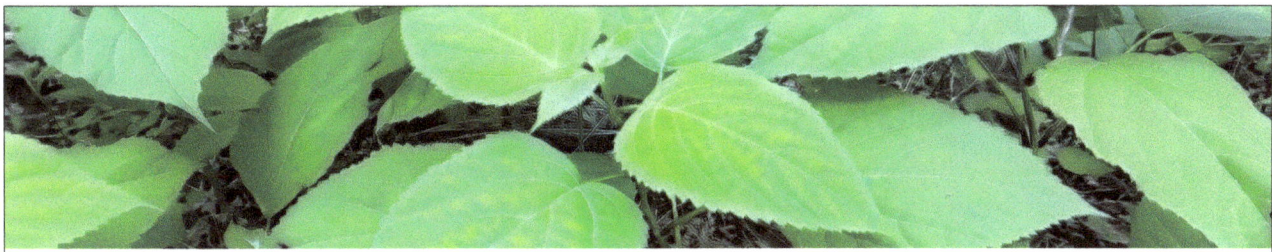

Stoneroot

COMMON NAME: Stoneroot

BOTANICAL NAME: *Collinsonia canadensis*

FAMILY: *Lamiaceae* (Mint)

OTHER NAMES: Preacher's Friend, Rich Weed, Horsemint, Horseweed, Horsebalm

RELATED SPECIES: Southern Horse Balm *(C. tuberosa)*, Whorled Horse Balm *(C. verticillate)*

DESCRIPTION: Stoneroot is an upright perennial, two to four feet high, with a square stem and opposite leaves. The leaves are three to four inches wide with serrated edges; lower leaves have a short stem or petiole, while the upper leaves attach directly to the stem. Lemon-scented flowers grow in racemes at the plant's top and bloom from July to August. The two-lipped flower is pale yellow; the lower lip has three lobes, with the middle lobe fringed and two prominent stamens protruding from the flower. The entire plant has a distinctive scent, faintly reminiscent of citronella, though some thought it reminded them of a sweaty horse, inspiring several of its common names.

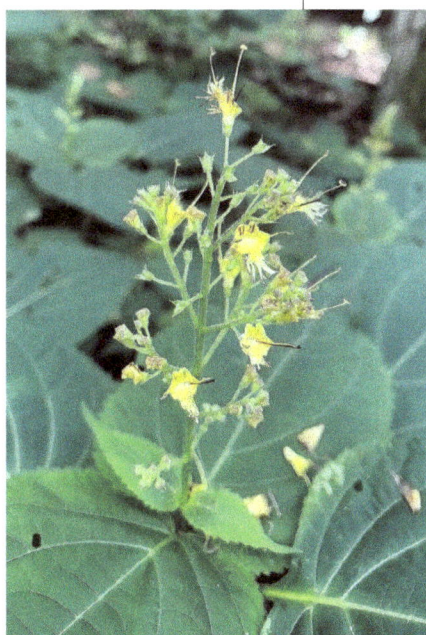

HABITAT: Grows in the deep shade of rich forests, usually in abundant colonies.

KEY ACTIONS: Anti-lithic, diaphoretic, circulatory stimulant, anti-inflammatory, vascular tonic

PART USED: Entire plant (in flower)

TRADITIONAL USES: American Indians used stoneroot as a poultice or a wash for painful swollen breasts, headaches, and rheumatic pains. The infusion was used to relieve kidney and heart problems and to cure listlessness in children. Flowers and leaves were rubbed on the skin as a deodorant.[1] It was considered one of the most valuable remedies for

---

[1] Moerman, *Native American Ethnobotany*, 171

hemorrhoids and other urinary tract problems. A poultice of the fresh leaves was used on bruises, sprains, and wounds.[2]

CURRENT USES: Stoneroot is used to relieve symptoms in several different parts of the body. It resolves vascular constriction in the pelvis and rectum, resulting in a sensation of bearing down or heaviness. It is a specific remedy for hemorrhoids, anal fistulas, rectal pain or inflammation and prostatitis. Its anti-inflammatory properties soothe sore throats and mouth ulcers and relieve laryngitis. As a tonic, stoneroot helps to prevent the formation of kidney stones and gallstones. It also acts as a gentle stimulant for the heart and is often combined with other vascular tonics, like hawthorn *(Crataegus spp.)* and motherwort *(Leonurus cardiaca)*.

CAUTIONS: None known.

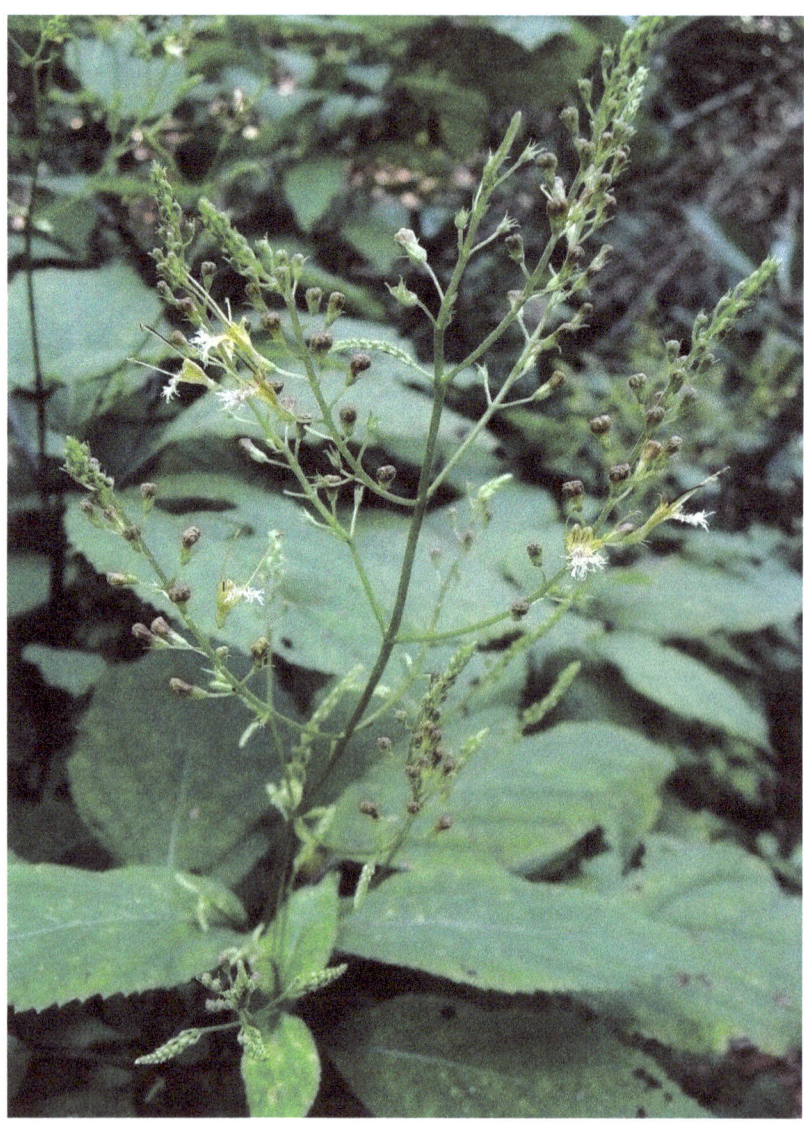

[2] O. P. Brown, *The Complete Herbalist*, 156

PREPARATIONS

Tincture should be prepared using the entire fresh plant (including roots). Except when used as a gargle for mouth and throat inflammation, stoneroot is almost always used as part of a formula to support other system specific herbs.

TINCTURE: Fresh – 1:2. Dried – 1:5, 50%.

DECOCTION: Use one tablespoon fresh or two tablespoons dried leaf and root for each eight ounces of water. Bring to a boil; cover and simmer for 15 minutes. Strain.

DOSAGES

Use as needed to relieve acute symptoms; for chronic conditions, use daily for a month or longer.

TINCTURE: For acute symptoms, one-half teaspoon every thirty minutes. As a tonic, a half teaspoon twice a day for a month or longer

DECOCTION: For acute symptoms affecting the pelvis and rectum, including gallstones and kidney stones, drink one to two quarts of decoction daily until symptoms improve. Use the decoction as a gargle for throat and mouth inflammation. Use as a compress or in a sitz bath for painful hemorrhoids and anal fistulas.

CAUTIONS: None known. Some sources report that high doses of stoneroot may cause nausea or vomiting, but this appears to be rare.

HARVESTING

Harvest the entire plant, including the root, while in flower in mid to late summer. Immediately clean the root and cut it into small pieces. Be prepared to use serious loppers or even a small hatchet to break up the fresh root as once it dries, even slightly, the implications of the common name "stoneroot" are evident.

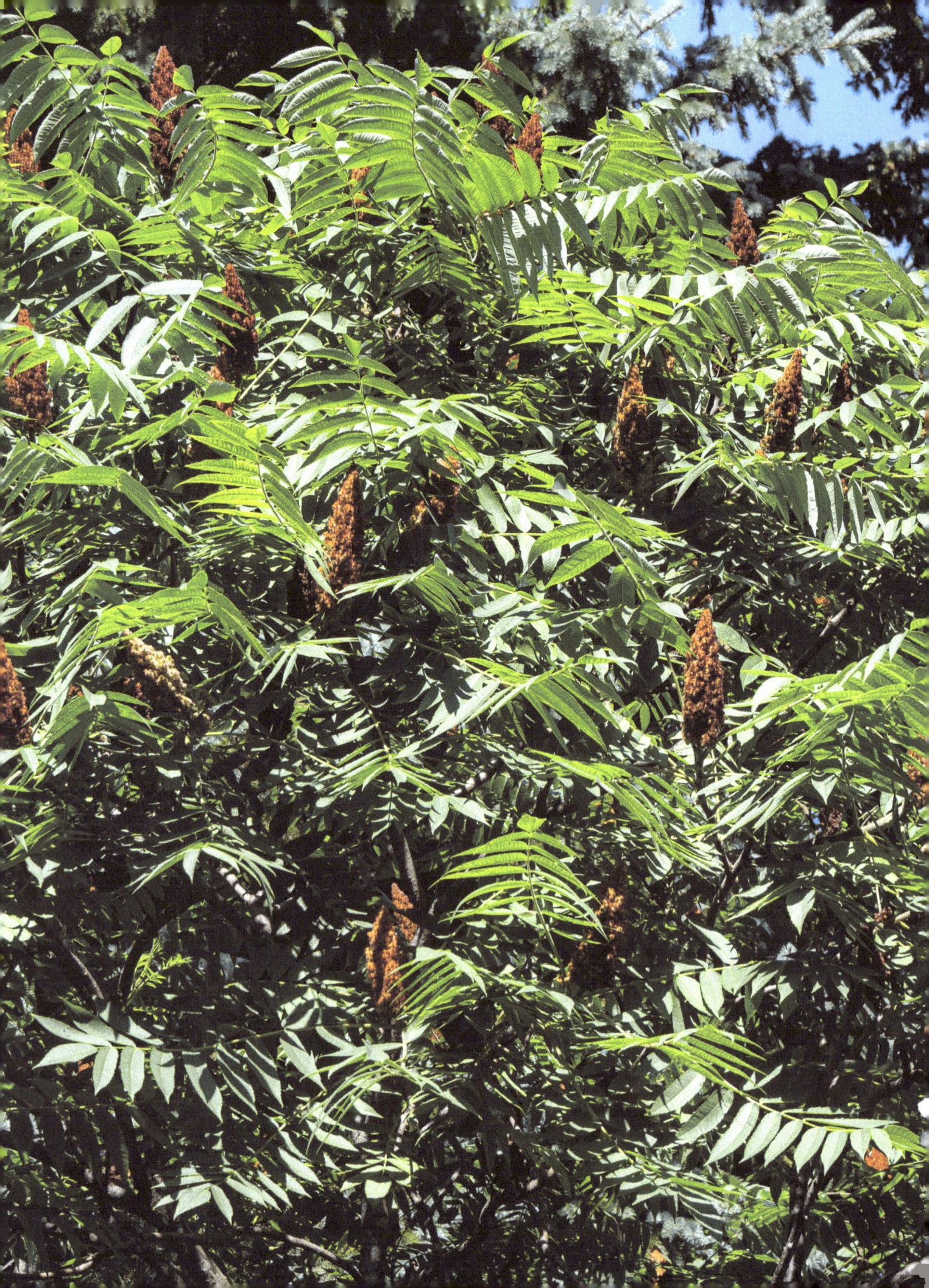

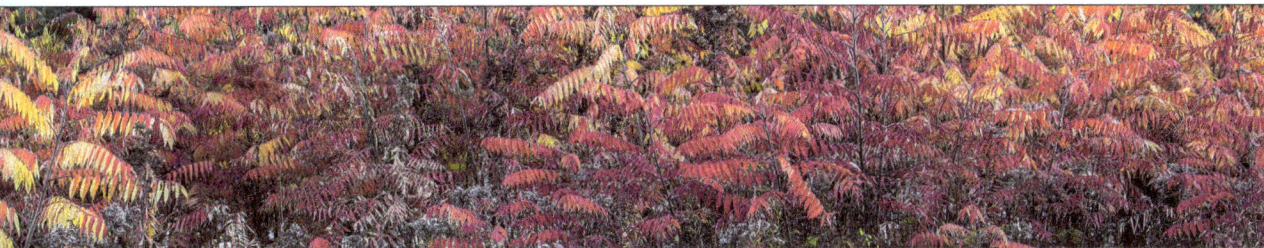

Sumac

COMMON NAME: Sumac

BOTANICAL NAME: *Rhus glabra*

FAMILY: *Anacardiaceae* (Cashew)

OTHER NAMES: Smooth Sumac

RELATED SPECIES: Flameleaf or Winged Sumac *(R. copallinum),* Staghorn Sumac *(R. typhina)*

DESCRIPTION: Three species of sumac with similar medicinal properties grow throughout the region. All are shrubs or small trees, four to twenty feet tall, which grow in thickets; each species differs slightly in appearance.

The compound leaves of smooth sumac *(R. glabra)* are composed of about thirteen sharply toothed leaflets, each about two inches long, with a red central rib and white undersides. The leaves and stalks are smooth and hairless. Those of flame leaf or winged sumac *(R. copallinum)* are shiny with a distinctive winged midrib along the stem between each leaflet. Staghorn sumac *(R. typhina)* has giant leaves — up to twenty-four inches long — with sharply toothed leaflets; both leaves and branches are covered with fine, downy hair.

In midsummer, all three species have clusters of tiny, upright, greenish-yellow flowers that ripen into hard, round, red berries covered with fine hair. As autumn progresses, sumac berries gradually turn from a brilliant scarlet to a muted rust color. At the onset of cold weather, the leaves of all three species turn a beautiful flame-red. The forked zigzag of bare sumac branches was thought to resemble a stag's horn silhouetted against the winter sky.

Poison sumac *(R. vernix)* is easily distinguished from the safe sumac species. It has toothless compound leaves with big spaces between the leaflets and hanging clusters of white berries. Contact with poison sumac results in severe skin rashes.

HABITAT: Common along roadsides and the edges of fields.

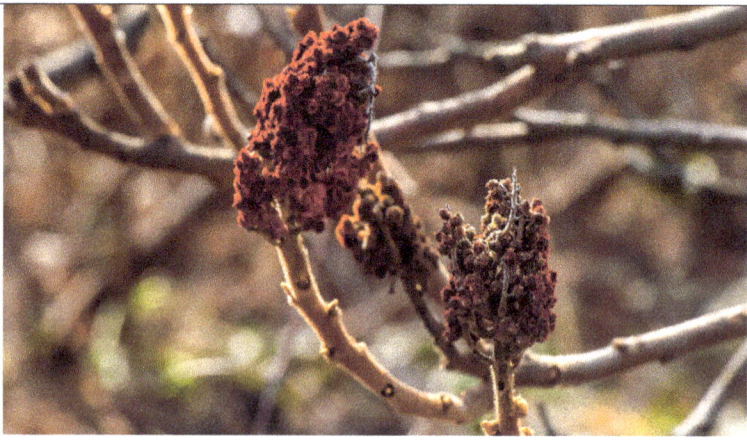

KEY ACTIONS: Astringent, styptic, refrigerant

PART USED: Leaf, berry, bark

TRADITIONAL USES: American Indians used almost every part of sumac. The leaves, bark, and berries were decocted or infused to make an astringent wash to treat burns, stop bleeding (internal and external), control diarrhea, and reduce fever. The leaves were also used to tan leather. The berries produce a rich black dye. After sumac leaves turned red in the fall, they were collected, dried, and mixed with tobacco in ceremonial smoking blends. Ripe berries were infused in water to make a cooling, lemony beverage.[1]

Alabama herbalist Tommie Bass considered the sumac berry a critical source of vitamin C. He recommended using berry tea as a gargle for sore throats or a compress for hemorrhoids.[2] During the Civil War, when access to supplies was limited, a black shoe polish called "shoemac" was made from the leaf.[3]

CURRENT USES: Sumac is not commonly used in herbal practice but is a potent folk remedy. Sumac berry or leaf infusions make an effective tea for relieving cold symptoms such as coughs and fevers. The tea is also a fast-acting remedy for diarrhea. Berry or leaf infusion is used topically to cool painful burns, clean wounds, stop bleeding, and as a douche to treat vaginal discharge. As a gargle, it treats sore throats, mouth sores or inflamed gums.

Powdered sumac berries are available commercially for culinary use; they are a traditional spice in Middle Eastern cooking. Wild food enthusiasts have made sumac berry lemonade a popular thirst-quenching trail beverage; see recipe on page 173.

CAUTIONS: None known. However, proper identification is needed.

---

[1] Moerman, *Native American Ethnobotany*, 471–473

[2] Patton, *Tommie Bass: Herb Doctor of Shinbone Ridge*, 135

[3] Porcher, *Resources of the Southern Fields and Forests*, 202

PREPARATIONS

Infusions of sumac berries or leaves are the most common way to use this plant as a medicine. Infuse sumac for the recommended times, or the mixture may be too astringent. Sumac leaves and berries can also be used to make cough syrup. See recipe on page 192.

INFUSION: Leaf—Use one-half cup of dried or one full cup of fresh, loosely packed leaves for each quart of boiling water. Cover and steep for ten minutes. Strain.

Berries—Use two clusters of crushed ripe berries for each quart of cool water. Crush berries by placing them in a medium-sized bowl and pressing them firmly with the back of a wooden spoon. Cover with cool water and steep for 10 minutes. Strain berry infusion through a colander lined with muslin to remove fine hairs from the berries before drinking.

DOSAGES

Because sumac is high in tannins, it should not be used internally for more than a few days by anyone with a history of kidney stones.

INFUSION: Drink one cup of infusion every hour until symptoms improve. Warm infusion may also be used as a gargle for throat inflammation and pain. Use a cool infusion as needed as a wash to treat burns and as a douche to relieve vaginal discharge.

HARVESTING

Harvest green leaves in midsummer just as the flower begins to bloom to make an astringent infusion. Gather sumac berries around the time of the first frost when the berries are bright red. When leaves turn red in the fall, gather them for smoking mixtures.

SUMAC BERRY LEMONADE

Sumac berry lemonade provides refreshing relief on hot summer afternoons. Sumac berry infusion can be heated before serving if it is used to relieve cold symptoms.

Place four to five clusters of fresh, ripe sumac berries in a gallon container. Crush the berries using a wooden spoon, then add one gallon of cool water. Swirl the berries around in the water for a few minutes. Steep for fifteen to twenty minutes or to taste. Strain the mixture through a colander lined with cotton muslin; straining is needed to remove the fine hairs from the berries. Sweeten the infusion with honey or mix it with fruit juices. In warm weather, you may want to chill before serving.

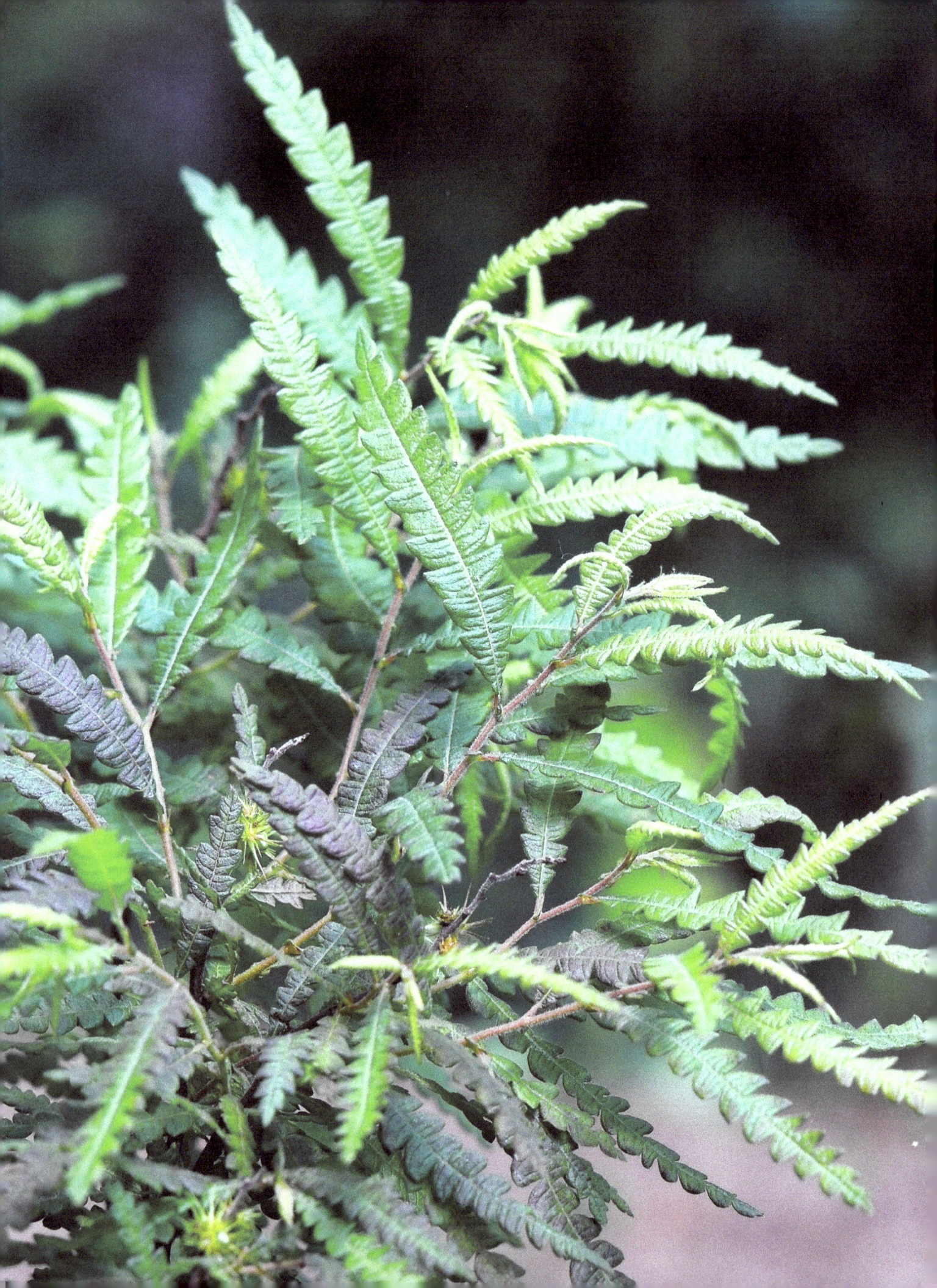

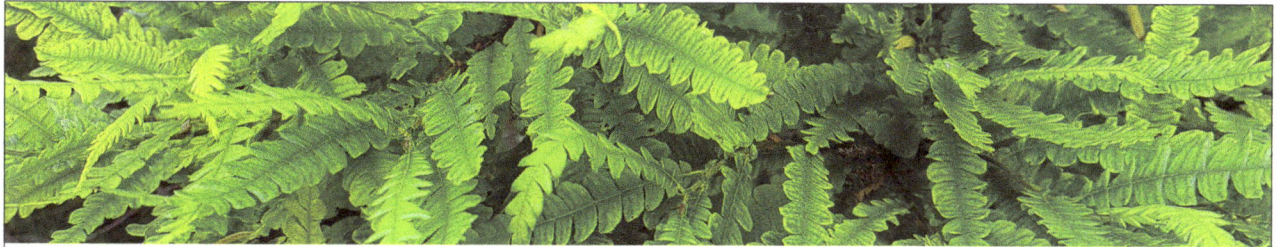

Sweetfern

COMMON NAME: Sweetfern

BOTANICAL NAME: *Comptonia peregrina*

FAMILY: *Myricaceae* (Wax Myrtle)

DESCRIPTION: Sweetfern is a small shrub, one to three feet tall, with a woody stem and fernlike appearance. Deep green, alternate leaves, lance-shaped with rounded teeth, appear late in the spring. When crushed, the leaves release an aromatic fragrance. When in bloom at midsummer, the inconspicuous green flowers are easy to miss. In the fall, sweetfern produces small burr-like seedpods enclosing tiny aromatic nuts.

HABITAT: Dry, open areas, often in poor soil.

KEY ACTIONS: Astringent, alterative, carminative

PART USED: Leaf

TRADITIONAL USES: American Indians frequently used the delightfully aromatic leaves of sweetfern: they were crushed and inhaled to relieve headaches, burned in religious ceremonies for purification, and wet leaves were laid on fire-heated rocks to create steam. Strong leaf infusions were applied as a wash to relieve itching from poison ivy.[1]

CURRENT USES: Though commercially unavailable, sweetfern enjoys a regional reputation as a reliable folk remedy. Sweetfern is easy to identify and abundant. Infusions used to treat gas, nausea, abdominal bloating, and diarrhea. Use strong decoctions as a wash to dry up poison ivy rash, cool sunburn, and reduce inflammation from eruptive skin conditions such as acne. And it is used as an astringent douche for vaginal discharge or as a gargle to treat inflamed gums or sore throats.

CAUTIONS: None known.

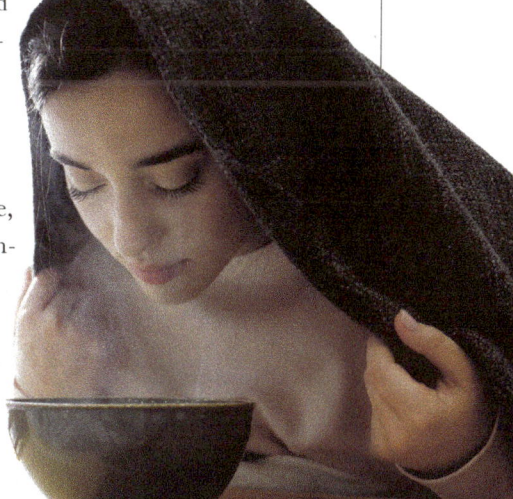

---

[1] Moerman, *Native American Ethnobotany*, 172

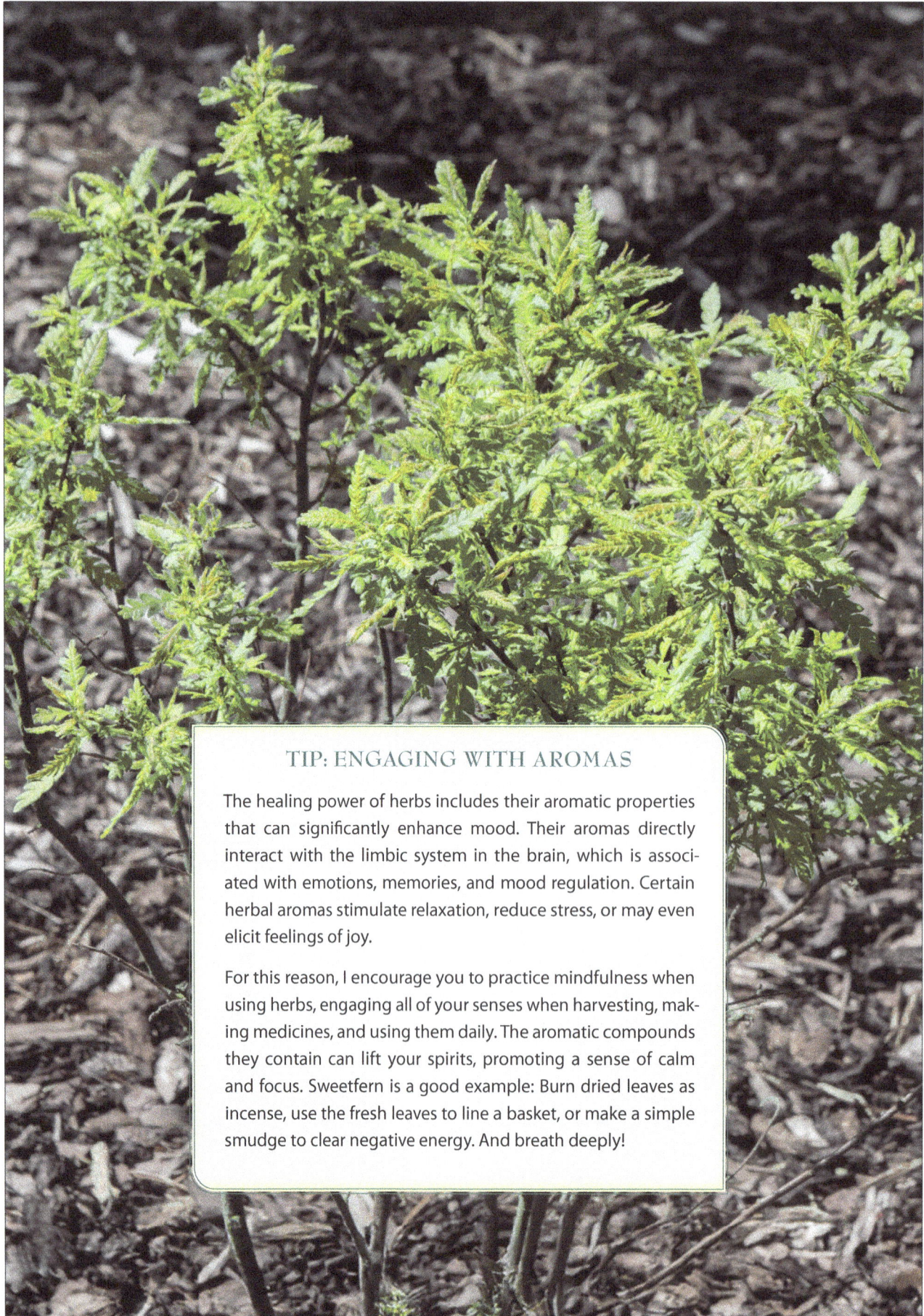

TIP: ENGAGING WITH AROMAS

The healing power of herbs includes their aromatic properties that can significantly enhance mood. Their aromas directly interact with the limbic system in the brain, which is associated with emotions, memories, and mood regulation. Certain herbal aromas stimulate relaxation, reduce stress, or may even elicit feelings of joy.

For this reason, I encourage you to practice mindfulness when using herbs, engaging all of your senses when harvesting, making medicines, and using them daily. The aromatic compounds they contain can lift your spirits, promoting a sense of calm and focus. Sweetfern is a good example: Burn dried leaves as incense, use the fresh leaves to line a basket, or make a simple smudge to clear negative energy. And breath deeply!

PREPARATIONS:

INFUSION: For internal use, make a cold infusion using one-half cup dried or one cup fresh chopped leaves with two cups of water. Use smaller leaves if possible and crush or crumble them first. Infuse for several hours. Strain and sweeten if desired.

DECOCTION: For external use, half a cup of dried or one cup of fresh leaves for two cups of water. Bring to a boil; cover and simmer for twenty minutes. Strain and let it cool before applying to affected area as often as needed.

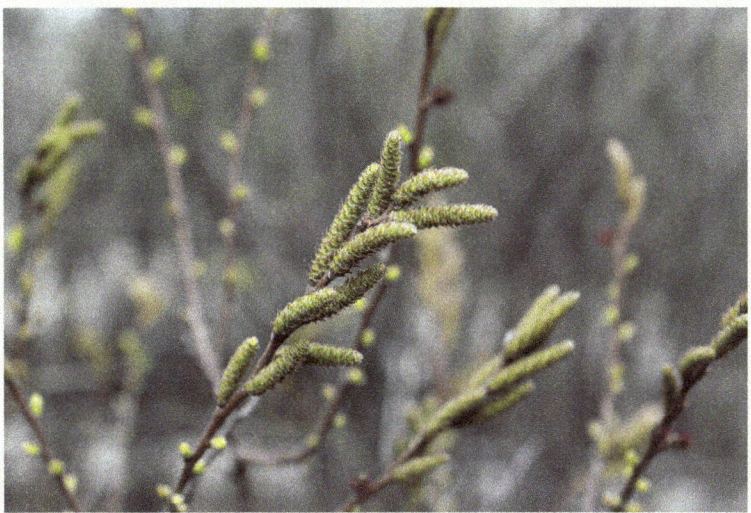

DOSAGES

Internal use of sweetfern is not recommended long term due to its astringency.

INFUSION: Drink one cup several times a day or as needed.

DECOCTION: Use the cool decoction as a skin wash, douche, or with a compress as often as needed. Gargle with the decoction several times daily to relieve sore throat or gum inflammation.

HARVESTING

Harvest leaves in the early summer before they are dried out from the heat. Larger leaves have strong astringent properties and are best used for topical preparations. Smaller, younger leaves contain less tannin and are best in teas. For the most potent aromatic properties, harvest sweetfern early in the day. Harvest several leaves from each plant, leaving most of the foliage. Sweetfern dries quickly, even in humid weather.

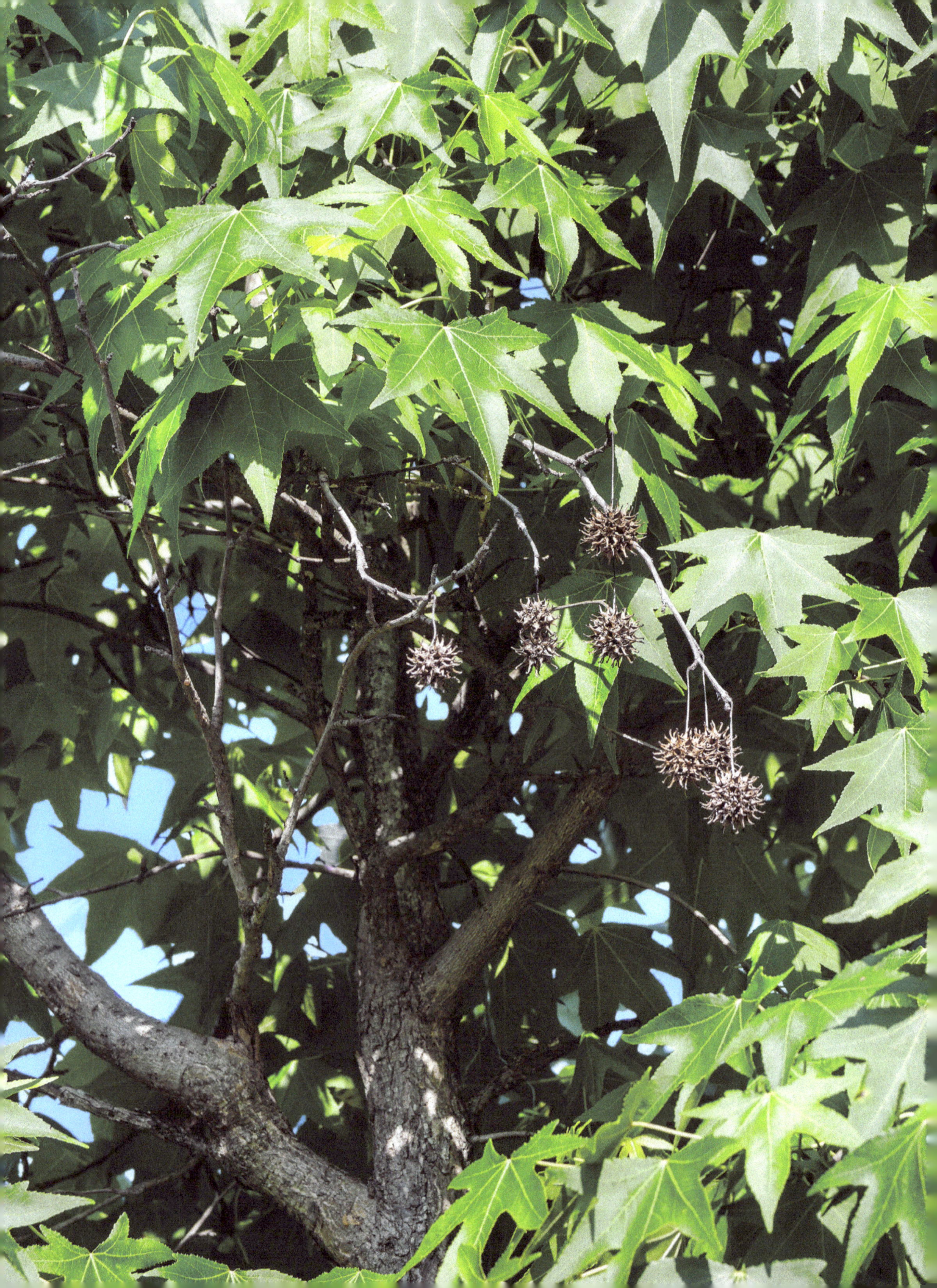

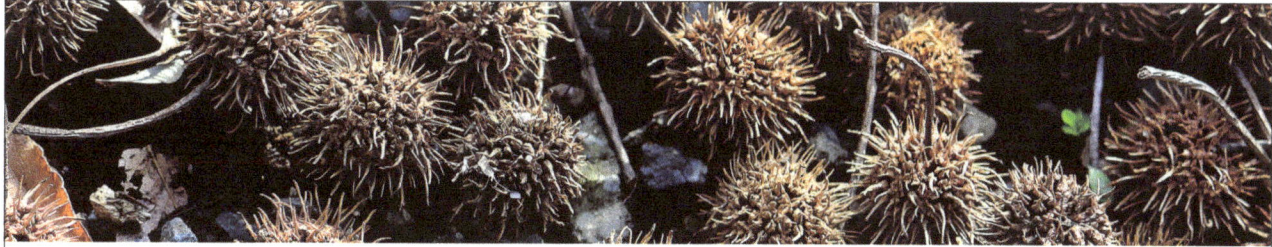

Sweetgum

COMMON NAME: Sweetgum

BOTANICAL NAME: *Liquidambar styraciflua*

FAMILY: *Hamamelidaceae* (Witch Hazel)

OTHER NAMES: Storax, Appalachian Frankincense

DESCRIPTION: Sweetgum is a large tree, sometimes over a hundred feet tall, with sharply palmate, star-shaped leaves with five to seven points. It has round fruits covered with short spikes encircling tube-like indentations, about one and a half inches in diameter; they are bright green in the spring and turn a dull brown as they ripen in the fall. After the leaves fall, the ripe fruits resemble ornaments dangling from the branches. Distinctive, wing-like ridges protrude from along the outermost sweetgum branches. You may notice brown sap oozing from the bark. In the Southern Appalachians, sweetgum is one of the first trees to change color in the fall. Crushed leaves have a piney scent.

HABITAT: Common. Frequently found along streams or in other wet areas.

KEY ACTIONS: Expectorant, anti-bacterial, anti-viral, astringent, sedative

PART USED: Sap (resin or gum), leaf, inner bark

TRADITIONAL USES: Among American Indians, sweetgum sap was used as an ingredient in skin preparations to treat itching, wounds, boils, and ulcers. The sap and inner bark were used to make an astringent tea for diarrhea and excessive menstrual bleeding. There is also some evidence that bark tea was used to relieve anxiety.[1]

---

[1] Moerman, *Native American Ethnobotany*, 309

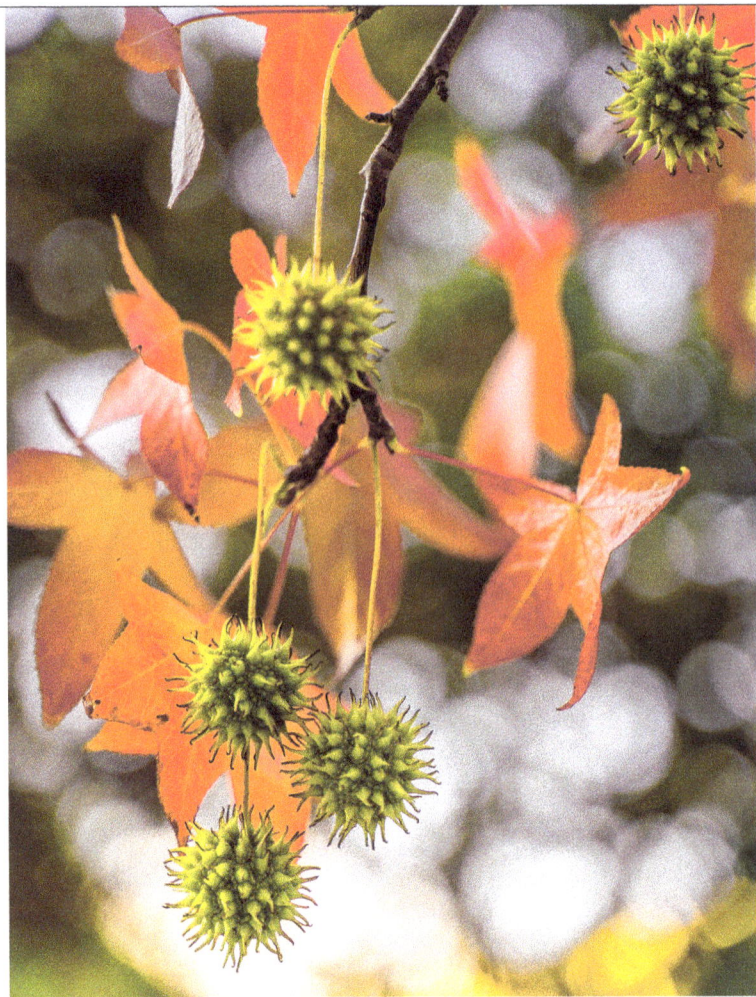

For generations, sweetgum sap has been a popular chewing gum.[2] Civil War doctors decocted the inner bark in milk to remedy diarrhea and dysentery. Alabama herbalist Tommie Bass burned sweetgum fruit and added the ash to lard or tallow to make a skin salve.[3]

CURRENT USES: Sweetgum sap is a valuable remedy to relieve respiratory congestion and chest colds, though it is rarely available on the commercial herb market. Sweetgum sap, leaf and bark are gentle expectorants used in cough syrups and tinctures. The sweetgum fruit or "gum balls" have strong anti-bacterial properties and may also be anti-viral. Small lumps of sap may be chewed to relieve sore throat pain and mouth (aphthous) ulcers. A decoction from the bark and leaf settles the stomach and reduces diarrhea. Traditionally, the bark was sometimes decocted in milk to stop diarrhea and soothe intestinal irritation. A salve is made with the tincture of the sap and used to heal wounds, eruptive skin conditions, persistent ulcers and itchy rashes.

CAUTIONS: None known.

---

[2] Porcher, *Resources of the Southern Fields and Forests*, 9

[3] Patton, *Tommie Bass: Herb Doctor of Shinbone Ridge*, 136

PREPARATIONS

DECOCTION: Use one-half cup of dried strips of the bark or one-fourth cup (about ten to fifteen fresh leaves, torn into pieces) to two cups of water. Bring to a boil, lower heat to a simmer, cover, and decoct for thirty minutes. Strain and sweeten if desired.

TINCTURE: Sap—Put two to three tablespoons of sap into a small jar and add enough grain alcohol to cover. Leave for two to three weeks; remember to shake daily. Strain through a fine mesh strainer.

Sweetgum fruit—Cut fresh green fruits in half. Add them to a jar and cover with grain alcohol. Leave for two to three weeks, shaking daily. Strain the tincture and discard the herb.

MILK TEA: Heat five or six fresh leaves, finely chopped, in one cup of milk over low heat for ten minutes, stirring often. Strain and sweeten with honey.

DOSAGES

All parts of sweetgum are used to treat acute symptoms. Frequent dosing for short periods is recommended for best results.

DECOCTION: Drink one-half cup of bark or leaf decoction twice to three times daily.

TINCTURE: Sap or fruit—One-fourth teaspoon tincture in a small amount of water two to three times daily.

MILK TEA: Drink one-half cup of warm tea every thirty minutes or as needed to relieve diarrhea.

SAP: Chew peanut-sized lumps of sweetgum sap to treat mouth sores or sore throat as needed.

HARVESTING: Sap—Collect from naturally occurring or intentional incisions in the bark. The fresh sap is honey-colored; it darkens as it ages. The best time to harvest sap is in the spring, when the weather is warm, just as the leaves emerge. However, you may collect the sap anytime it appears. Use a small hatchet or serious knife to scrape off a vertical strip of the bark about four inches long. Create a little trough by loosening the bark along the bottom edge of the exposed inner trunk. The sap oozes out slowly, and you should collect it every few days. Use a knife to scrape sap off the tree. If you get some bits of tree bark, that is fine, as they are also medicinal. Store sap in a small jar until you have enough to make a tincture (two to three tablespoons).

Bark—Collect bark in the spring. Look for sweetgum saplings, often abundant anywhere you find a mature tree. Trim smaller branches from the main trunk, strip the leaves and reserve for infusions. Use a sharp knife to scrape off the outer bark.

Leaf—Gather leaves in spring or early summer.

Sweetgum fruit—Collect while still green and process fresh. Use a small hatchet or cleaver to split fruits in half before processing.

SWEETGUM SALVE

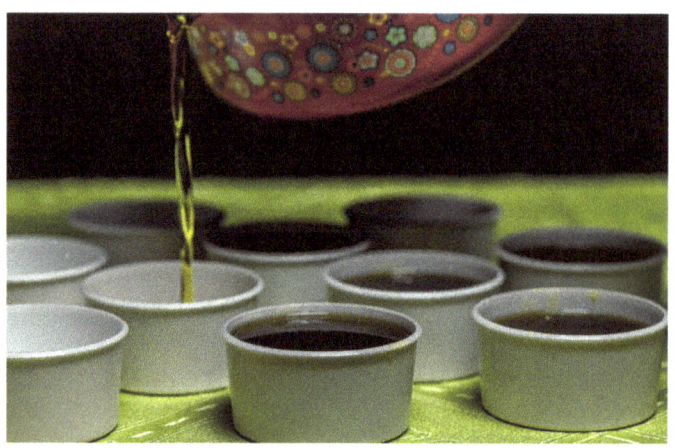

Like many medicinal resins, sweetgum sap is a potent anti-bacterial that may also have anti-viral properties. It effectively heals infected wounds, relieves itching and promotes healing. Several steps are required to make this salve, but it is a worthwhile task.

First, collect at least two to three tablespoons of sweetgum sap, following the directions under Harvesting. Then, make a simple tincture by steeping the sap in undiluted grain alcohol for several weeks; see Tincture directions above. Shake daily so that most of the sap dissolves in the alcohol. Strain out any lumps that remain.

Mix one part sap tincture with two parts olive oil in a small saucepan. Warm the mixture over low heat, stirring occasionally until all the alcohol has evaporated, leaving behind the sap-infused olive oil. As you stir the mixture, you will see the two liquids. Watch until all tincture has evaporated and only the oil remains. Use this oil to make a standard salve. Apply salve to the skin as needed.

TIP: HOW TO HARVEST BARK SUSTAINABLY

Bark is generally collected in early spring as the sap rises and leaves begin to emerge. During the growing season, positively identify the tree or shrub and mark it in some way. I like to use a small piece of survey tape or yarn and a note to myself in my foraging journal with the plant's name. Wild cherry bark, an exception to the spring harvesting rule, is best harvested in the fall, around the time of the first few frosts.

Technically, we use the tree or shrub's inner bark, which resembles a spongy pale green or whitish membrane inside the outer protective bark.

Good wildcrafting should follow wise pruning practices. Never harvest bark from a tree's trunk; instead, collect branches. This bark is just as potent, much easier to collect, and less stressful for the tree. There are two ways to cut branches: either flush with the tree (a thinning cut) or just after the first place leaves emerge on the branch (a heading cut). Before cutting, observe the tree. Are there branches crowded together? Trimming a few of these will benefit the others, allowing them to receive more sunlight. If it is a tall tree, choose lower branches within reach. As always, avoid harvesting more than you need or can use.

After harvesting the branches, you must strip the bark unless the branch is about the thickness of your thumb or smaller. Cut these thinner branches crosswise into thin slices. There is no need to strip the outer bark from these branches. When working with thicker branches, clip off any leaves and smaller branches, then cut the branch into manageable lengths, usually about one or two feet long. Hold a sharp, strong knife at an angle, insert it under the outer bark and slide it (with some effort) between the inner woody center and the outer bark. You may get long strips or smaller pieces; both are fine.

The bark, either in strips or slices, dries easily. Spread it on a screen for a few days in a well-ventilated place or dehydrate it for a few hours at a low temperature (120°). Thoroughly dried bark should be rigid and snap into pieces easily. Store in jars or process.

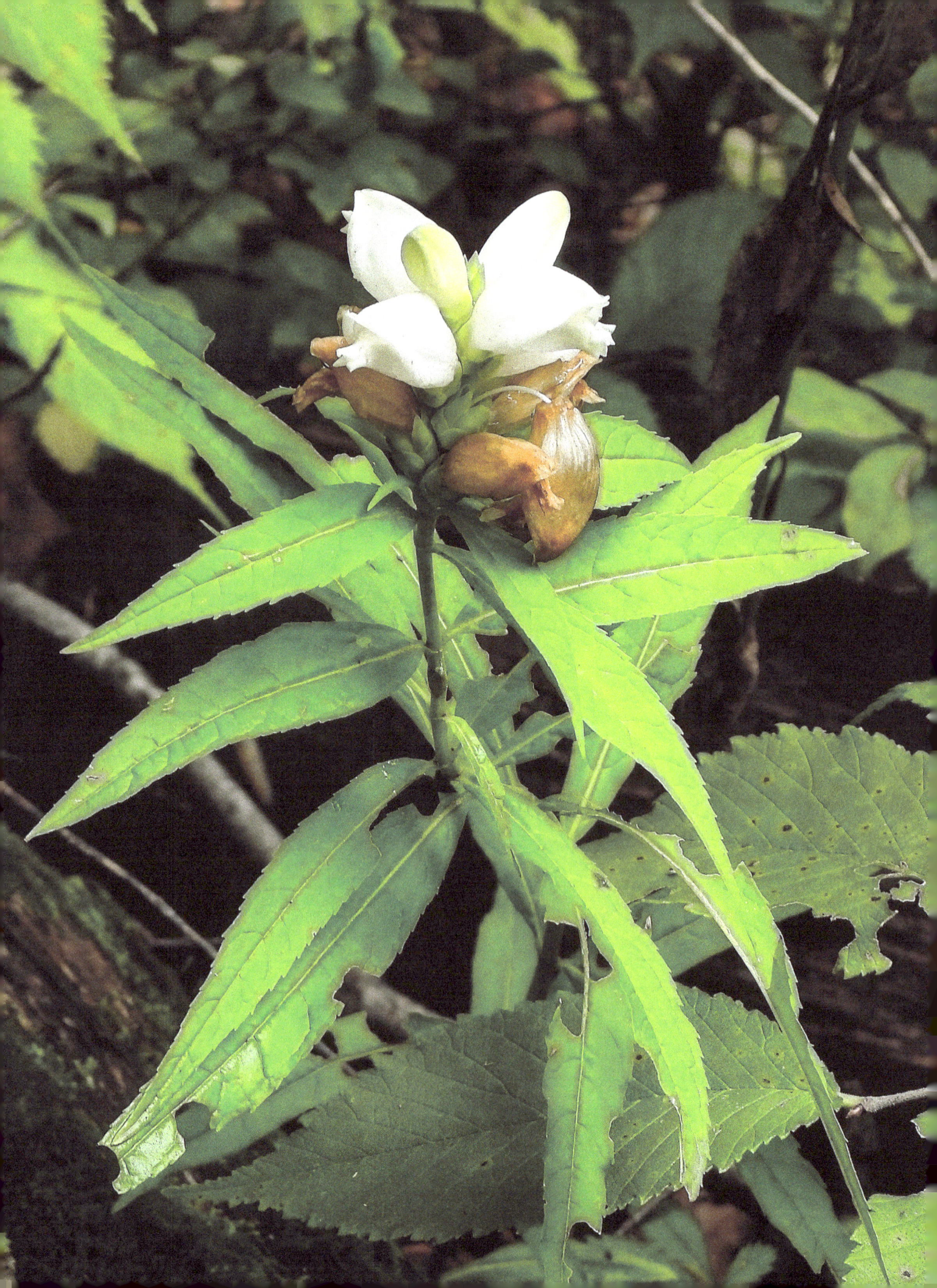

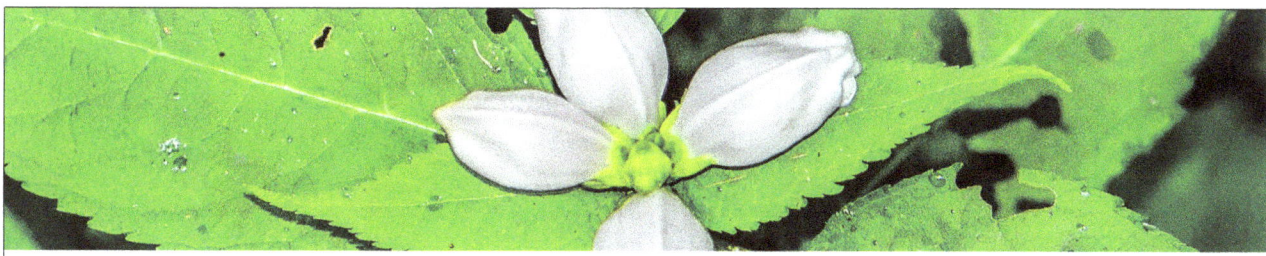

Turtlehead

COMMON NAME: Turtlehead

BOTANICAL NAME: *Chelone glabra, C. lyonii*

FAMILY: *Plantaginaceae* (Plaintain)

OTHER NAMES: White Turtlehead *(C. glabra)*, Pink Turtlehead *(C. lyonii)*, Balmony, Snakehead, Turtlebloom

DESCRIPTION: Turtlehead is an upright perennial, one to three feet tall, with opposite, lance-shaped, serrated leaves on short stems and a square stem. The distinctive two-lipped pale pink *(C. lyonii)* or white flowers *(C. glabra)* resemble a turtle's head and are clustered together in a terminal spike. *C. glabra* flowers are sometimes tinged with pink. Blooms from late summer into early autumn.

HABITAT: Turtlehead grows along creeks, ponds and branches. It prefers damp, shady areas, often with cardinal flowers *(Lobelia cardinalis)* and jewelweed nearby.

KEY ACTIONS: Hepatic, cholagogue, bitter stimulant, mild laxative, anti-inflammatory, anti-helminthic, cathartic

PART USED: Aerial (in flower)

TRADITIONAL USES: American Indians used both species of turtlehead to stimulate the appetite, as a mild laxative, and to expel parasites. Some tribes believed the herb had contraceptive properties.[1]

During the Civil War, turtlehead was used to treat "impure conditions of the blood" such as jaundice, hepatitis, and constipation. Small doses of infusion were used as a general digestive system tonic. Turtlehead was considered a specific remedy for indigestion, bloating, poor digestion, and constipation. Larger doses were used as a cathartic to expel parasites. The leaves were also used topically to heal ulcers and reduce breast inflammation, hemorrhoids, and other inflammatory skin conditions.

---

[1] Moerman, *Native American Ethnobotany*, 172

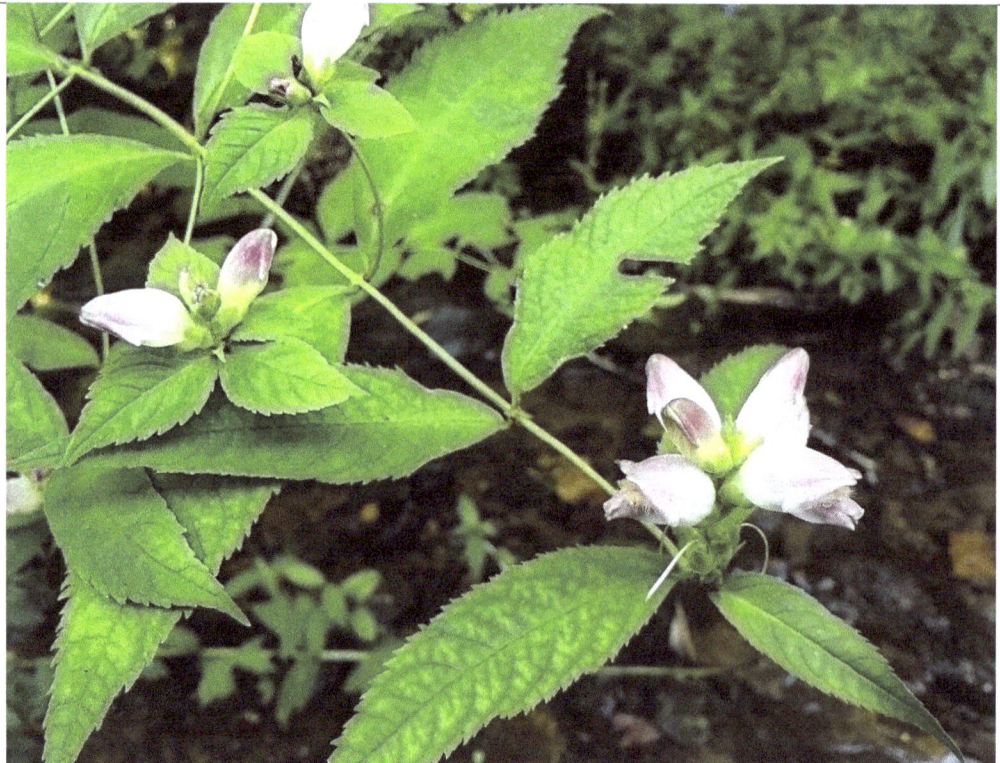

CURRENT USES: Turtlehead is an underused but effective remedy, though it is widely used in Europe, where it is known by the common name "balmony."

Turtlehead's primary action is on the liver. Use it for symptoms associated with liver congestion, including indigestion, gastric upset, bloating, constipation, and lethargy after meals. It is a specific remedy for relieving gallbladder inflammation and is often part of formulas for jaundice and hepatitis. Small doses act as an appetite stimulant and general digestive system tonic.

As a fresh leaf poultice, turtlehead relieves painful, inflamed skin and ulcers, boils, hemorrhoids and fibrocystic breasts. Dried or fresh leaves can be added to salves for astringency.

CAUTIONS: Avoid during pregnancy; it is not suitable for babies or children. Doses larger than those recommended may cause nausea, vomiting, or diarrhea.

PREPARATIONS

INFUSION: Use two teaspoons of dried or one tablespoon fresh turtlehead for each cup of water. Cover and infuse for twenty minutes. Strain.

TINCTURE: Fresh – 1:2, 95%. Dried – 1:5, 40%.

POULTICE: Prepare a poultice by pounding the fresh leaves in a mortar and pestle until juicy. If needed, add a small amount of water or aloe vera gel.

SALVE: Make a standard salve with infused turtlehead oil.

DOSAGES

To reap the full benefits of turtlehead on liver function, the bitter flavor must register on the tongue. Hold a small amount of tincture or infusion in your mouth for several seconds before swallowing. Do not add sweeteners. Large doses may have a laxative effect. Start with the lowest recommended dose and gradually increase as needed.

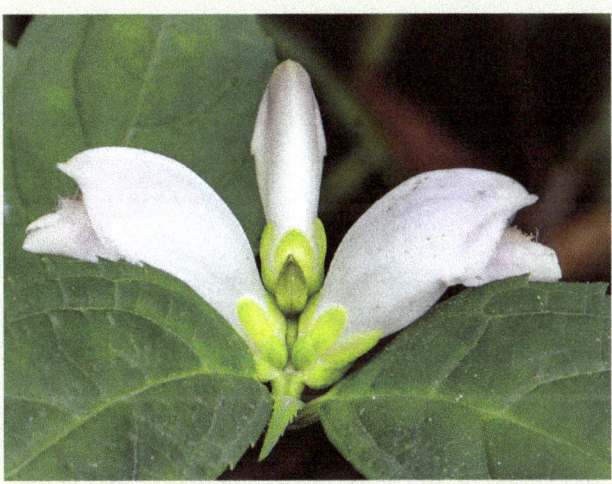

INFUSION: Drink one cup of warm infusion after meals to stimulate digestion. Drink one cup of infusion twice daily for one month or longer as a tonic.

TINCTURE: Take ten to thirty drops in warm water after meals to relieve indigestion and bloating. Take a half teaspoon two or three times a day for several months as a tonic.

POULTICE: Apply to inflamed skin as needed to relieve symptoms.

SALVE: Apply to inflamed skin as needed to relieve symptoms.

HARVESTING

Collect the aerial parts in flower in late summer.

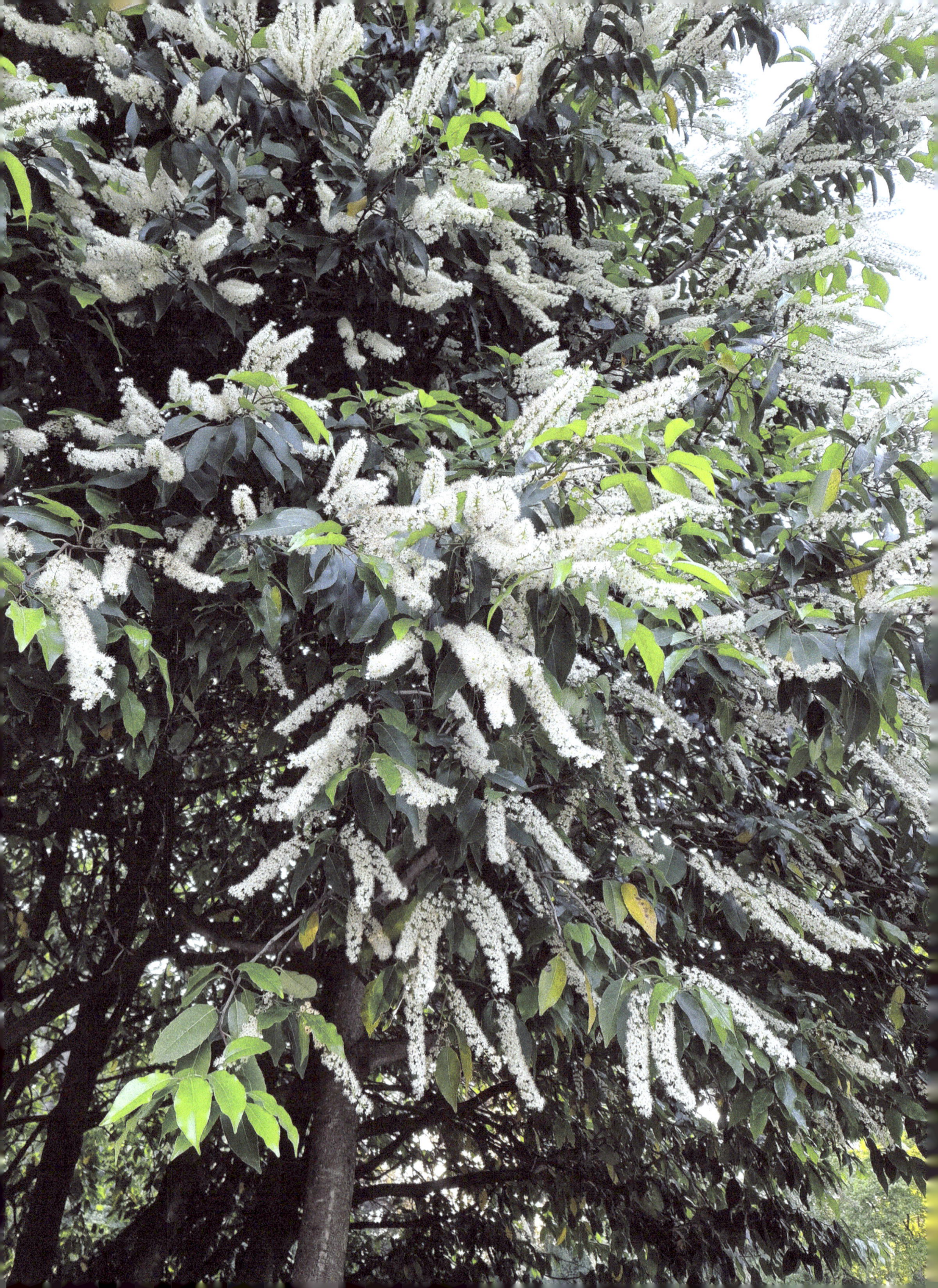

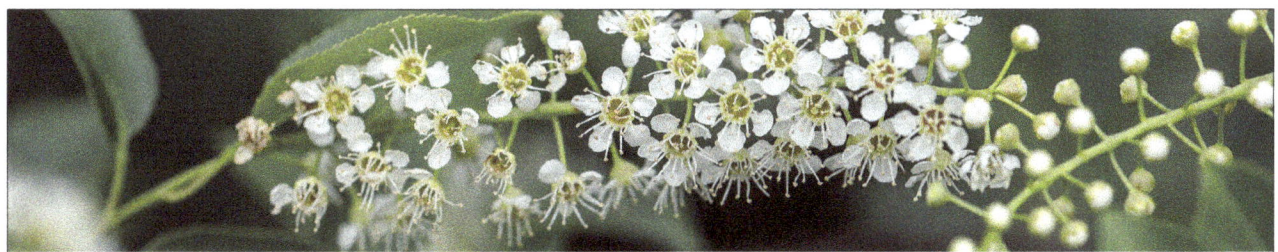

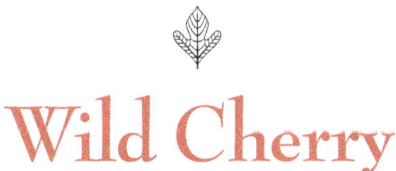

Wild Cherry

COMMON NAME: Wild Cherry

BOTANICAL NAME: *Prunus serotina*

FAMILY: *Rosaceae* (Rose)

OTHER NAMES: Black Cherry, Wild Black Cherry

RELATED SPECIES: Choke Cherry *(Prunus virginiana)*

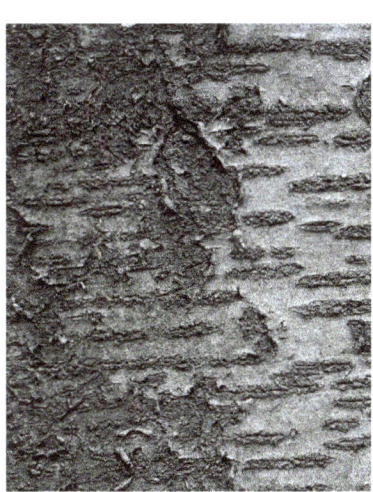

DESCRIPTION: Wild cherry is a twenty to forty-foot tall deciduous tree with distinctive dark shiny bark marked with horizontal raised lines or lenticels. Oval leaves with sharply toothed edges are smooth on top, while the undersides are pale with fine hair along the midrib. Clusters of small white flowers bloom between April and June in finger-sized racemes hanging down at the terminal end of the branches. In late summer, look for dark blue-black pea-sized cherries with large seeds. The bark has a distinctive bitter almond smell.

HABITAT: Common in wooded areas throughout the region.

KEY ACTIONS: Stimulating expectorant, antispasmodic, astringent, diaphoretic, sedative

PART USED: Bark, fruit

TRADITIONAL USES: Wild cherry bark is a time-honored remedy used by the Cherokee and others to relieve coughs, fevers, and sore throats. Wild cherry bark infusion was used as a uterine tonic and sedative at the onset of labor and as a wash for skin or eye irritation. Cooked berries were used to relieve acute diarrhea symptoms. Dried berries were mixed with nuts and animal fats to make pemmican, a winter food.

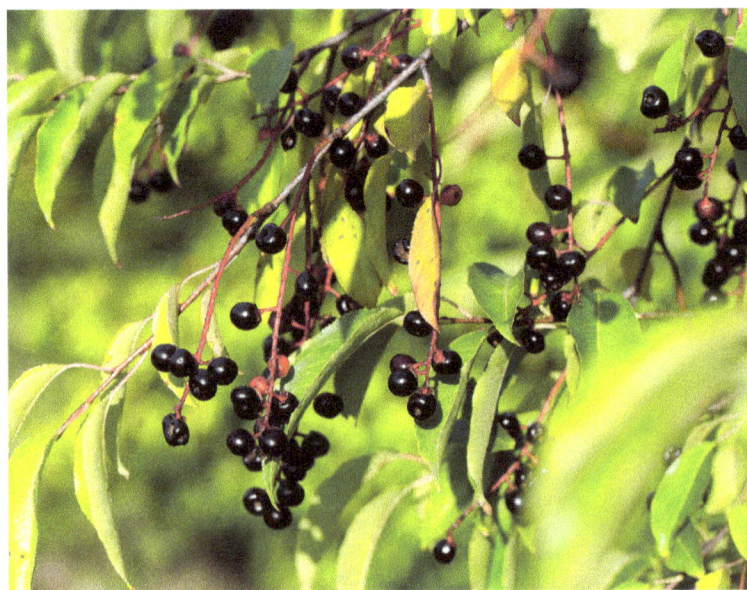

CURRENT USES: Wild cherry bark is a stimulating expectorant for lung congestion and coughs. It relieves inflammation of the lower respiratory system from colds, bronchitis, and pneumonia and reduces fevers. Wild cherry soothes irritation of the mucus membranes in the respiratory system, as well as the stomach and urinary tract. It is a mild sedative that can be used for heart palpitations, restlessness and insomnia. Use the decoction as a wash to soothe skin and eye irritation.

CAUTIONS: Avoid during pregnancy. Only suitable for short-term use. Wild cherry contains prussic acid, a toxic substance that gives its distinctive, almond-like fragrance, and is most concentrated in the leaves, which should never be used. Use fresh or completely dry cherry bark as medicine. The leaves and bark are also highly toxic to animals who should not be allowed to graze on wild cherry.

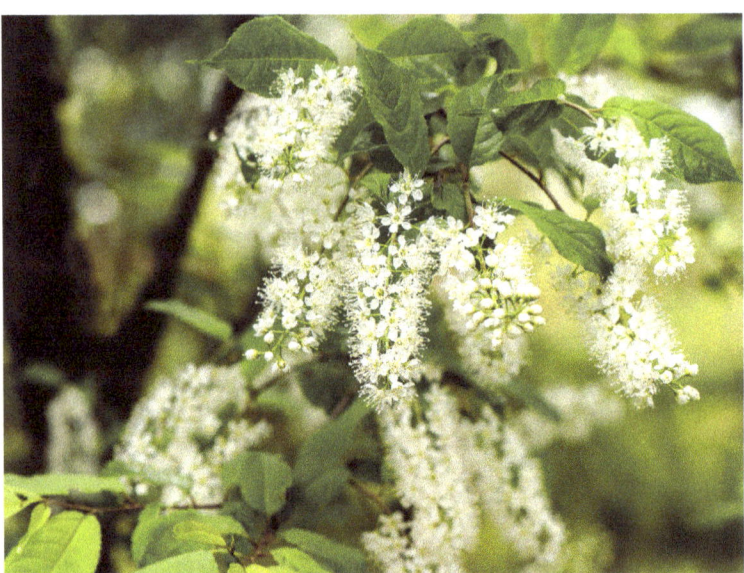

PREPARATIONS

Unlike most barks, wild cherry bark should be prepared as a cold infusion for internal use. The decoction is recommended as a wash for external use.

Traditionally, wild cherry bark is an essential ingredient of cough syrup, along with other lung herbs such as mullein *(Verbascum thapsus)*, to treat coughs and lung congestion. A simple brandy tincture may be used as a sedative and to improve digestion.

INFUSION: Use one-half ounce of dried bark for each pint of cool water. Chop bark into small pieces and steep for three to four hours. Strain.

DECOCTION: Use one teaspoon of dried bark for each cup of water. Bring to a boil; cover and simmer for fifteen minutes. Strain. (For external use only.)

DOSAGES

Wild cherry should never be used for more than two weeks due to potentially toxic compounds it contains; see Cautions.

INFUSION: Drink one cup three to four times daily or as needed.

DECOCTION: Use cool decoction as a wash for skin or eye irritation as needed.

HARVESTING

Wild cherry bark should be collected in the fall after the first frost. Look for younger trees and cut thicker branches. Use a knife to remove long strips of the bark and slice or chop the bark into small pieces. Pick berries when fully ripe, usually in late July. Cook the berries and strain out the seeds before using in wild foods recipes (with lots of sugar or other sweeteners). Wild cherry leaves are toxic.

WILD CHERRY COUGH SYRUP

Some variations of this syrup, inspired by a recipe used by Tommie Bass, should be in every home before winter arrives. Most herbs can be easily gathered fresh if you make this in August or September.

INGREDIENTS

Three ounces fresh or six ounces dried, chopped wild cherry bark
Three ounces fresh or six ounces dried, chopped sweetgum bark
Two bunches of ripe sumac berries stripped from the stem and rinsed
One ounce fresh or a half ounce dried bloodroot root
Two ounces fresh or four ounces dried black cohosh root
Four or five fresh sweetgum balls cut in half
Plus approximately four cups of chopped, fresh herbs: any combination of boneset, goldenrod, rabbit tobacco, spicebush leaf, sweetgum leaf and sumac leaf.

Put the sweetgum bark in a pot with two quarts of water; cover and simmer for twenty minutes. Remove from heat; add all other herbs. Use a spoon to push all the herbs down into the water. Steep overnight. In the morning, strain out the herbs and discard them.

Measure the strained mixture and place it in a clean pot. Bring to a boil; reduce heat to a simmer. Cook, uncovered, until the total volume is reduced by half (about one quart). While the decoction is still hot, stir in one pint of honey or to taste. Mix well. Pour into sterilized bottles and store in the refrigerator.

Take one to two tablespoons of syrup for coughs and sore throat. The syrup may be added to hot tea. Use as often as needed.

Note that this recipe is open to endless variation depending on the herbs you have on hand. Other herbs include coltsfoot *(Tussilago farfara)*, elderflowers, elderberries, elecampane *(Inula helenium)*, horehound *(Marrubium vulgare)*, mullein *(Verbascum thapsus)*, sage *(Salvia officinalis)*, and thyme *(Thymus vulgaris)*.

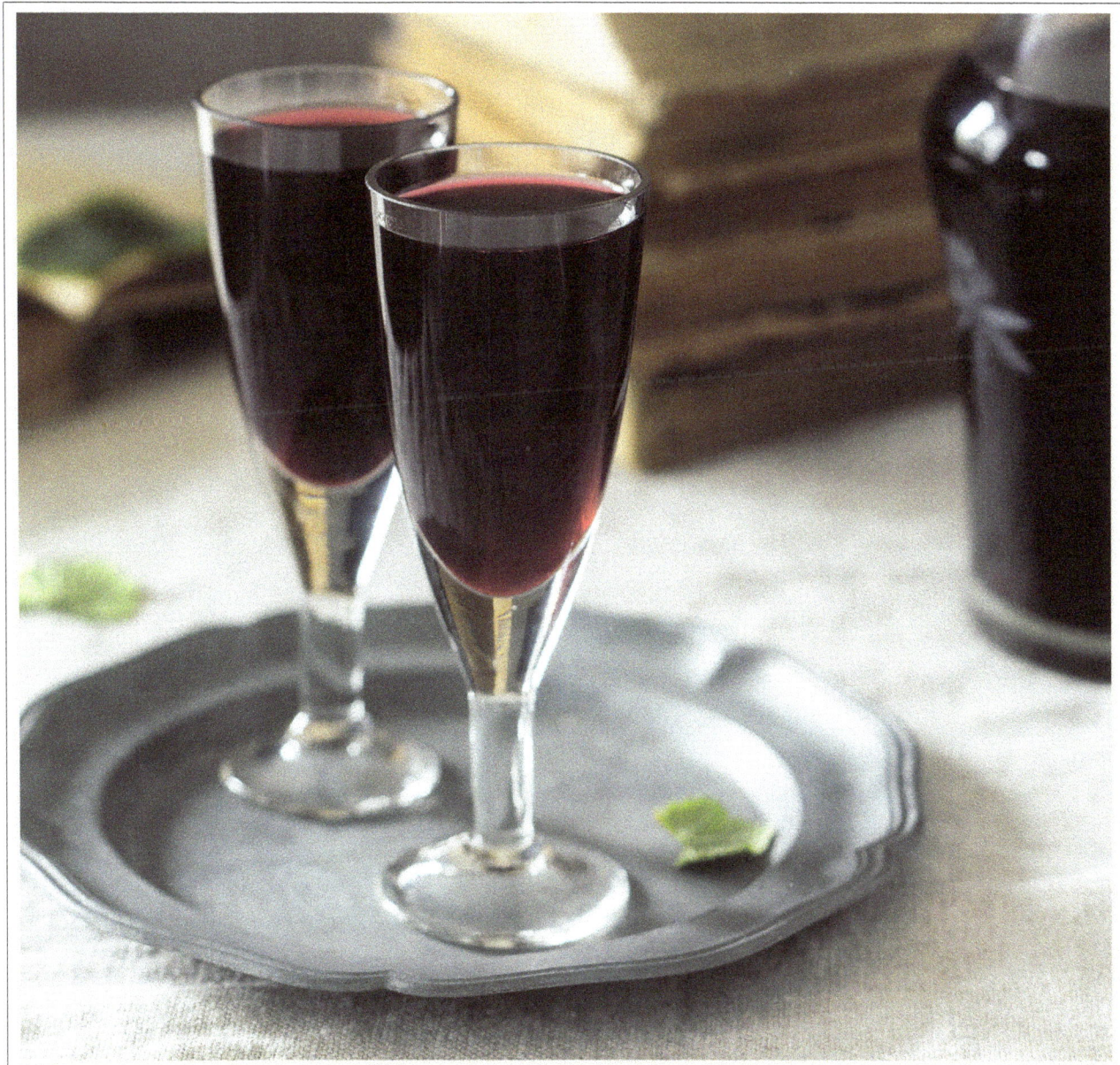

WILD CHERRY BRANDY

Fill half of a quart jar with ground or finely chopped dried cherry bark and add good-quality brandy to fill the jar. Cover and store in a cool, dark place for two weeks, shaking daily. Strain and discard the bark.

Take one teaspoon after meals to relieve digestive discomfort as a sedative or to relieve coughs.

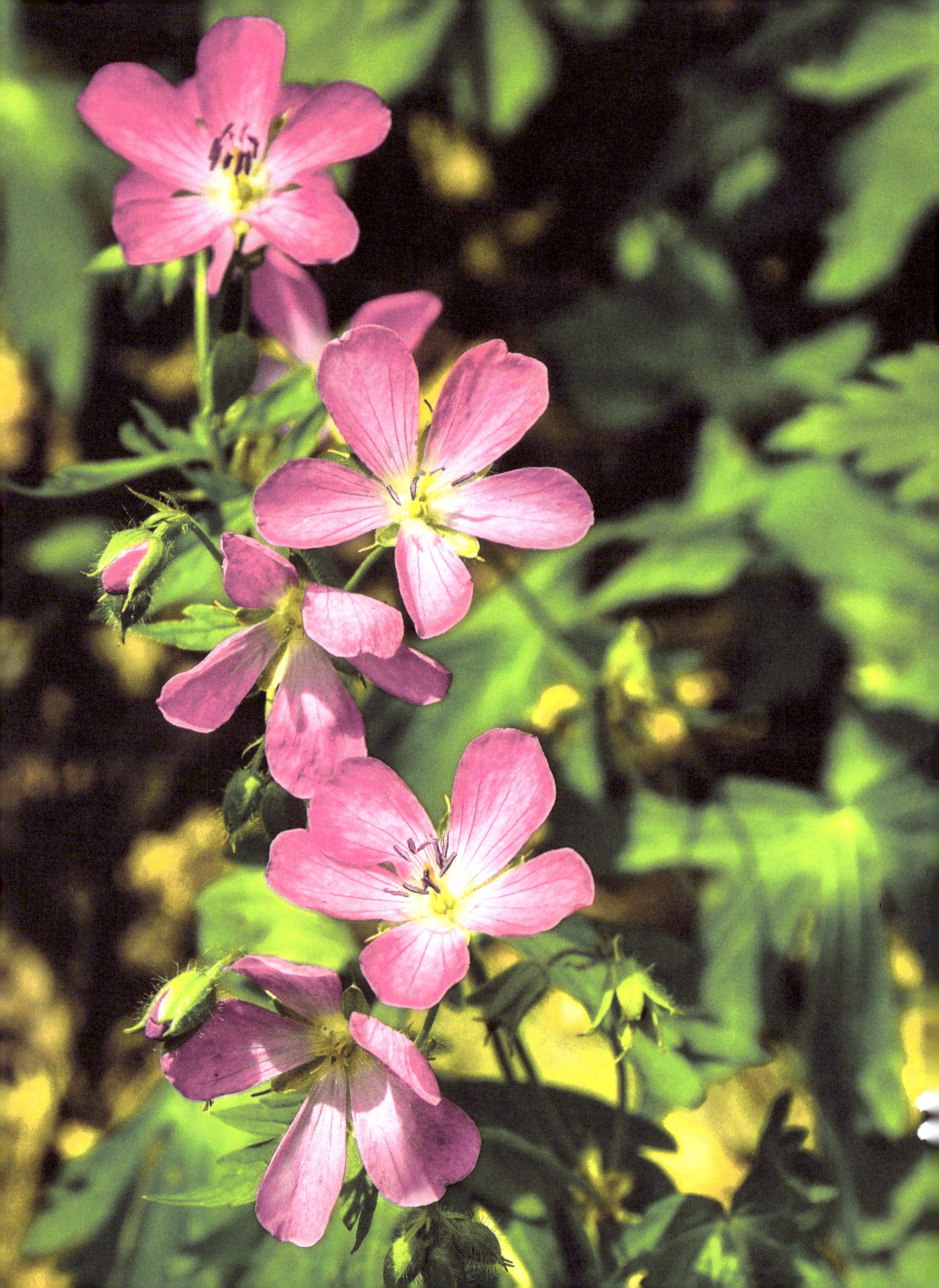

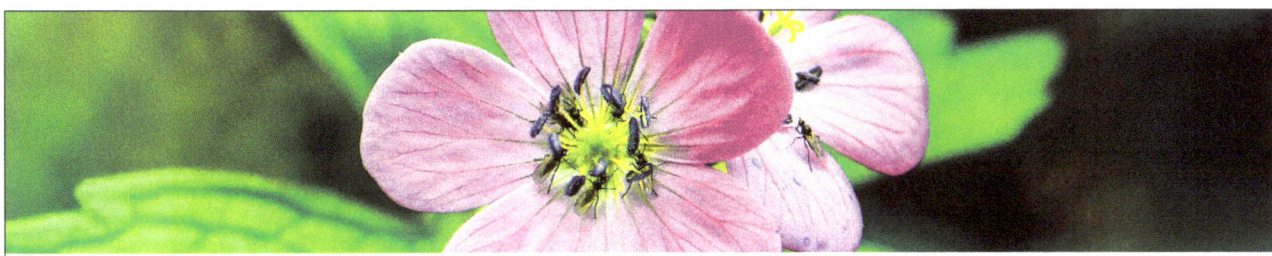

Wild Geranium

COMMON NAME: Wild Geranium

BOTANICAL NAME: *Geranium maculatum*

FAMILY: *Geraniaceae* (Geranium)

OTHER NAMES: Cranesbill, Alumroot, Stork's Bill, American Tormentil

RELATED SPECIES: Carolina Cranesbill *(G. carolinianum)*, Herb Robert *(G. robertianum)*

DESCRIPTION: Wild geranium is a gangly spring perennial, one to two feet tall. The leaves are deeply cleft into three to five segments with roughly-toothed edges at the tip. Delicate pinkish-purple flowers with five petals bloom between April and June. The seed-pod, shaped like a long pointed beak, resembles a crane's bill.

Carolina cranesbill *(G. carolinianum)* is a slightly smaller plant with intricately cut leaves and toothed margins. Flowers are pinkish-purple, with all the petals fused at the base to form a short tube. The entire plant has a pungent aroma.

A less common introduced European species, Herb Robert *(G. robertianum)* is used interchangeably with *G. maculatum*.

HABITAT: In moist areas in deep shade throughout the region. Often found with foam flower *(Tiarella cordifolia)*.

KEY ACTIONS: Astringent, styptic, anti-inflammatory

PART USED: Entire plant (root, leaf and flower)

TRADITIONAL USES: Wild geranium is a powerful, all-purpose astringent used by American Indians for excessive bleeding, debilitating diarrhea, and excessive discharges anywhere in the body. Typical uses include the treatment of thrush, canker sores, ulcers, vaginal discharge, diarrhea, and heavy menstrual bleeding.

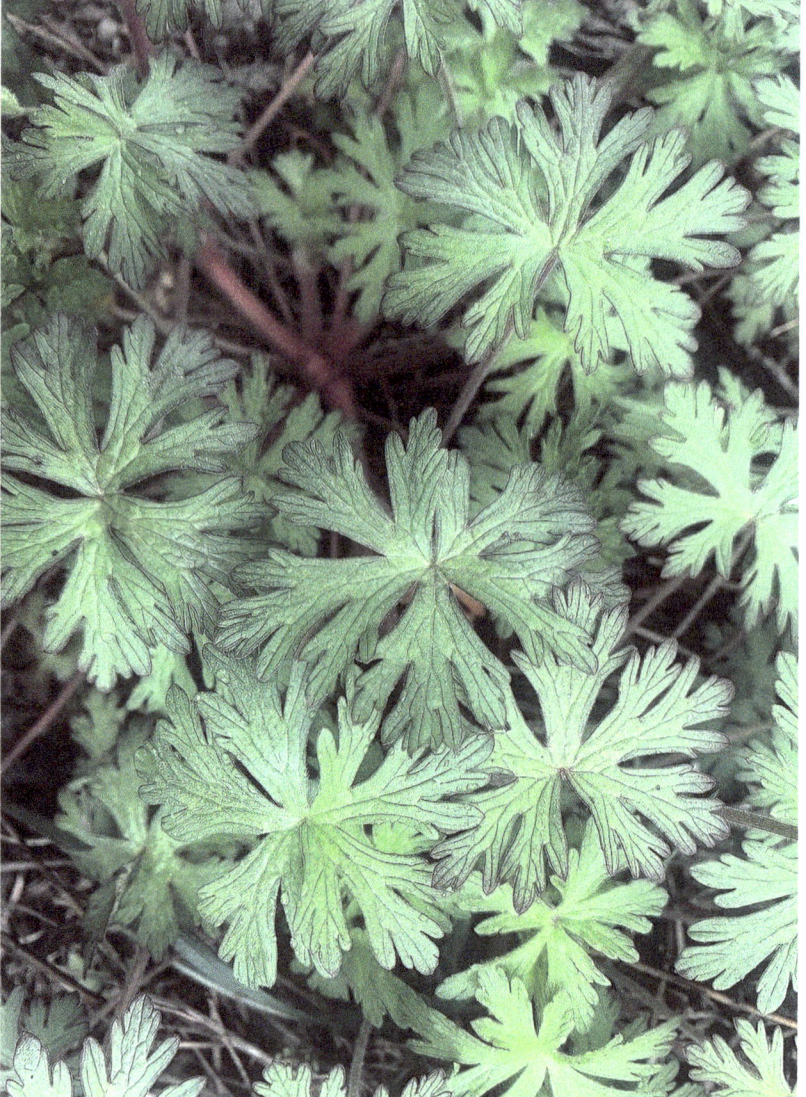

CURRENT USES: Wild geranium is a fast-acting astringent remedy that reduces excessive discharges without causing symptoms of dryness. It is used internally and externally. Use a tincture or tea internally to treat stomach ulcers, excessive diarrhea, and to reduce heavy menstrual flow. A warm beverage of fresh or dried plant simmered in milk soothes irritation in the digestive system. Gargle with the tea to heal canker sores, cold sores, thrush, and sore throat. An infusion used as a douche will reduce vaginal discharge, and as a wash to soothe skin inflammation and conjunctivitis. Add wild geranium to salves to shrink hemorrhoids or treat skin infections. The dried powdered herb placed directly into a wound stops bleeding.

CAUTIONS: None known.

PREPARATIONS

TINCTURE: Fresh – 1:2. Dried – 1:5, 40%.

INFUSION: Use one tablespoon of dried herb or two tablespoons of fresh herb, chopped or crushed, for each cup of water. Cover and steep for ten to fifteen minutes.

DECOCTION: Use one tablespoon dried or two tablespoons fresh herb for each cup of water. Bring to a boil; cover and simmer for ten to fifteen minutes. Strain.

MILK TEA: Like many other astringent herbs that treat severe diarrhea, wild geranium is often simmered in milk to make a fast-acting, soothing remedy. Use one tablespoon of dried herb or two tablespoons of fresh herb in one cup of milk. Slowly heat to a simmer; cook for fifteen minutes, stirring frequently. Strain and sweeten. Drink while warm.

INFUSED OIL/SALVE: Make a standard salve using infused oil of fresh wild geranium.

DOSAGES

Small, frequent doses of wild geranium are most effective in relieving acute symptoms.

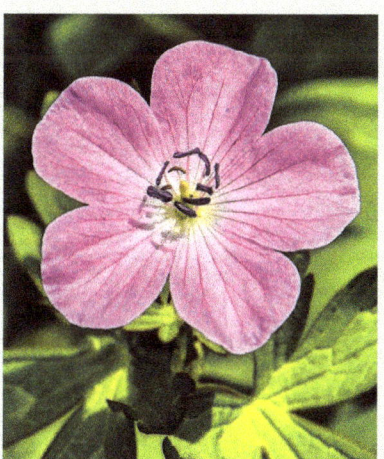

INFUSION/DECOCTION: Drink one cup every thirty minutes or as needed. Use as a gargle or skin wash three times a day.

TINCTURE: Take one half teaspoon every thirty minutes until symptoms improve.

MILK TEA: Drink one cup of warm tea every hour or as needed.

SALVE: Apply to the skin as often as needed.

HARVESTING

Collect the entire plant (root, leaf and flower) in the spring. The root is considered the most potent part of the plant, while the leaf is a slightly milder astringent; combine them for best results.

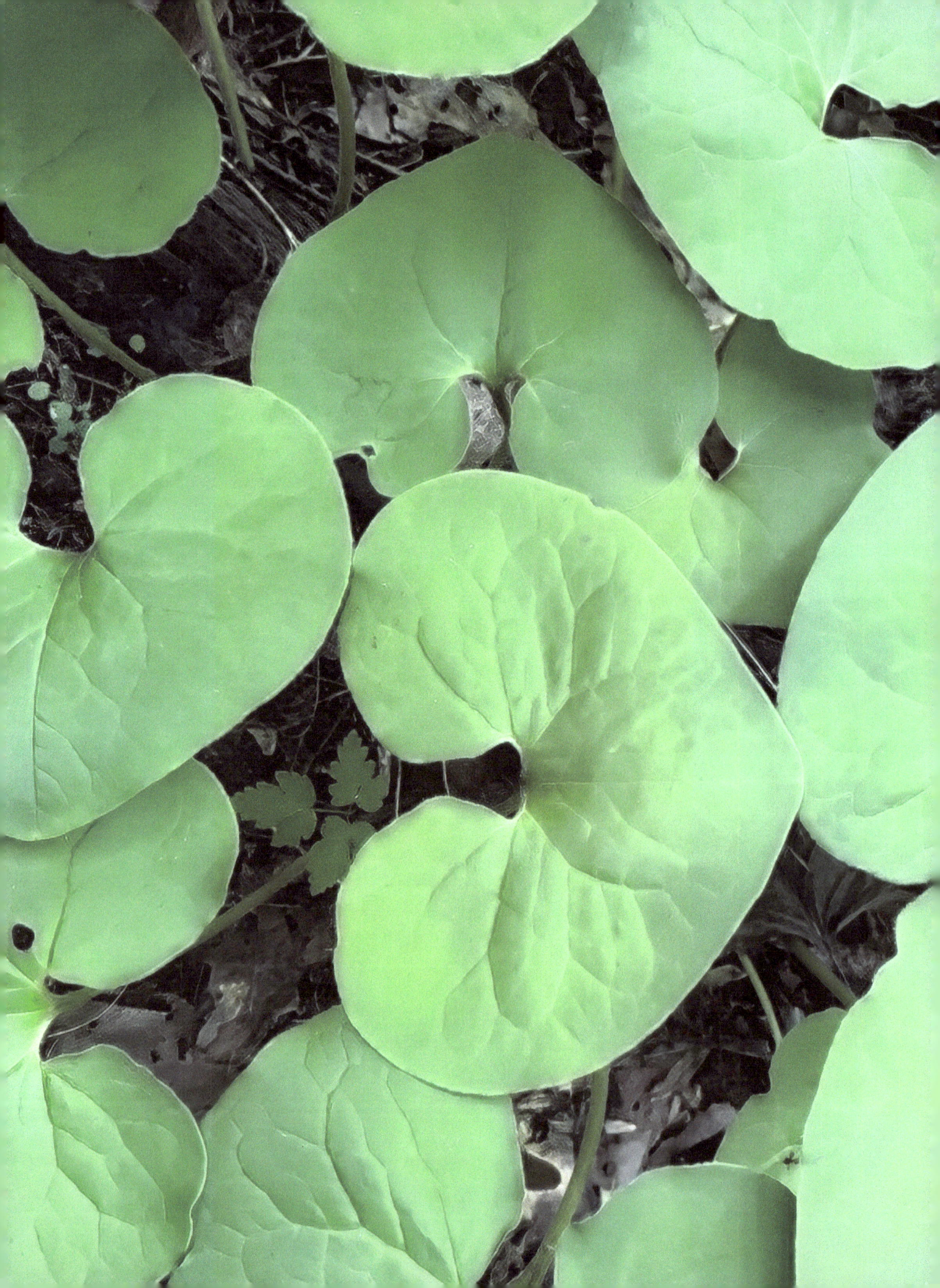

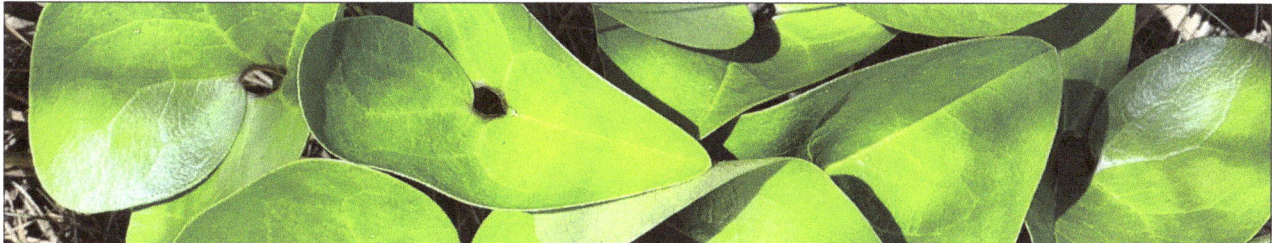

Wild Ginger

COMMON NAME: Wild Ginger

BOTANICAL NAME: *Asarum canadense*

FAMILY: *Aristolochiaceae* (Birthwort)

RELATED SPECIES: Little brown jug *(Hexastylis arifolia)*, heartleaf *(H. virginica)*

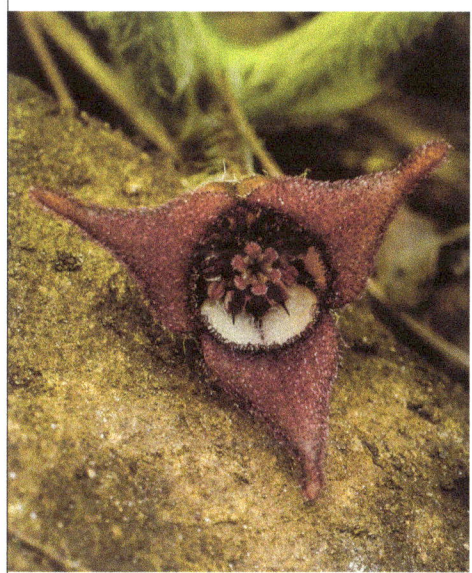

DESCRIPTION: Wild ginger is a low-growing deciduous perennial, four to five inches tall, with thick, glossy, kidney-shaped leaves, one on each stem. The single maroon-brown flower, about one inch long, with a white interior, blooms at the base of the leaves in April and May. The flower is shaped like an upright bell with three long pointed lobes.

Two other members of the Birthwort family go by the common name wild ginger and sometimes as little brown jug *(H. arifolia)* or heartleaf *(H. virginica)*, and both are evergreen. *H. arifolia* has glossy triangular leaves, and its flowers resemble a jug, while *H. virginica* flowers have a mottled maroon and white color, a darker interior and three prominent triangular lobes. *H. virginica* leaves are rounded and kidney-shaped, similar to those of *A. canadense*. Flowers of both species bloom at ground level at the base of the leaves. *H. arifolia* and *H. virginica* are used interchangeably with wild ginger.[1]

HABITAT: In the deep shade of deciduous forests.

KEY ACTIONS: Carminative, mild diaphoretic, antispasmodic

PART USED: Root and leaf

TRADITIONAL USES: The Cherokee used wild ginger tea internally to bring on delayed menses, relieve stomach and breast pain, lower fevers,

---

[1] Crellin and Philpott, *A Reference Guide to Medicinal Plants*, 452–453

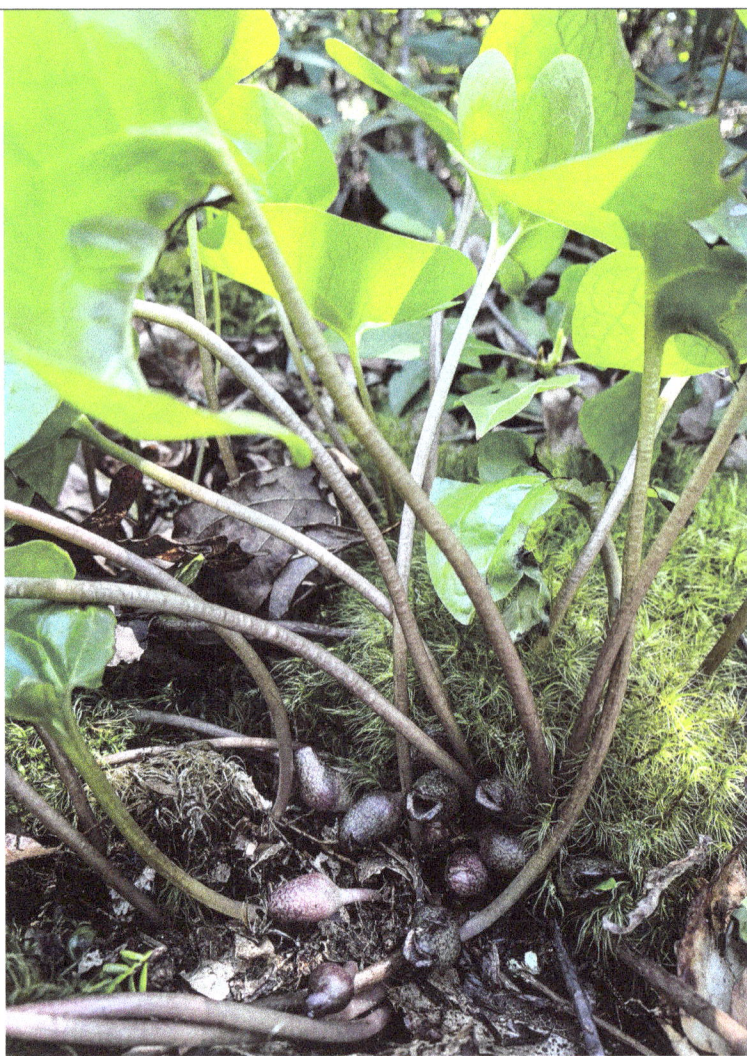

and soothe coughs. More potent preparations were used to induce vomiting and to expel worms. A poultice of the fresh leaves was applied to wounds. Dried root was used as a snuff to relieve headaches and sinus congestion.[2] Wild ginger has been used throughout the region as a mild folk remedy for stomach upset, colic, coughs, and delayed menses.

CURRENT USES: A gentle, aromatic remedy, wild ginger relieves nausea, soothes menstrual cramps, and reduces fevers or coughs. Its actions are milder than commercially grown tropical ginger *(Zingiber officinale)*.

CAUTIONS: Contraindicated in pregnancy and while nursing. Because wild ginger contains aristolochic acid, a compound that may damage the kidneys, it should not be used regularly or for longer than a week. Large or frequent doses may cause nausea.

---

[2] Moerman, *Native American Ethnobotany*, 105

PREPARATIONS

Both fresh and dried wild ginger can be used for any of these preparations.

INFUSION: Use one tablespoon of dried or two tablespoons of fresh herb for each cup of water. Cover and steep for fifteen minutes. Strain.

TINCTURE: Fresh – 1:2. Dried – 1:5, 50%.

DOSAGES

Tincture shold be prepared using the fresh root.

INFUSION: Drink a half cup of warm infusion every half-hour or as needed to relieve symptoms.

TINCTURE: Take a half teaspoon in a small amount of warm water every half-hour or as needed. For cramps, fever and coughs, add to hot tea to increase potency.

HARVESTING

Harvest *A. canadense* anytime in the summer when the leaves are present. *Hexastylis spp.*, an evergreen herb, can be harvested anytime.

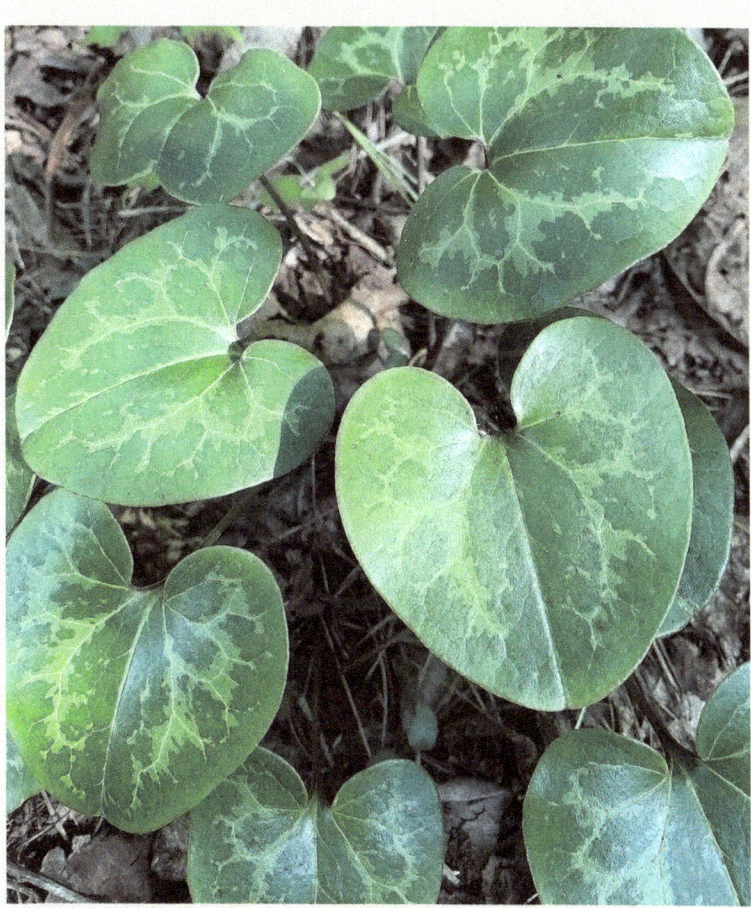

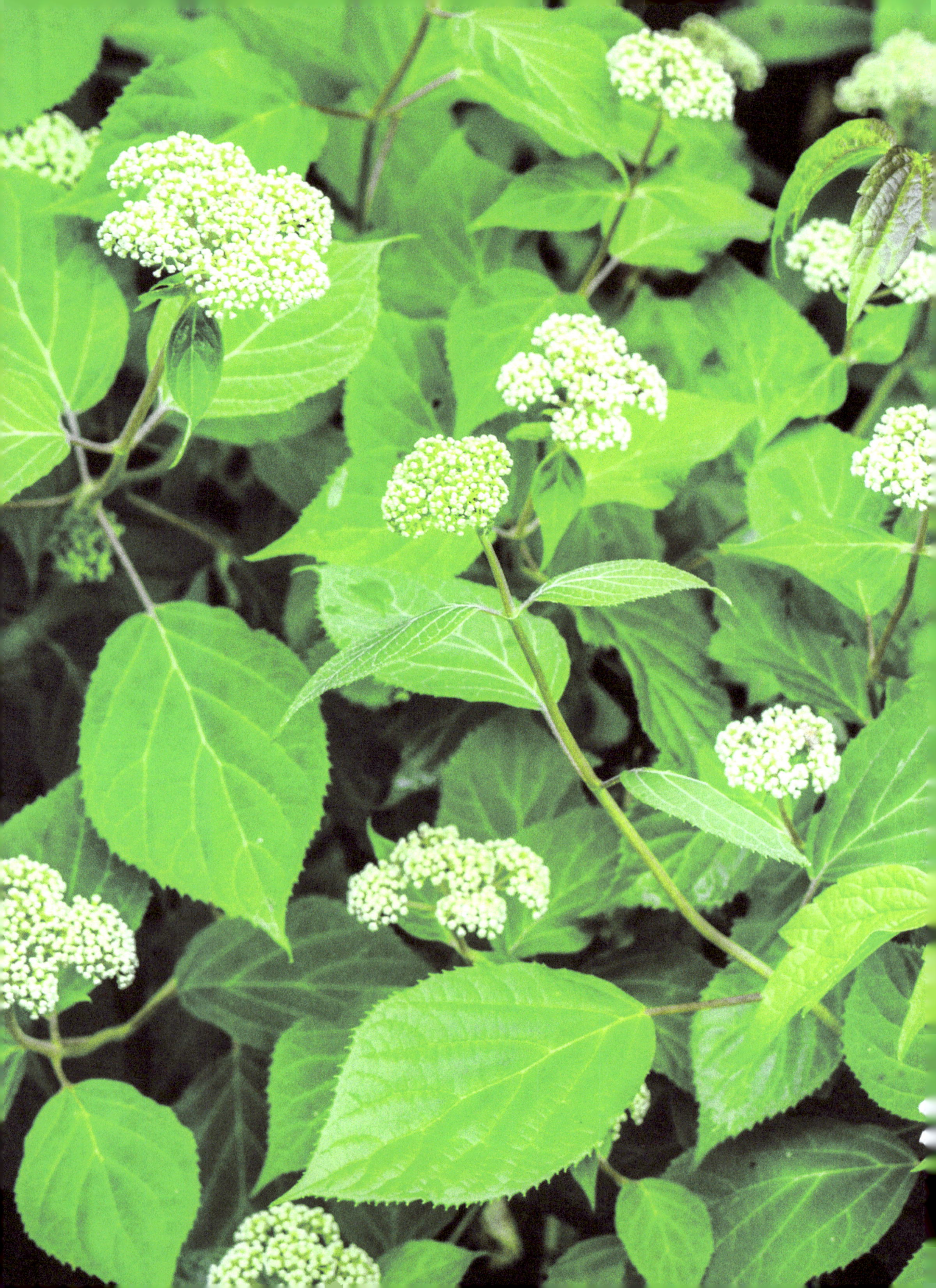

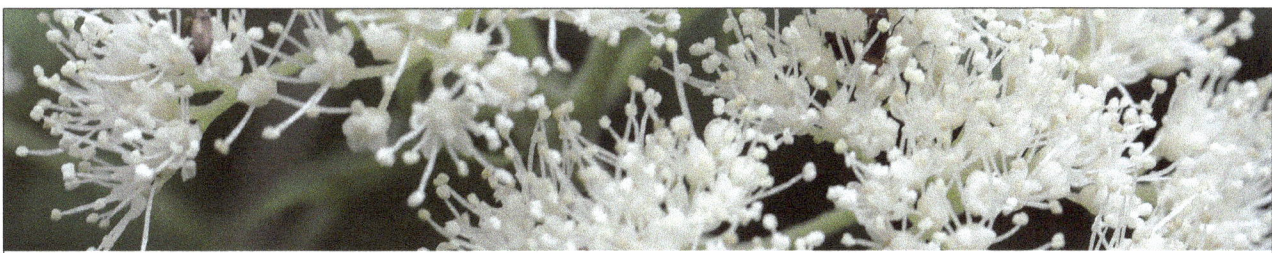

Wild Hydrangea

COMMON NAME: Wild Hydrangea

BOTANICAL NAME: *Hydrangea arborescens*

FAMILY: *Saxifragaceae* (Saxifrage)

RELATED SPECIES: Silver leaf hydrangea (*H. radiata*) and ashy hydrangea *(H. cinerea)*

OTHER NAMES: Sevenbark

DESCRIPTION: Wild hydrangea is a small round shrub, four to six feet tall, with oval leaves with sharply pointed tips and serrated edges. Tiny white flowers in round terminal clusters, with five petals and eight to ten prominent stamens, bloom between June and August. Irregularly lobed, sterile flowers with papery, white petals surround the actual flowers in the center; they attract pollinators to the otherwise unremarkable fertile flowers. The bark on older shrubs peals back in thin layers along the branches. Wild hydrangea is often challenging to differentiate from several native Viburnums with similar leaves and flowers. For positive identification, look closely at the stamens; wild hydrangea has eight to ten stamens, while Viburnum look-alikes have five.

HABITAT: Common understory shrub in deciduous forests.

KEY ACTIONS: Diuretic, anti-lithic, analgesic

PART USED: Root bark

TRADITIONAL USES: American Indians used wild hydrangea root bark as a poultice for burns, ulcers, and rashes. The bark was chewed to relieve high blood pressure and stomach problems. In folk medicine, wild hydrangea was used extensively to treat kidney symptoms, including blood in the urine, kidney stones and kidney infections. Herbalist Tommie Bass relied heavily on wild hydrangea to treat gallbladder problems, kidney stones, rheumatic inflammation, gout, and liver congestion.[1]

---

[1] Crellin and Philpott, *A Reference Guide to Medicinal Plants*, 392

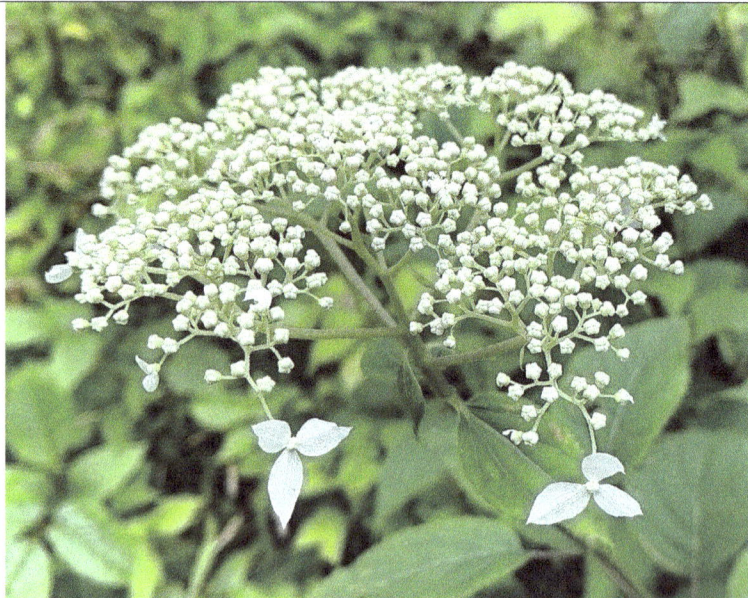

CURRENT USES: Wild hydrangea effectively reduces acute inflammatory and pain caused by interstitial cystitis or an enlarged prostate gland. It also relieves pain associated with acute urinary tract infections, including lower back pain and painful urination. As a daily tonic, wild hydrangea may help eliminate and prevent kidney stones. For an effective formula to help eliminate and prevent kidney stones, combine wild hydrangea with Joe Pye weed and pipsissewa. See Cautions before using wild hydrangea for any of these symptoms.

CAUTIONS: Some acute symptoms listed above may indicate a life-threatening kidney infection, especially if accompanied by sharp pain in the lower back and fever. If in doubt, immediately seek an accurate diagnosis from a medical professional trained to diagnose kidney infections before attempting to treat these symptoms with herbs.

PREPARATIONS

DECOCTION: Add two tablespoons fresh or one tablespoon of dried root to each cup of water. Bring to a boil, cover, and simmer for twenty minutes. Strain.

TINCTURE: Fresh – 1:2, 95%. Dried – 1:5, 50%.

DOSAGE

DECOCTION: Drink a cup of warm decoction every two to three hours or as needed.

TINCTURE: Take one-half teaspoon of tincture in a small amount of water three times daily. Increase the dosage by up to two teaspoons of tincture per dose if needed to relieve pain and reduce inflammation.

HARVESTING

Dig the roots in late summer or early autumn after the flowers have bloomed. Wash the roots and remove the outer bark by scraping it with a sharp knife and immediately cut into small pieces.

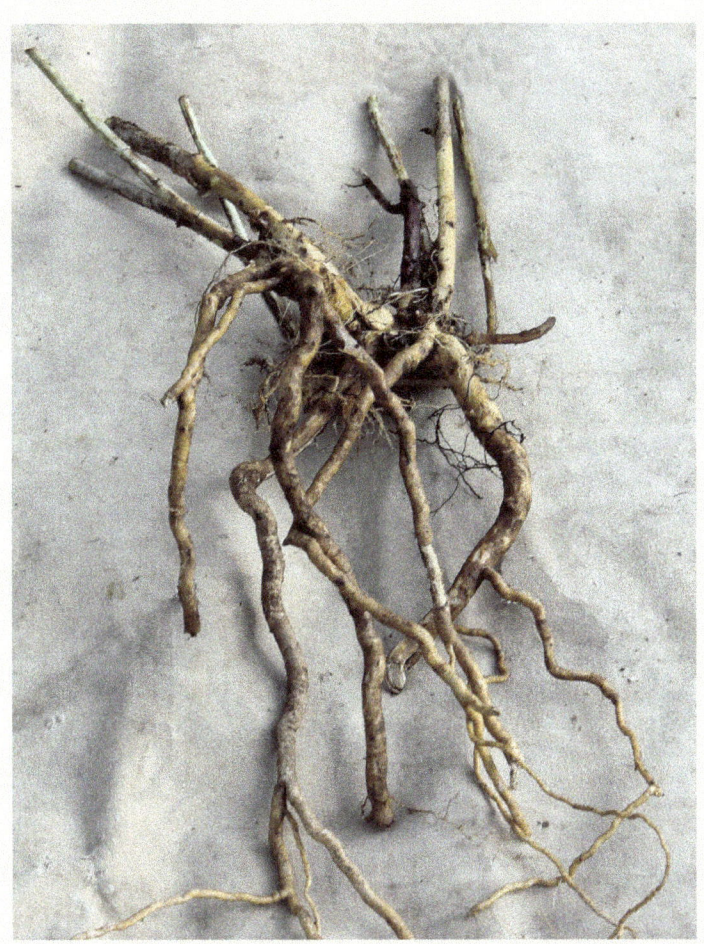

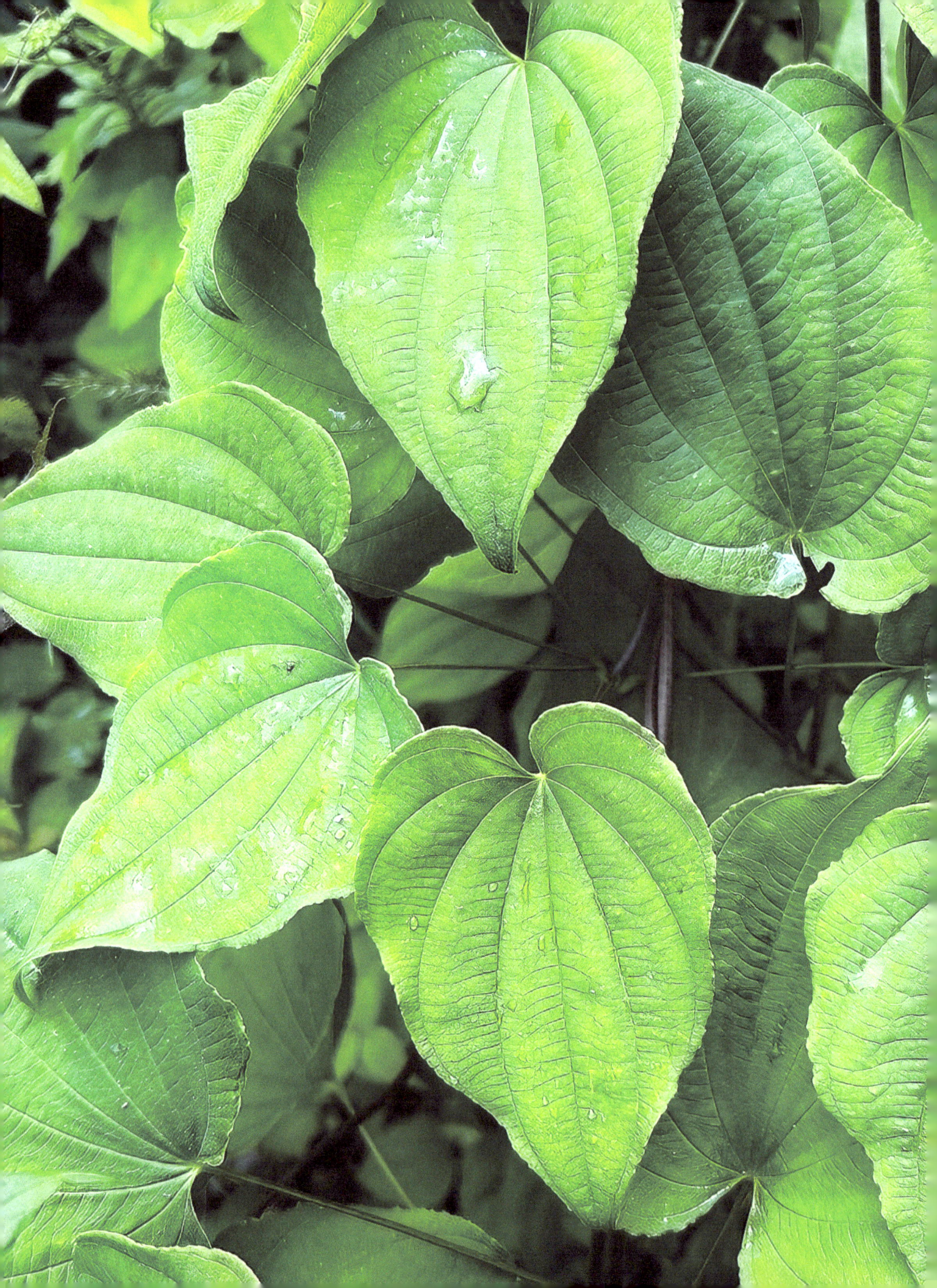

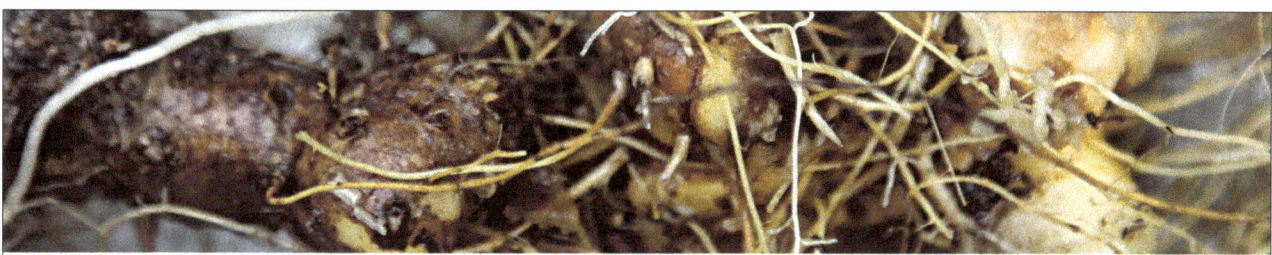

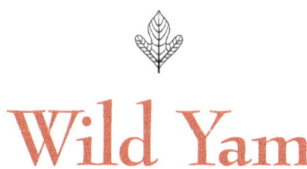

Wild Yam

COMMON NAME: Wild Yam

BOTANICAL NAME: *Dioscorea villosa*

FAMILY: *Dioscoreaceae* (Yam)

OTHER NAMES: Colic Root, Rheumatism Root

RELATED SPECIES: *D. quaternata*

DESCRIPTION: Wild yam is a non-woody, perennial vine five to ten feet long. The heart-shaped leaves have distinctive, parallel veins that run evenly from the base to the tip. Small, inconspicuous, green flowers bloom on female plants from May to July, producing dangling triangular seed capsules. The young wild yam plant is upright, with the first set of leaves arranged in whorls of four to eight. After this, leaves are alternate along the length of the vine.

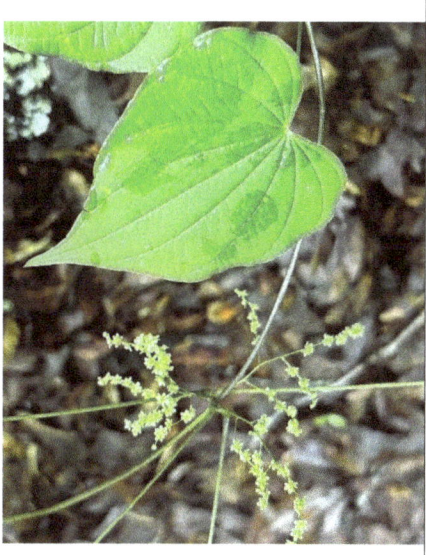

HABITAT: Common in shady, damp areas in deciduous woods.

KEY ACTIONS: Anti-inflammatory, antispasmodic

PART USED: Root

TRADITIONAL USES: American Indians used wild yam to relieve labor pains. It has a long history in traditional folk medicine for colic, intestinal cramps, morning sickness and arthritic and rheumatic pain.

CURRENT USES: Wild yam is a fast-acting remedy that relieves painful spasms and cramps and reduces inflammation. Small, frequent doses relieve intestinal spasms related to Irritable Bowel Syndrome, diverticulitis, and colic. It is a specific remedy for relieving menstrual cramps. Wild yam also reduces inflammation to alleviate pain caused by rheumatoid or osteoarthritis. I have also used it for traumatic injuries with extensive bruising and swelling. In pregnancy, wild yam may ease morning sickness and relax uterine spasms that could lead to miscarriage.

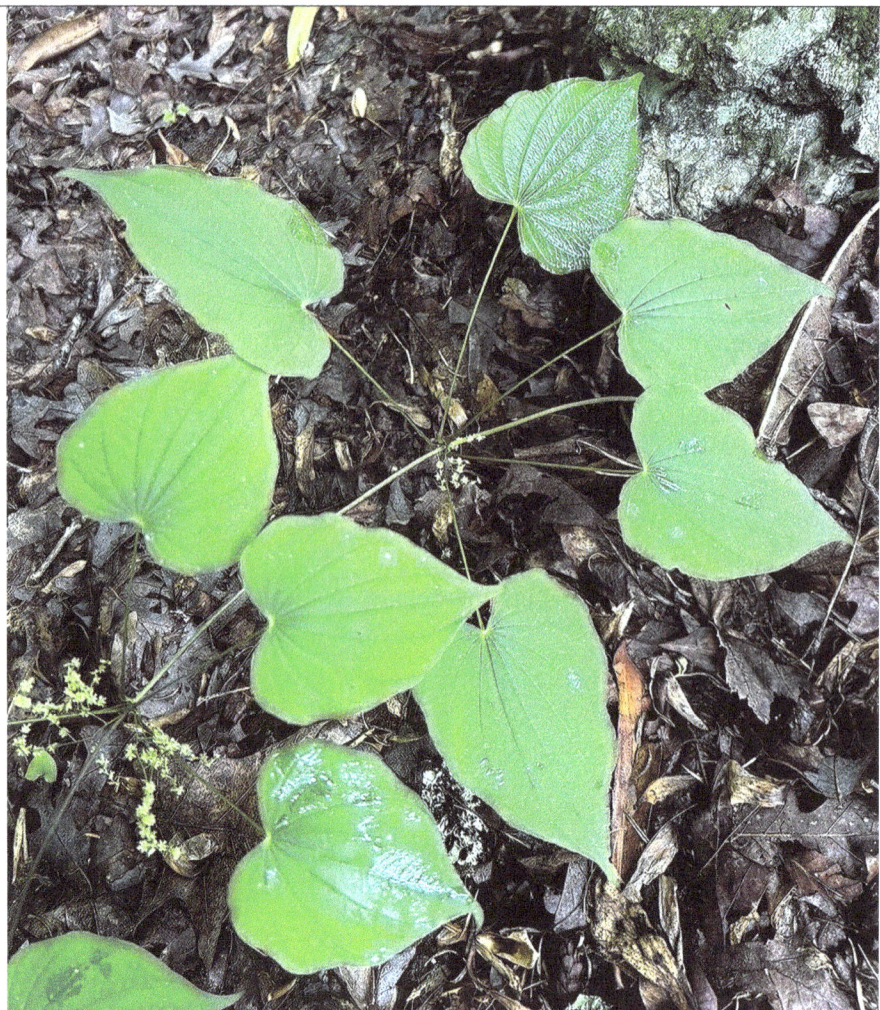

CAUTIONS: None known. The root contains diosgenin and other phytohormones that were synthesized to create the first birth control pill and are frequently found in hormonal creams used to balance progesterone and estrogen levels in perimenopausal and menopausal women. Wild yam roots have no birth control properties.

PREPARATIONS

All wild yam preparations are made with dried root.

DECOCTION: Use one tablespoon of dried root for each cup of water. Bring water to a boil; cover and simmer for fifteen to twenty minutes. Strain.

TINCTURE: Dried root – 1:5, 50%.

DOSAGES

Wild yam requires frequent dosing every fifteen to thirty minutes until the intensity of the symptoms decreases. As symptoms improve, the time between doses can be increased to control spasms and cramping.

DECOCTION: Drink half a cup of decoction every thirty minutes or as needed to relieve symptoms. If you don't see improvement after two or three doses, increase the dosage to one cup every fifteen minutes.

TINCTURE: Take one-half teaspoon every thirty minutes or as needed to relieve symptoms. If you don't see improvement after two or three doses, increase the dosage to one teaspoon.

HARVESTING

Dig roots in the early fall. Clean and immediately cut roots into small pieces using strong clippers or a small hatchet. Once wild yam root dries, it is as hard as a stone and almost impossible to cut or grind, so don't wait to process the fresh root.

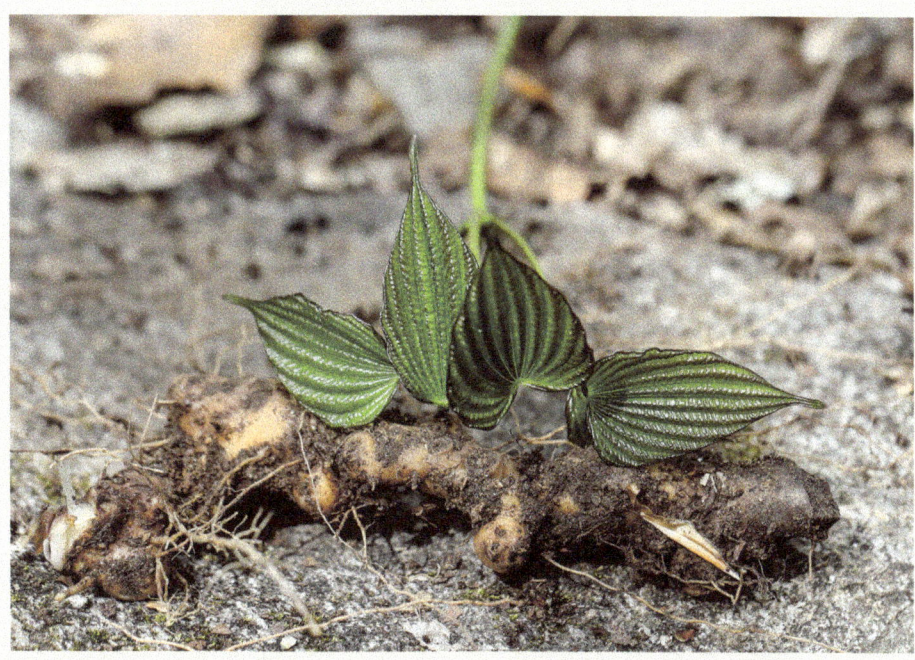

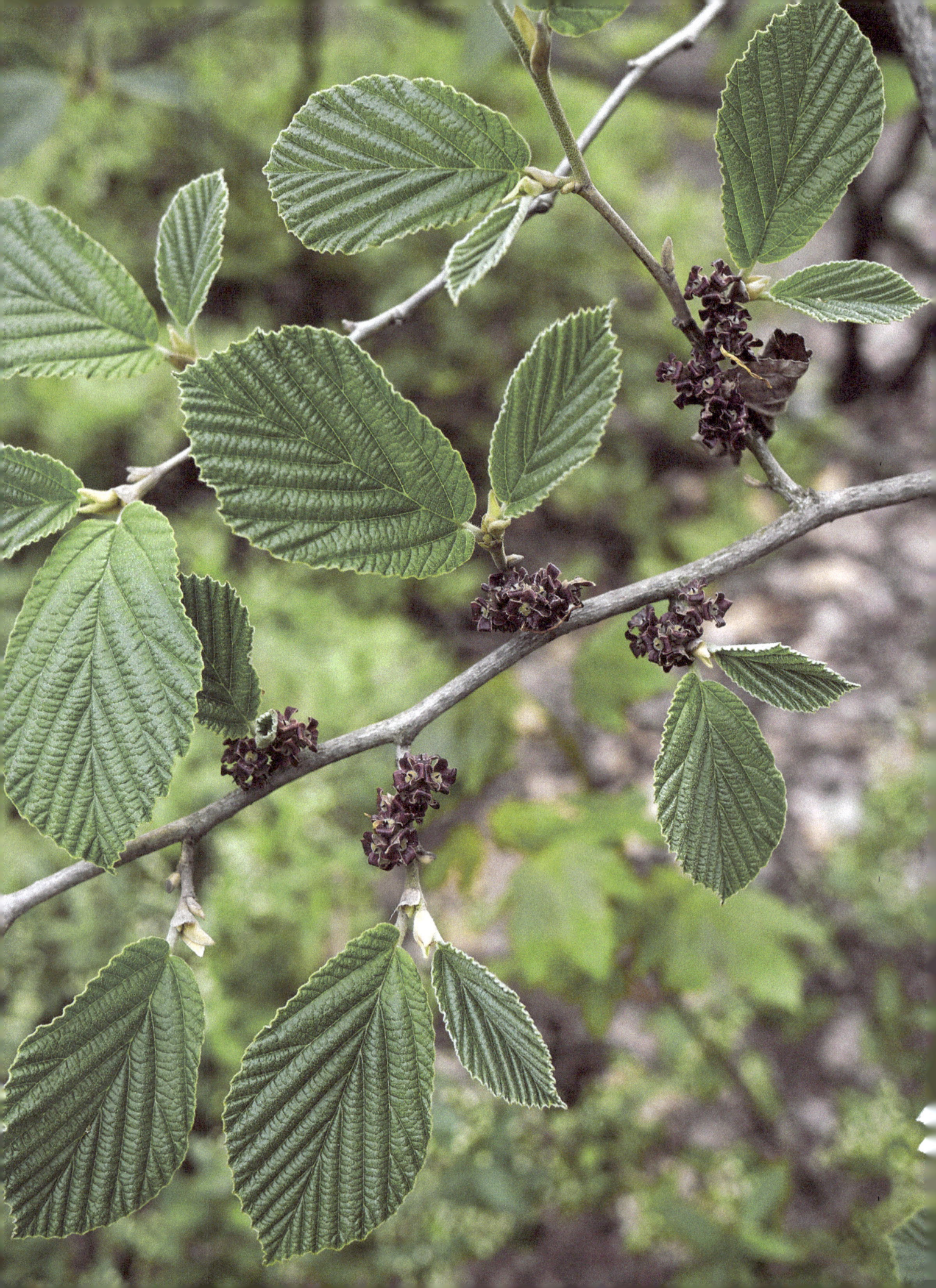

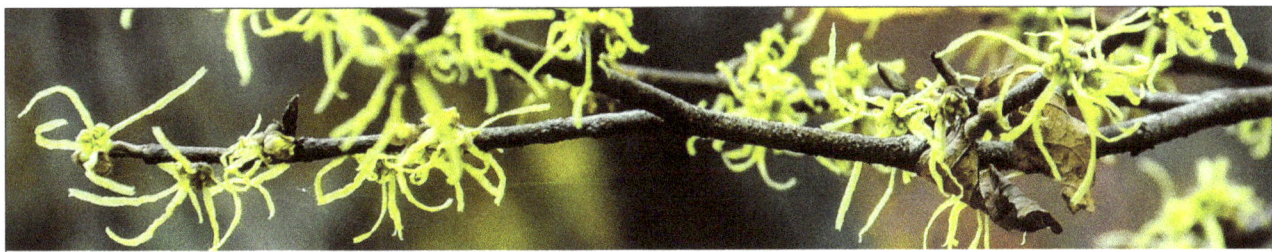

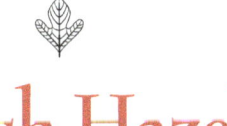

Witch Hazel

COMMON NAME: Witch Hazel

BOTANICAL NAME: *Hamamelis virginiana*

FAMILY: *Hamamelidaceae* (Witch Hazel)

DESCRIPTION: Witch hazel is a small deciduous tree, ten to fifteen feet tall, with alternate, ovate leaves that are irregular in shape, asymmetrical at the base and wider at the tip, with wavy edges. Delicate small yellow flowers with four narrow petals resembling thin shreds of crepe paper bloom between October and December, providing a late-season food source for insects. An insect gall (an abnormal growth caused by an insect feeding or laying eggs on the leaf) is responsible for witch hazel's common name; look for small protrusions on the leaf surface that resemble the point of a witch's hat.

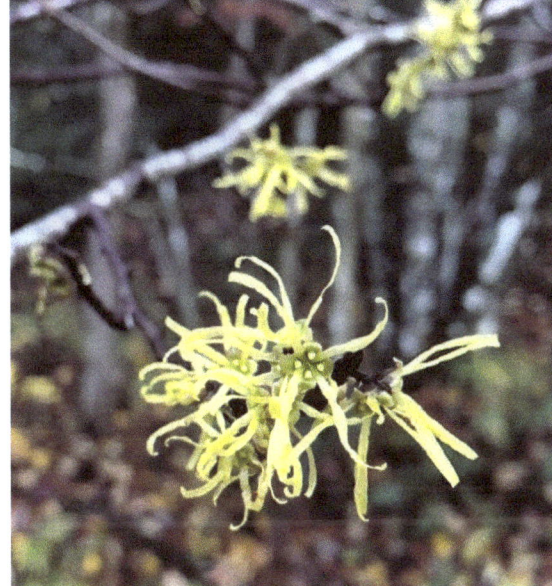

HABITAT: Deciduous forests. Witch hazel is often abundant in transition zones at the edge of forests, in open sunny areas, and along waterways.

KEY ACTIONS: Astringent, anti-inflammatory

PART USED: Leaf, bark

TRADITIONAL USES: The Cherokee rubbed the fresh leaves on the skin to treat scratches and used an infusion of the leaves to wash for sores and skin abrasions. Witch hazel decoction was taken internally to relieve menstrual pain, fever, sore throats, and diarrhea.[1] Distilled witch hazel, a time-tested home remedy, has been a staple in North American medicine chests for several hundred years. It has been used widely to relieve pain and inflammation from varicose veins, sprains, bruises, cuts, abrasions, hemorrhoids, smashed fingers and toes, shaving rash, and insect bites.

---

[1] Moerman, *Native American Ethnobotany*, 270

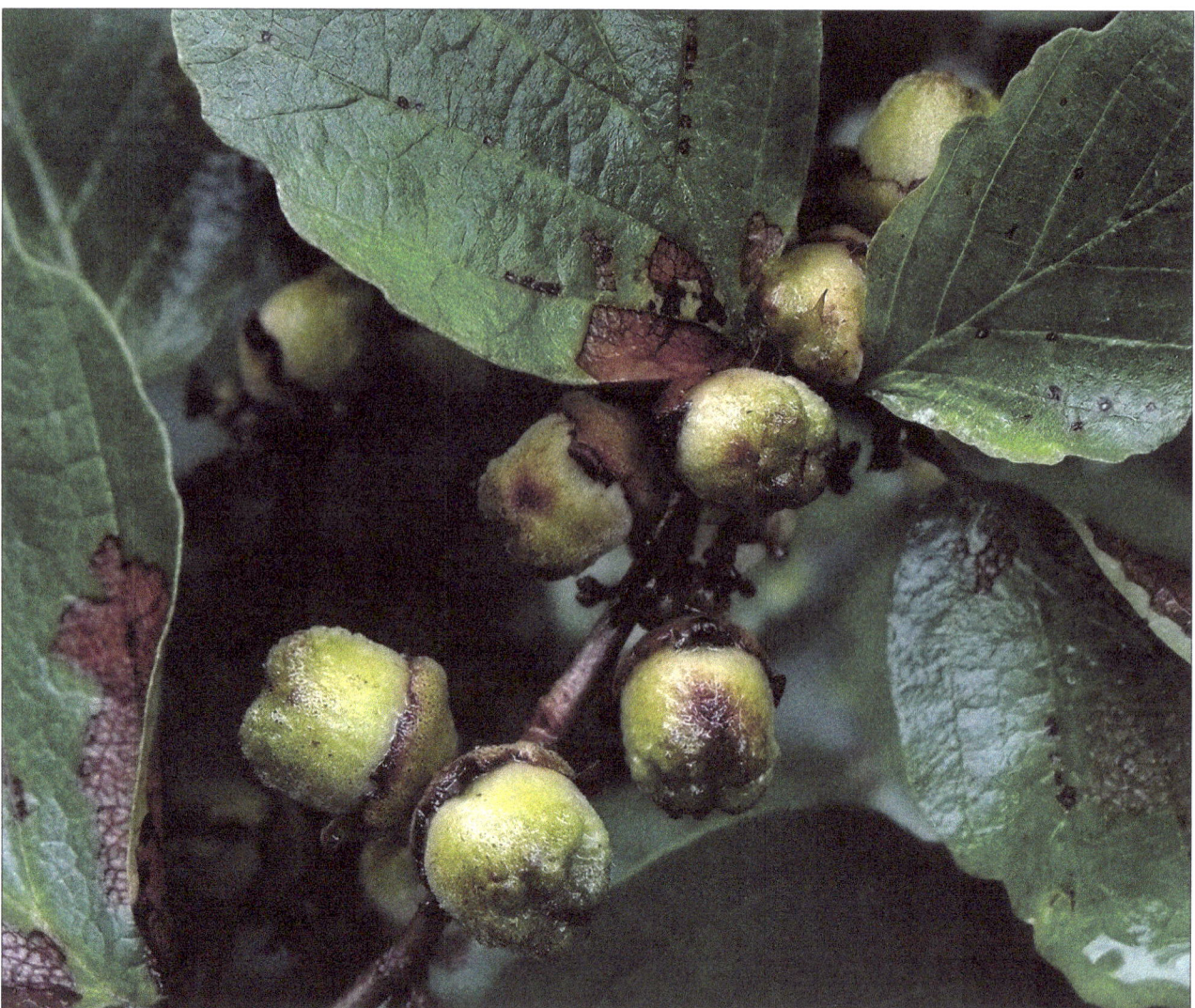

CURRENT USES: Witch hazel is a reliable remedy that deserves a place in every first aid kit. Witch hazel decoction or tincture is used internally to control severe diarrhea and reduce excessive menstrual bleeding. The decoction can also be used as a wash for the eyes and a gargle for sore throat. Saturate cotton balls with witch hazel decoction and apply directly to hemorrhoids, burns, varicose veins, bug bites, sprains, aching muscles, backaches, and bruises for immediate relief. Dowsers use the forked branch of a witch hazel tree to locate underground water.

CAUTIONS: None known. Occasional reports of stomach discomfort from internal use.

PREPARATIONS

Use fresh leaf and bark for best results. Although distilled witch hazel (for external use) is readily available in most drugstores, an effective home remedy can be made by steeping fresh leaves and bark in rubbing alcohol. When making witch hazel tincture, you should add a small amount of vegetable glycerin to the menstruum to extract the tannins.

DECOCTION: Use one-fourth cup of dried leaf and bark or one-half cup of fresh leaf and bark for each cup of water. Cover and simmer for fifteen minutes. Strain.

TINCTURE: Fresh leaf and bark – 1:2, 65% alcohol and 10% vegetable glycerin. Dried bark and leaf – 1:5, 50% alcohol and 10% vegetable glycerin.

LINIMENT: Fill a quart jar with fresh leaves and bark coarsely chopped. Pour in enough rubbing alcohol to cover the herb completely. Steep for two weeks, shaking the jar daily. Strain and label: For External Use Only.

DOSAGES

For external use, witch hazel decoction and liniment can be used interchangeably with commercially distilled witch hazel. All three preparations are excellent astringents for relieving inflammation and sore muscles.

DECOCTION: Drink one cup two to three times a day. The decoction is also used as a compress, wash, or douche as needed.

TINCTURE: Take one-quarter teaspoon of tincture in a small amount of water three times a day.

LINIMENT: Soak cotton balls or gauze in liniment and apply to the skin to treat sore muscles. Do not use it on broken skin or open wounds.

HARVESTING

Collect young leaves and twigs in the spring and early summer. Cut branches, strip the leaves and reserve, and peel off the outer bark using a knife. Thin branches less than one-half inch in diameter can be chopped into small pieces without removing the bark.

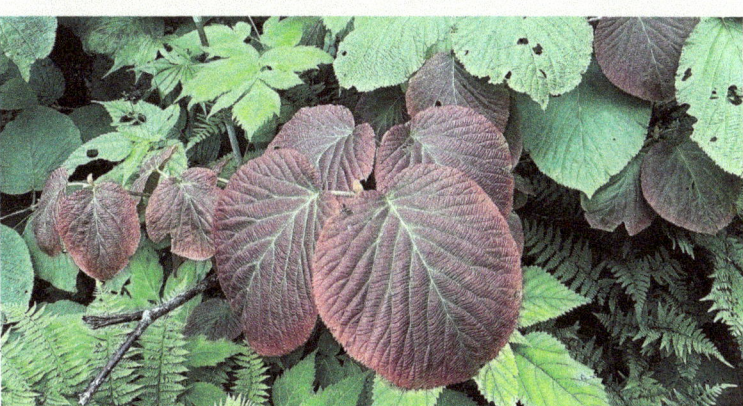

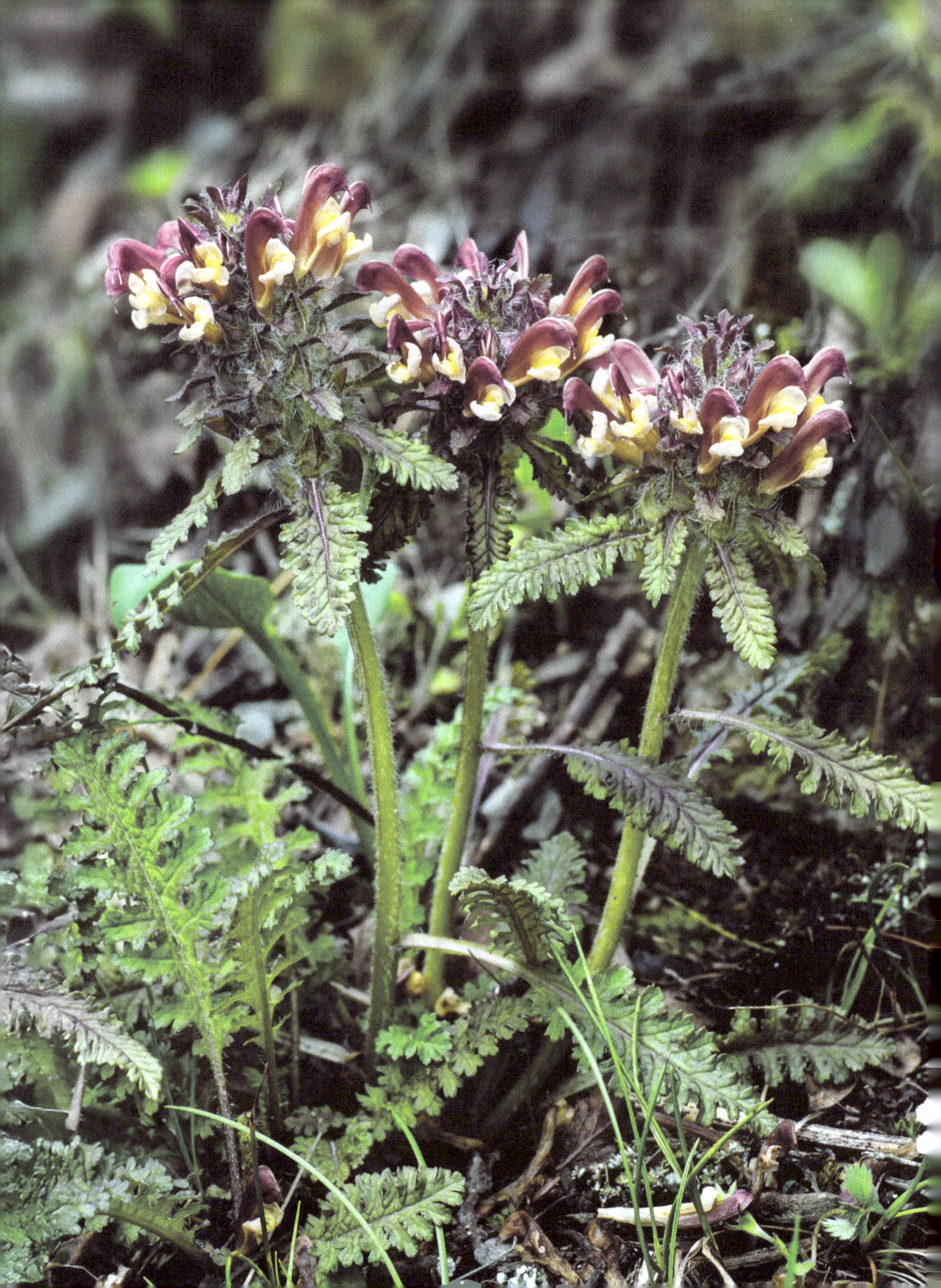

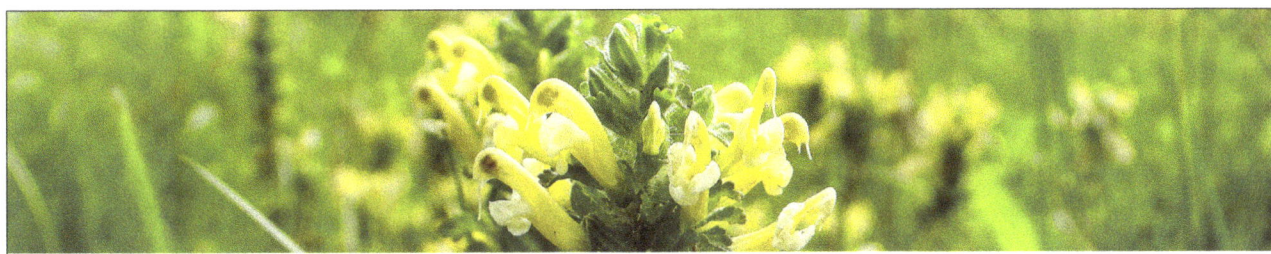

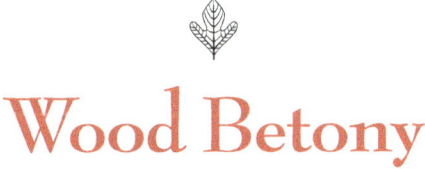

Wood Betony

COMMON NAME: Wood Betony

BOTANICAL NAME: *Pedicularis canadensis*

FAMILY: *Orobanchaceae* (Broomrape)

OTHER NAMES: Lousewort. Note: Wood betony is also the common name for *Betonica officinalis*, also known as *Stachys officinalis*, a plant native to Europe. They have similar actions as muscle relaxants but are not considered interchangeable.

DESCRIPTION: Wood betony is an upright perennial, eight to twelve inches tall, that grows in colonies. Its two to six inches long leaves are pinnately lobed and resemble ferns. Leaves are basal, then alternate, and become smaller towards the top of the plant. Irregular two-lipped flowers, usually with a lower lip yellow and upper lip a rusty maroon color, or sometimes all yellow, grow in whorls at the terminal end and bloom in May. Wood betony is symbiotic with a root fungus that it uses to absorb nutrients, in addition to using photosynthesis.

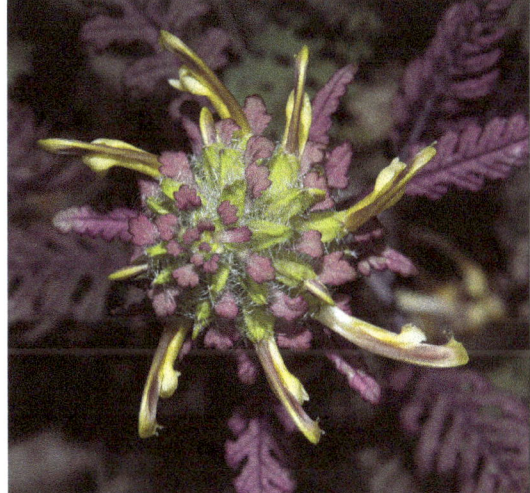

HABITAT: Shady, dry woodlands.

KEY ACTIONS: Antispasmodic, anti-inflammatory

PART USED: Leaf

TRADITIONAL USES: Wood betony was a common remedy for flux (bloody diarrhea) caused by bacterial infections from contaminated food and water. In Europe, it was known as Lousewort, and it was believed that if farm animals fed on wood betony plants, they would attract lice. American Indians used wood betony in love charms to attract a lover or foster harmony in love relationships.[1]

---

[1] Moerman, *Native American Ethnobotany*, 380

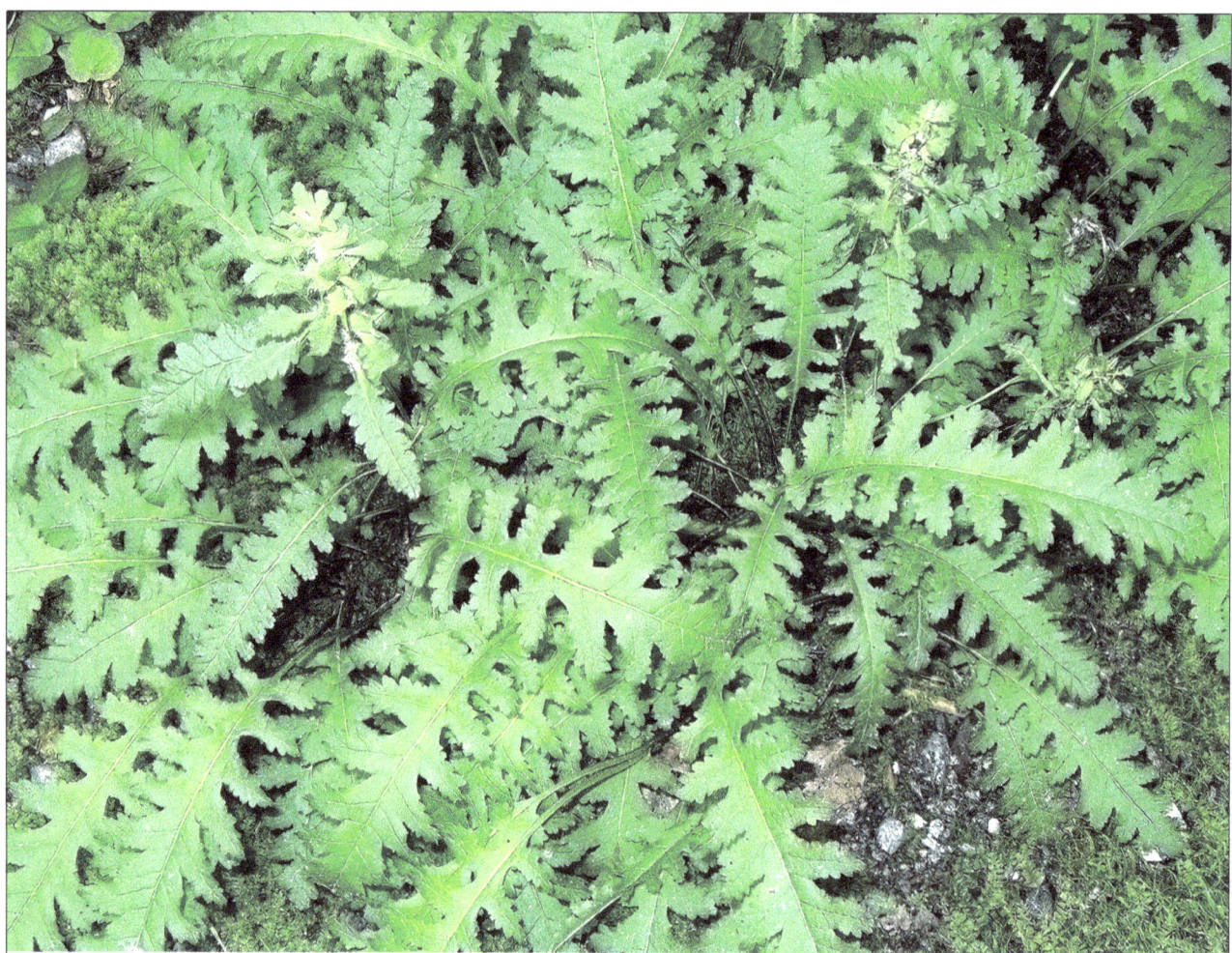

CURRENT USES: Wood betony excels at relaxing skeletal muscles to relieve spasms, tension and pain caused by trauma injuries. It can be used for chronic back and neck pain and sprained or torn ligaments and tendons. Wood betony also relieves stomach aches caused by inflammation and soothes intestinal pain from diarrhea. It can also be used in formulas to relieve sore throats, dry coughs, laryngitis and other inflammatory symptoms in the upper respiratory system.

CAUTIONS: Contraindicated in pregnancy or while nursing. Large doses may cause nausea and vomiting; careful attention to dosing is recommended.

PREPARATIONS

Use wood betony leaves fresh or dried.

INFUSION: Use one tablespoon of dried or two tablespoons of fresh herb for each cup of water. Infuse for 20 minutes.

TINCTURE: Fresh – 1:2. Dried – 1:5, 50%.

DOSAGES

Use small, frequent doses until symptoms improve, then increase the time between doses.

INFUSION: Drink a half cup every thirty minutes.

TINCTURE: Take a half teaspoon every thirty minutes.

HARVESTING

Gather leaves in early summer, being careful not to disturb or dislodge the roots. Wood betony is common but not abundant, so only harvest from well-established colonies.

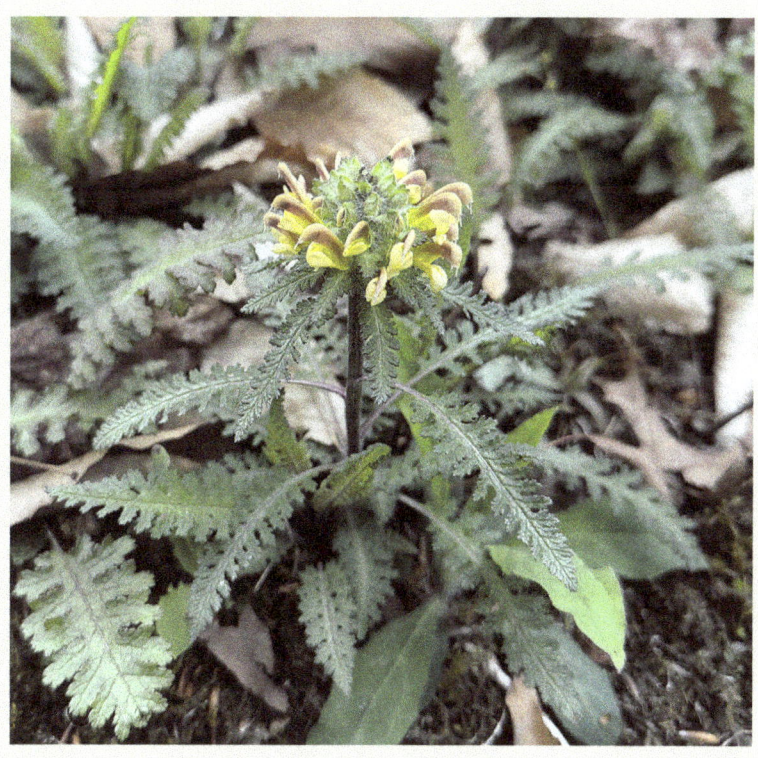

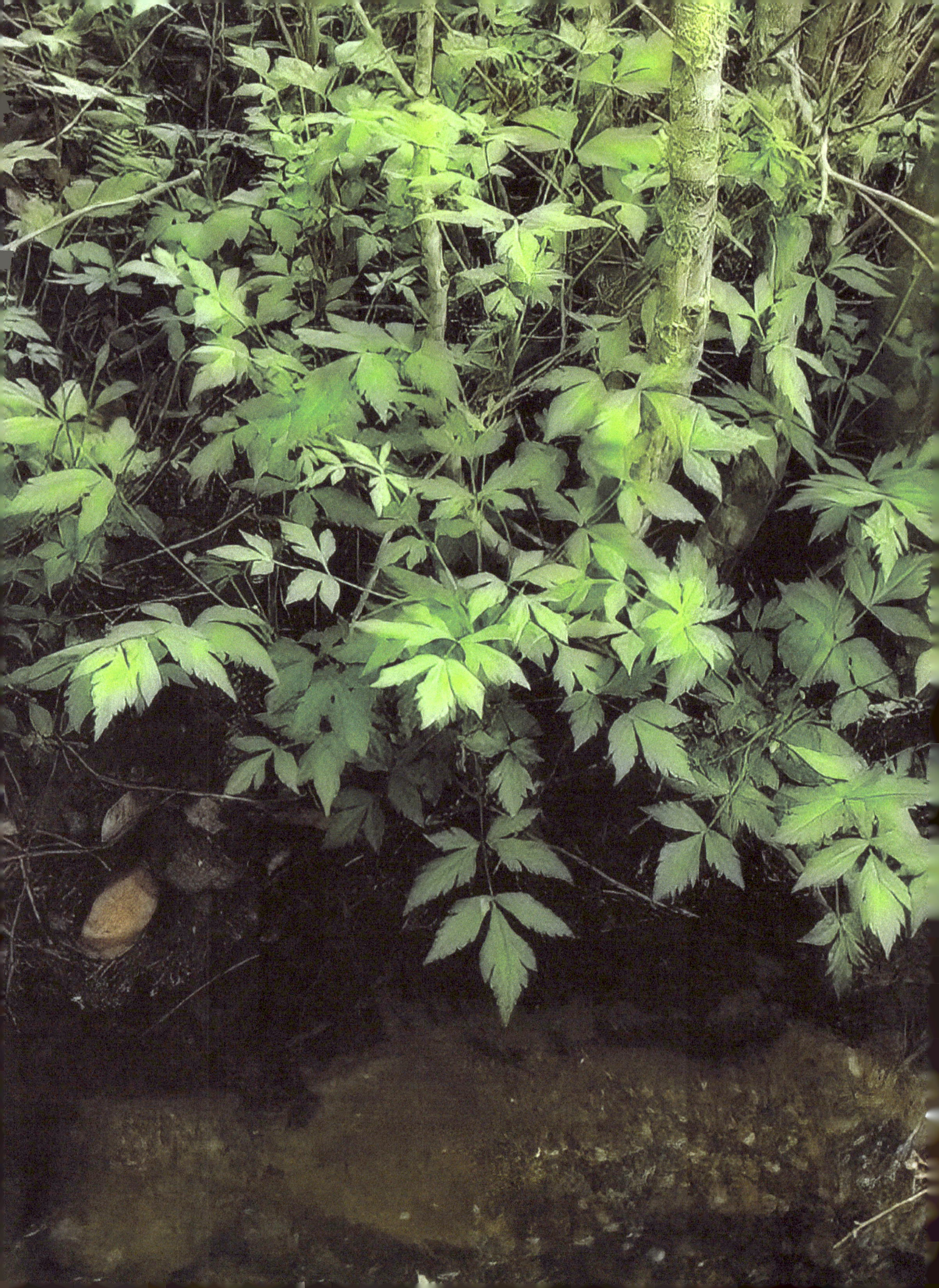

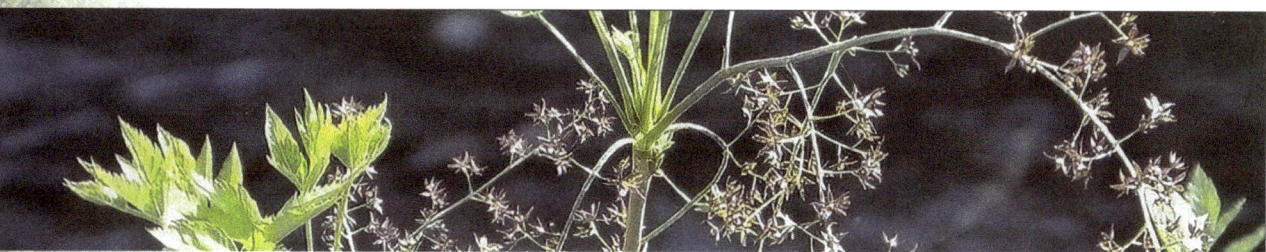

Yellowroot

COMMON NAME: Yellowroot

BOTANICAL NAME: *Xanthorhiza simplicissima*

FAMILY: *Ranunculaceae* (Buttercup)

OTHER NAMES: Redneck Goldenseal

DESCRIPTION: Yellowroot is a woody shrub, one to three feet tall, with compound leaves with three to five deeply cleft, toothed leaflets on each stalk. The brown outer bark of the main stems easily peels away to reveal the bright yellow inner bark. Small greenish-brown flowers are composed of five sepals, as yellowroot is without actual petals. They emerge before the leaves are fully unfurled and later can be found under the leaves in a drooping spray of small green stars. As the season progresses, the flowers slowly turn a dark brown-maroon color. Look for blooms from April to August. The yellow roots are woody and fibrous and have an acrid smell.

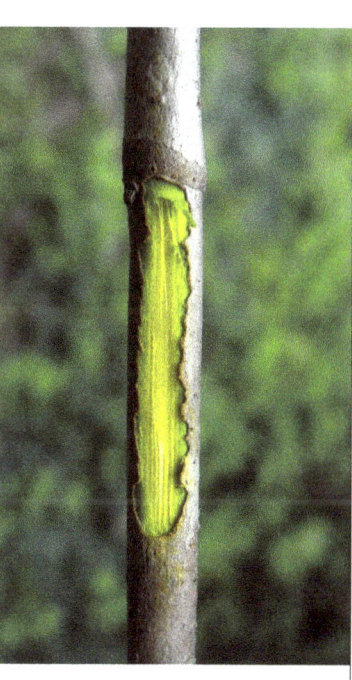

HABITAT: Grows in dense thickets along streambeds and other damp, shady areas. Yellowroot is endemic to the southern Appalachian Mountains.

KEY ACTIONS: Digestive bitter, astringent, anti-microbial, anti-bacterial, anti-fungal, abortifacient

PART USED: Root and stem

TRADITIONAL USES: Yellowroot was used by the Cherokee to treat jaundice, hepatitis, and chronic liver problems, as well as to heal persistent ulcers. In Southern folk medicine, yellowroot is considered a general tonic to improve overall health and remedy indigestion, ulcers, and heartburn. Yellowroot can still be found for sale at farm stands and markets in the South. The root was decocted to make a wash used to treat sties, thrush, gum disease, toothaches, and skin rashes. It was also used to create a yellow dye.

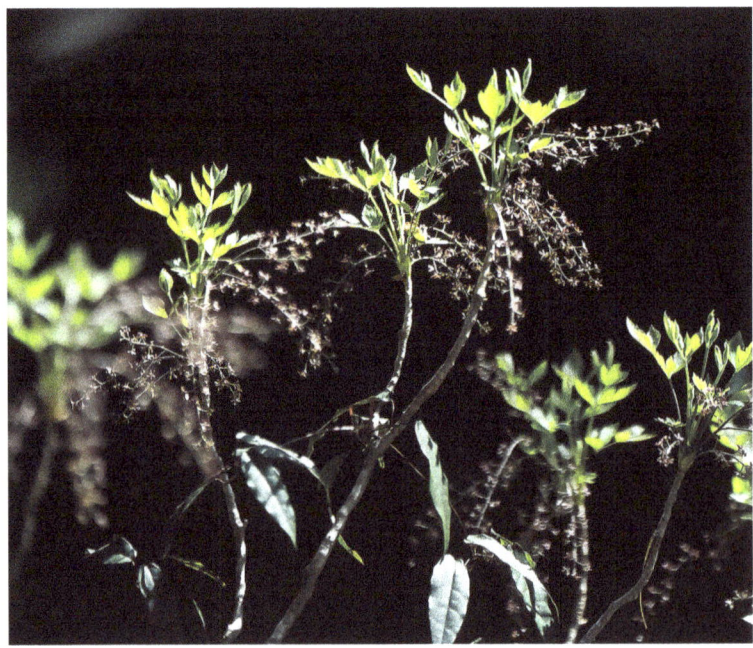

"More people is taking it now for ulcers...it's absolutely the real stuff. We've got so many people smiling after taking that, now, that ain't no joke."

Tommie Bass, (1989) A Reference Guild to Medicinal Plants

CURRENT USES: Like goldenseal *(Hydrastis canadensis)*, yellowroot contains the alkaloid berberine, which gives both plants their yellow color, bitter flavor and antibacterial properties. Though yellowroot is a much milder herb, it is an effective bitter tonic that improves digestion and elimination. It is a specific remedy for healing stomach ulcers caused by Helicobacter pylori.

Use yellowroot decoction as a wash to clean wounds, a gargle and mouthwash for sore throats, thrush, aphthous ulcers (canker sores) and bleeding gums, and as a nasal flush for sinus infections. As a douche, it is one of the best remedies for vaginitis and yeast infections. Apply the salve to bedsores, persistent ulcers, fungal infections, and for general wound healing.

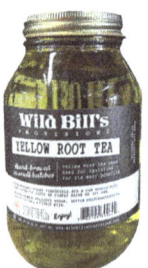

CAUTIONS: Not for use in pregnancy or while nursing. Yellowroot may cause nausea if used in high doses, so pay careful attention to dosing recommendations.

PREPARATIONS

The moisture content of fresh and dried yellowroot is very similar, so I prepared them both as if they were dry.

DECOCTION: Use one teaspoon of fresh or dried root and stem for each cup of water. Bring to a boil; cover and simmer for 20 minutes. Strain.

TINCTURE: Fresh or dried root and stem – 1:5, 60%.

DOUCHE: Prepare a decoction as described.

SALVE: Make a standard salve using infused yellowroot oil.

DOSAGE

Be forewarned: Yellowroot is a very acrid, bitter herb. However, the taste of bitterness on the tongue is essential when treating digestive system symptoms. For this reason, it may not be the best remedy (internally) for anyone unconvinced of the benefits of herbal medicine.

DECOCTION: Slowly sip one-fourth cup over about ten minutes. If this is unbearable, you can take a dose and immediately follow it with a swig of juice or water. Repeat three to four times daily.

TINCTURE: Take a half teaspoon in a small amount of water three to four times daily.

SALVE: Apply to affected areas once or twice a day. For fungal conditions, wash and completely dry the skin before each application.

DOUCHE: Use a douche bag filled with warm decoction daily for five to seven days. Wait a day, and if you still have symptoms, repeat the douche for five to seven days until symptoms are gone.

HARVESTING

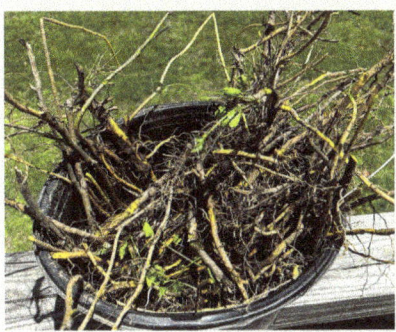

Roots and stems can be collected at any time during the growing season. Clean the root carefully and immediately cut it into one inch pieces. Yellowroot typically grows along streams and branches, so try to minimize soil disturbance as you collect the roots.

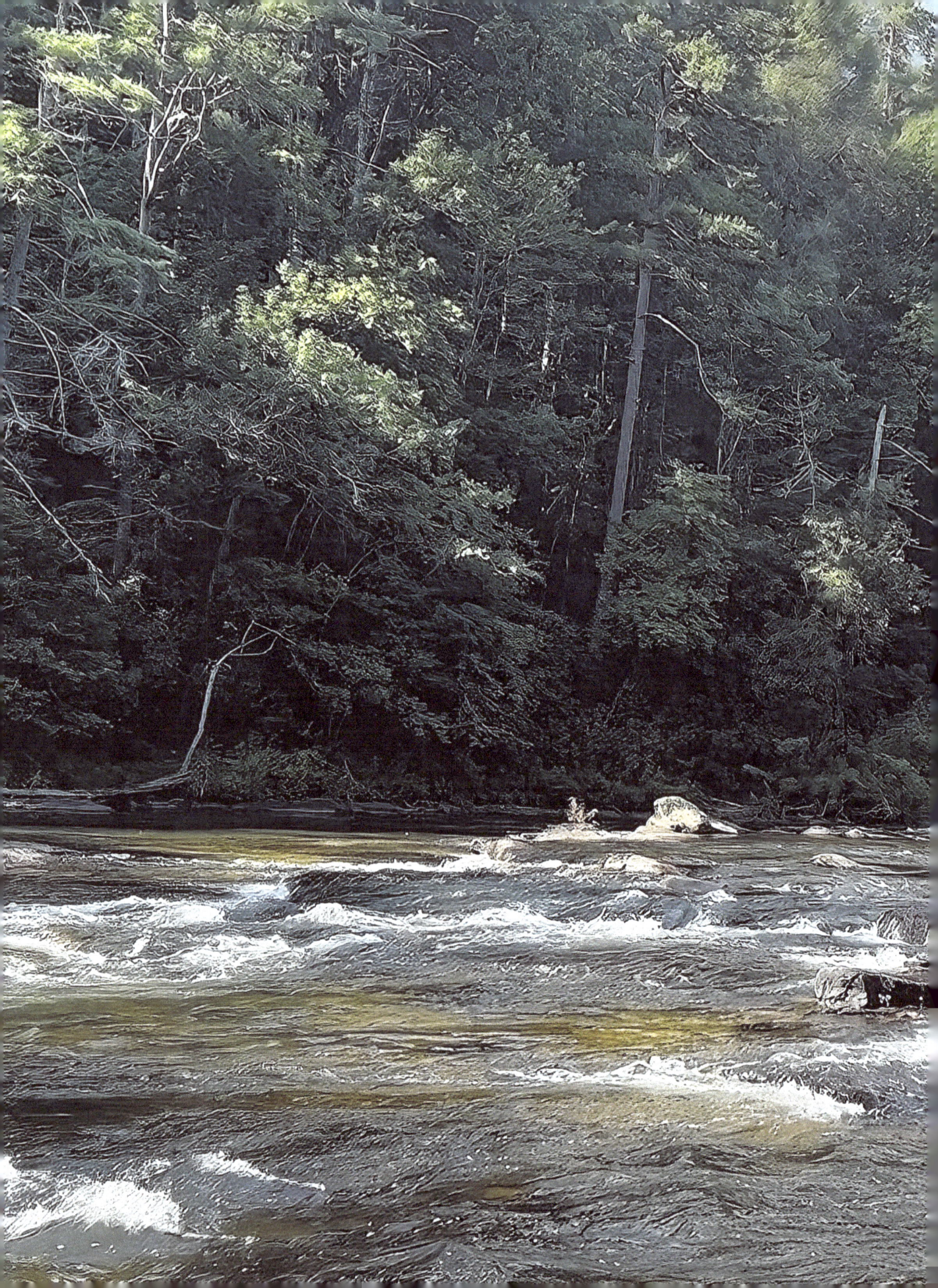

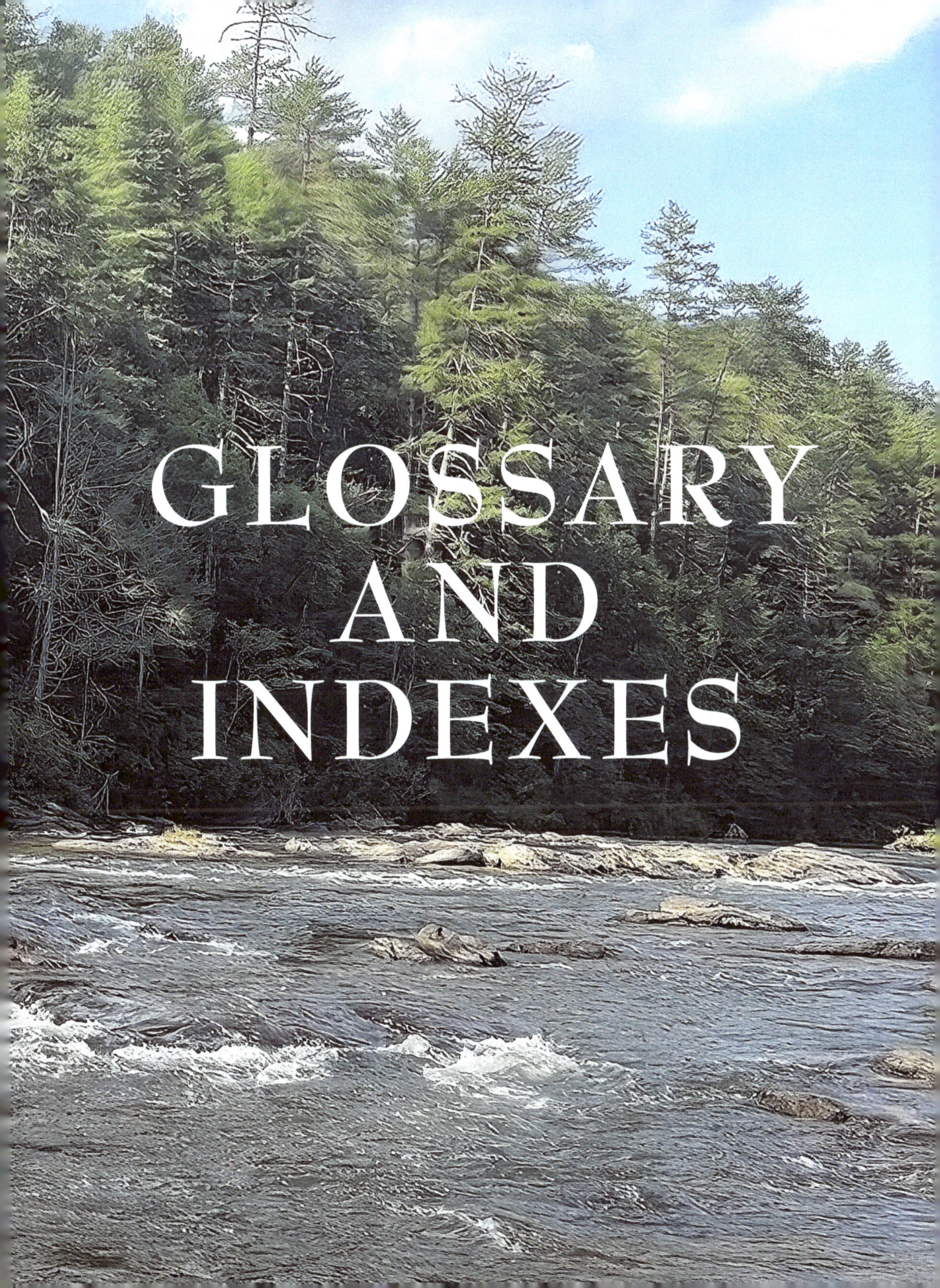

GLOSSARY AND INDEXES

Bloom Calendar

COMMON NAME	JAN	FEB	MAR	APR	MAY	JUNE	JUL	AUG	SEPT	OCT	NOV	DEC
Bee Balm							■	■	■			
Black Cohosh						■	■					
Black Haw				■	■							
Black Walnut					■	■						
Bloodroot			■	■								
Blue Cohosh				■	■							
Boneset							■	■	■			
Devil's Walking Stick							■	■				
Edler						■	■					
Evening Primrose							■	■	■			
Fringetree					■	■						
Gentian								■	■	■		
Ginseng, American						■	■					
Goldenrod								■	■	■		
Jewelweed							■	■	■			
Joe Pye Weed							■	■	■	■		
Lobelia							■	■	■	■		
Mountain Mint						■	■	■				
Partridgeberry						■	■					
Passionflower						■	■	■				
Pipsissewa						■	■	■				
Pleurisy Root						■	■	■	■			
Poke Root						■	■	■				

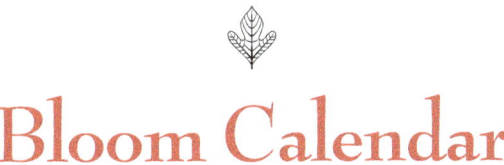

Bloom Calendar

COMMON NAME	JAN	FEB	MAR	APR	MAY	JUNE	JUL	AUG	SEPT	OCT	NOV	DEC
Rabbit Tobacco								■	■	■		
Ragweed								■	■	■		
Red Root						■	■					
Sarsaparilla					■	■						
Sassafras				■								
Skullcap						■	■	■	■			
Solomon's Seal					■							
Spicebush			■	■								
Stoneroot							■	■	■			
Sumac					■	■	■	■	■	■		
Sweetfern					■							
Sweetgum					■	■						
Turtlehead								■	■			
Wild Cherry					■	■						
Wild Geranium					■	■						
Wild Ginger			■	■	■	■						
Wild Hydrangea						■	■	■				
Wild Yam					■	■						
Witch Hazel										■	■	■
Wood Betony					■	■						
Yellowroot				■	■							

Harvest Calendar

COMMON NAME	PART USED	JAN	FEB	MAR	APR	MAY	JUNE	JUL	AUG	SEPT	OCT	NOV	DEC
Bee Balm	Aerial in flower							■					
Black Cohosh	Root										■		
Black Haw	Bark					■	■						
Black Walnut	Hulls									■	■		
Bloodroot	Root									■			
Blue Cohosh	Root										■		
Boneset	Aerial in flower									■			
Devil's Walking Stick	Bark, berry				bark				berry				
Edler	Leaf, flower, berry					leaf	flower		berry				
Evening Primrose	Aerial in flower							■					
Fringetree	Root bark (dried)												
Gentian	Aerial in flower								■	■			
Ginseng, American	Root									■	■		
Goldenrod	Aerial in flower								■	■			
Jewelweed	Aerial							■	■				
Joe Pye Weed	Root										■		
Lobelia	Aerial in flower							■	■				
Mountain Mint	Aerial in flower							■	■				
Partridgeberry	Aerial	■	■	■							■	■	■
Passionflower	Aerial in flower								■				
Pipsissewa	Aerial	■	■	■							■	■	■
Pleurisy Root	Root										■		
Poke Root	Root, berry										■		

Harvest Calendar

COMMON NAME	PART USED	JAN	FEB	MAR	APR	MAY	JUNE	JUL	AUG	SEPT	OCT	NOV	DEC
Rabbit Tobacco	Aerial in flower								■	■	■		
Ragweed	Aerial in flower								■				
Red Root	Root										■		
Sarsaparilla	Root										■		
Sassafras	Bark			■	■								
Skullcap	Aerial in flower							■	■	■			
Solomon's Seal	Root									■	■		
Spicebush	Bark, leaf, berry				bark, leaf			berry					
Stoneroot	Entire plant						■						
Sumac	Berry							■					
Sweetfern	Leaf						■	■	■				
Sweetgum	Bark, resin, seeds			bark, resin					seeds				
Turtlehead	Aerial in flower								■				
Wild Cherry	Bark, fruit							fruit		bark			
Wild Geranium	Entire plant						■						
Wild Ginger	Root						■		■				
Wild Hydrangea	Root bark								■				
Wild Yam	Root					leaf and bark	■						
Witch Hazel	Leaf, bark											■	
Wood Betony	Aerial in flower												
Yellowroot	Bark	■	■								■	■	■

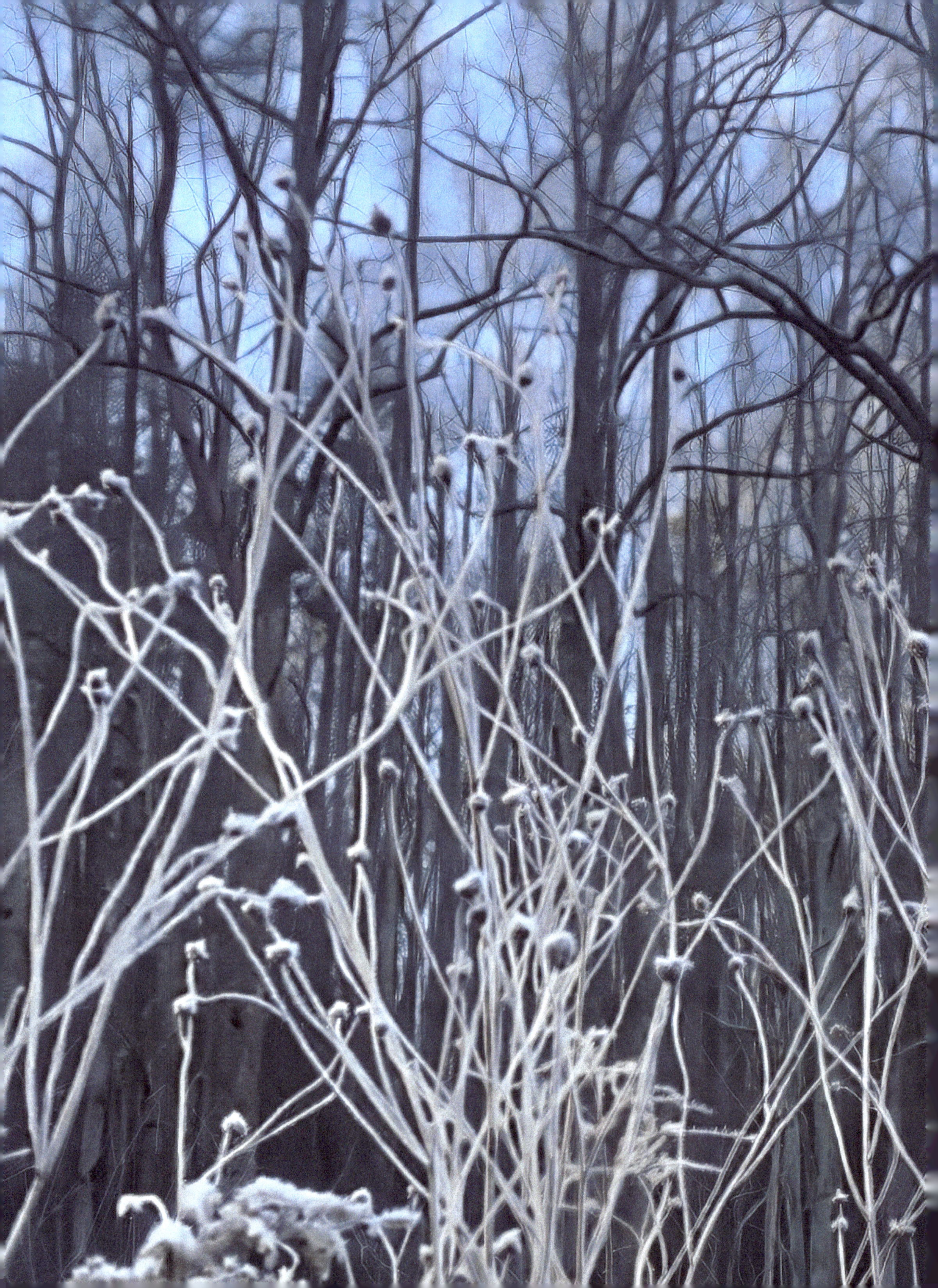

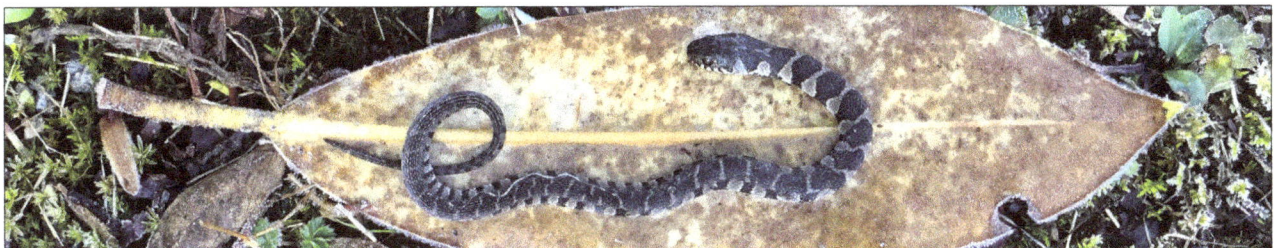

Glossary

Acute—A symptom that appears suddenly, usually resolves itself reasonably quickly, often accompanied by severe symptoms.

Adaptogen—Herb with a non-specific action that increases the overall ability to respond and adapt to physical and mental stress.

Aerial—All parts of a plant above ground, i.e., stem, leaves, flowers, seeds or fruits.

Alkaloid—A chemical that contains nitrogen as part of a heterocyclic ring structure and usually causes a strong reaction in the body.

Alterative—A general term used to describe the action of certain herbs to increase the efficiency of the lymphatic system, kidneys, liver, and skin and enhance their ability to remove and eliminate toxins and waste.

Alternate (leaves)—Single leaves that grow on alternate sides along the stem.

Amenorrhea—Lack of menses.

Analgesic—Herb that relieves pain without altering consciousness.

Annual—A plant that lives for only one growing season.

Anodyne—Herb that relieves pain and may cause drowsiness.

Anther—The part of the stamen that produces pollen.

Anti-helmintic—Herb that kills and often helps purge certain worms or parasites.

Anti-bacterial—Herb that inhibits the growth of bacteria.

Anti-catarrhal—Herb that reduces inflammation and congestion of mucus membranes in the respiratory system.

Anti-depressant—Herb that relieves symptoms of depression.

Anti-emetic—Herb that prevents or stops vomiting.

Anti-inflammatory—Herb that relieves inflammation.

Anti-fungal—Herb that kills fungal growth and may prevent fungal infections.

Anti-lithic—Herb that breaks up stones, or calculi, in the gallbladder or kidney. See also lithotropic.

Anti-microbial—Herb that kills microorganisms.

Anti-rheumatic—Herb that relieves rheumatic pain and inflammation.

Antiseptic—Herb that prevents or stops the growth of microorganisms.

Antispasmodic—Herb that relieves muscle spasms and relaxes tight muscles, ligaments and tendons.

Aromatic—Herb that contains high amounts of volatile oils. See also carminative and diaphoretic.

Asthma—Obstruction of the airways caused by spasms of the bronchi.

Attention Deficit Disorder (ADD)—A mental condition characterized by persistent difficulty in maintaining attention and concentration. See also Attention Deficit/ Hyperactivity Disorder.

Attention Deficit/Hyperactivity Disorder (ADHD)—It is the same as ADD but with hyperactive physical behavior.

Axil—The angle formed at the point where a leaf attaches to the stem.

Basal—Leaves crowded around the base of the plant stem.

Basal rosette—Describes how basal leaves look when many of them are crowded together at the base of the plant.

Biennial—Plants having a two-year growing cycle; the first year's growth is limited to a taproot and leaves. During the second year, the plant produces flowers and seeds.

Bitter—Taste or flavor that stimulates bile and other secretions.

Bisexual (flowers)—Flowers composed of both pistils and stamens.

Bract—Very small or modified leaf that appears near a flower.

Bronchitis—Inflammation of the bronchial tubes.

Calyx—A collection of sepals that encloses the flower bud. After the flower opens, the calyx forms the outer whorl of the flower itself. The calyx is composed of individual sepals. In some flowers, what looks like petals are sepals, such as black cohosh.

Cambium—The inner layer of a woody plant. This tube-like tissue that conducts fluids and nutrients from the roots to the leaves.

Candidiasis—Systemic fungal infection caused by Candida albicans.

Canker Sore—Ulcers in the mouth.

Cardiotonic—Regulates and strengthens heart function.

Carminative—Stimulates digestion; relieves flatulence, spasms, and bloating.

Catkin—A dangling spike of pistillate (lacking stamens) or staminate (lacking pistils) flowers on the branches of certain trees. Wind-pollinated.

Cathartic—Herb that acts as an irritant to cause a dramatic evacuation of the large intestine.

Cholagogue—Stimulates secretions from the gallbladder.

Chlorophyll—A green pigment in plants that indicates photosynthesis.

Circulatory stimulant—Increases blood circulation; may increase heart rate.

Cold Sore—Sore on the lip or mouth caused by the herpes simplex virus.

Colic—Abdominal contractions and pain. Often accompanied by nausea and vomiting.

Conjunctivitis—Bacterial or viral infection of the conjunctiva, or lining of the eyelid, with inflammation, discharge, and irritation. Highly contagious.

Compound (leaf)—A leaf composed of distinct leaflets, usually arranged and attached to the stem at a common point, with one single leaf at the terminal end.

Compress—A cloth saturated with a hot or cold herbal infusion or decoction applied to the skin to relieve pain, congestion, inflammation or infection.

Contraindicated—Not to be used when specific symptoms are present.

Cystitis—A type of urinary tract infection. Symptoms include pain and a frequent, urgent need to urinate.

Deciduous—Plants that lose their leaves at the end of the growing season.

Deciduous forest—A forest dominated by trees that lose their leaves at the end of the growing season.

Decoction—A water-based herbal extract made by boiling or simmering herbs in water for a specific amount of time.

Deep immune activator—Increases immune response; stimulates the production of blood, T-cells, phagocytes, and other immune responses. Long-term use strengthens the immune system's ability to recognize and eliminate pathogens and other actions.

Demulcent—Soothes irritated inflamed tissues. See also Emollient.

Diabetes—Abnormally high blood sugar levels caused by low levels of insulin.

Diaphoretic—Induces sweating; reduces or relieves fevers.

Diuretic—Stimulates the kidneys to increase urine output and reduce excess fluids in the tissues (edema).

Diverticulitis—Inflammation of the diverticula or sac-like pockets in the large intestine.

Dysentery—Severe diarrhea with intestinal inflammation caused by bacterial or parasitic infections. Symptoms include abdominal pain, vomiting, fever, nausea, and cramps. Potentially life-threatening, especially with infants, children and the elderly.

Eclectic (physician)—Physicians from a school of medicine that flourished in the United States in the late 19th and early 20th centuries who researched and promoted medicinal plants native to North America.

Edema—Swelling caused by a build-up of fluid in the tissues. Symptoms include swelling of the legs, ankles and feet. Also known as dropsy.

Emetic—Herb that induces vomiting.

Emmenagogue—Herb that stimulates the onset of menses and may be abortifacient in large doses.

Emollient—Herb that soothing and moistening to external tissues. See also demulcent.

Endemic (plant)—A plant only found growing within a specific region.

Endometriosis—A disorder caused by endometrial tissues (usually found only in the uterine lining) outside of the uterus in other parts of the pelvis. Symptoms include severe cyclical pain, excessive menstrual bleeding, and infertility.

Escharotic—A folk remedy that kills diseased tissues or unwanted growths (warts, skin tabs, tumors), usually in the form of a corrosive salve applied topically.

Ethnobotany—Study of how specific groups of people use plants for food, medicine, etc.

Evergreen—Plants with leaves that remain throughout all or most of the year.

Expectorant—Herb that increases the elimination of mucus from the lungs.

Febrifuge—Herb that reduces fevers. See also diaphoretic.

Fibromyalgia—A group of disorders characterized by symptoms that may include pain and stiffness throughout the body, poor sleep, fatigue, depression, and Irritable Bowel Syndrome.

Fistula, anal—A crack or fissure in the mucus membrane of the anus.

Flu—A highly contagious viral infection that affects the respiratory system. Symptoms include fever, body aches and excessive congestion. Also known as Influenza.

Folk method—A simple method of preparing herbal tinctures that involves macerating herbs in 80 or 100-proof alcohol without measuring or weighing the ingredients.

Fibrocystic Breast Disease—Disease of the breast with symptoms that include cyclical pain and non-cancerous lumps and cysts.

Galactagogue—Increases the flow of breast milk.

Gastritis—Inflammation of the stomach lining. May lead to infections and peptic ulcers.

Gout—A disorder caused by deposits of crystals (sodium urate) in the joints due to high uric acid levels in the blood. Symptoms include joint pain and inflammation, usually in the feet, especially the big toe.

Hemorrhoids—Dilated or inflamed veins in the rectum or anus. Symptoms include pain and bleeding.

Hepatic—An herb that tonifies and detoxifies the liver.

Hepatitis—Inflammation of the liver caused by the hepatitis virus, alcoholism, or pharmaceutical drug use.

Hormonal balancer—Herb that nourishes the endocrine system and helps regulate hormonal secretions.

Hypnotic—Herb that acts as powerful sedative to relax the nervous system and help promote sleep.

Hypotensive—Herb that reduces blood pressure.

Indigenous—Native to the local area, usually applied to groups of people.

Influenza—A highly contagious viral infection that affects the respiratory system. Symptoms include fever, body aches and excessive congestion. Also referred to as the flu.

Infusion—Tea or water extract made by steeping fresh or dried herbs in hot or cold water for a specific amount of time.

Inhalation—Herbal steam used to treat the congestion and inflammation of the respiratory system.

Interstitial cystitis—Painful inflammation or ulceration of the bladder with no evidence of infection. Symptoms include pain and frequent, urgent need to urinate.

Irritable Bowel Syndrome—A disorder that causes abdominal pain, cramping and explosive diarrhea, sometimes alternating with constipation. Possible causes include food allergies, overeating, eating too quickly, and fatty foods.

Jaundice—Abnormally high levels of bilirubin in the body caused by an obstruction of the bile duct, liver disease, or an excessive breakdown of red blood cells. Symptoms include yellowing of the skin and eyes.

Labor tonic—An herbal preparation used during the last three weeks of pregnancy to prepare for childbirth.

Laxative—Herb that stimulates bowel movements.

Lithotropic—Herb that breaks up stones (calculi) in the kidney or gallbladder; may prevent recurrence.

Lymphatic—Herb that stimulates lymphatic drainage and reduces swelling of the lymph nodes.

Leaf nodes—The places along a stem where leaves or leaf buds emerge.

Leaflet—Leaf segments that together form a compound leaf.

Leucorrhea—Vaginal discharge.

Lobed—Leaf margin with a rounded shape, like an ear lobe.

Macerate—The process of steeping a plant in a menstruum (solvent) to extract active compounds.

Marc—The spent plant matter that remains after a tincture is pressed.

Menstruum—A liquid solvent used to make a tincture. Typical menstruums are a mixture of alcohol and water.

Mucolytic—Dissolves mucus, primarily in the respiratory system.

Naturalized—An introduced plant that is now well-established and common.

Naturopathy—System of natural healing that does not rely on drugs or surgery. Instead, it uses herbs, vitamins, hydrotherapy, diet and other methods to promote healing.

Nervine—Herb that strengthens, relaxes or stimulates the nervous system.

Opposite (leaves)—Leaves grow in pairs opposite from each other along the stem.

Oxalic acid—An acid found in many plants and vegetables, it is toxic in large amounts.

Oxytocic—Herb that stimulates uterine contractions and promotes labor.

Palmate—Shaped like the palm of the hand.

Panacea—Cure-all.

Perennial—A plant with a growth cycle of three or more growing seasons.

Peripheral vasodilator—Herb that expands peripheral blood vessels, increases blood circulation and may reduce blood pressure.

Petiole—The stalk of a leaf.

Pinnate (leaf)—Three or more leaflets arranged on two sides along a stalk with a terminal leaf resembling the shape of a pine tree.

Pistil—Female reproductive organ of the flower. It consists of the stigma that receives the pollen and the style, a tube-like structure that connects the stigma to the ovaries and the ovules (seeds).

Pith—The spongy center within a woody branch's bark and cambium layers.

Pleurisy—Inflammation of the pleura, a membrane surrounding the lung, caused by respiratory infections and other lung diseases.

Pollinator—An insect or animal that visits flowers for nectar and, in the process of moving from flower to flower, distributes pollen, resulting in fertilization.

Post-partum—Occurring after childbirth.

Poultice—A soft mass of fresh or dried herbs moistened and applied to the skin to promote cellular healing, increase circulation, or relieve pain and infections.

Prostatitis—A condition that involves inflammation or infection of the prostate gland, a small gland located below the bladder in males. Symptoms include painful or difficult urination.

Psoriasis—Chronic, scaly skin condition with inflammation and itching.

Pulmonary edema—Accumulation of fluid in the lungs that causes breathing difficulties. Usually due to cardiac weakness.

Purgative—Herb that causes dramatic evacuation of the bowels. See also cathartic.

Raceme—A non-branching flower stalk with flowers on small stems or petioles.

Resin—Aromatic sap produced by trees to protect damaged bark.

Rheumatism—Chronic inflammation and pain in the joints. May also refer to rheumatoid arthritis, an autoimmune disease that causes deformed joints.

Rhinitis—Inflammation of the nose with mucus discharge.

Rhizome—An underground stem that usually grows horizontally just below the ground's surface, with small roots or rootlets emerging along its length.

Rootlet—Small root.

Rubefacient—Increases blood circulation by causing localized skin irritation. Used externally.

Salve—Medicinal preparation made from vegetable oil infused with herbs and thickened with beeswax. Used topically.

Sciatica—Pain caused by a compressed or injured sciatic nerve. Symptoms include pain radiating from the lower back down the buttocks and into one leg. Other symptoms may include a tingling, burning sensation in the hip and leg weakness.

Sedative—Herb that slows heart and respiratory rate to reduce nervousness and anxiety and promote restful sleep.

Sepals—The individual parts of a flower's calyx, or outer whorl. Usually green, though some sepals may resemble flower petals.

Serrated (leaf)—Sharply toothed edges that point upward toward the leaf tip.

Sessile—A leaf attached directly to the main stem, without a stem or petiole
Sialagogue—Stimulates the production of saliva, may increase appetite and improve digestion.
Simple (leaf)—A single leaf growing directly from the stem.
Stamen—Male reproductive organs of a flower. Consists of the filament and the pollen-producing anther.
Stigma—Part of the flower's pistil or female reproductive organ, located at the terminal end of the pistil. The stigma receives the pollen grains.
Styptic—Stops blood flow from wounds. Used externally.
Surface immune activator—Increases defensive responses of the skin and mucus membranes against invading pathogens.
Syrup—A sweet preparation is usually made by combining a concentrated herbal decoction with honey.
Taproot—A long root that grows vertically into the ground, like a carrot.
Terminal—Growing at the end of a stem.
Thrush—Fungal infection of the mouth.
Tincture—A medicinal extract made by steeping or macerating herbs in a solvent for specific amount of time. Most tinctures are made with a solvent or menstruum that combines alcohol and water.
Tonic—An herb with restorative properties used to strengthen or regulate organ function. Most tonics are used for long periods.
Umbel—Flowers arranged on stems or petioles radiating from the same point. Viewed from below, this arrangement of flower stems resembles the spines of an umbrella.
Understory plants—Plants that thrive in the shade of deciduous forests. This term usually applies to shrubs and small trees.
Urethra—The channel that carries urine from the bladder out of the body.
Urethritis—Inflammation of the urethra.
Uterine tonic—Tonifies and strengthens the uterus; may increase fertility.
Vaginitis—Inflammation of the vagina, often due to fungal infections.
Vermifuge—Herb that kills and purges parasites.
Vulnerary—Promotes tissue healing by stimulating cell regeneration. It may be used internally or externally.
Whorled (leaves)—Three or more leaves arranged in a circle.
Whooping cough—Bacterial infection of the air passages causes inflammation and coughing spasms, resulting in a loud whooping inhalation. Highly contagious. Also known as pertussis.

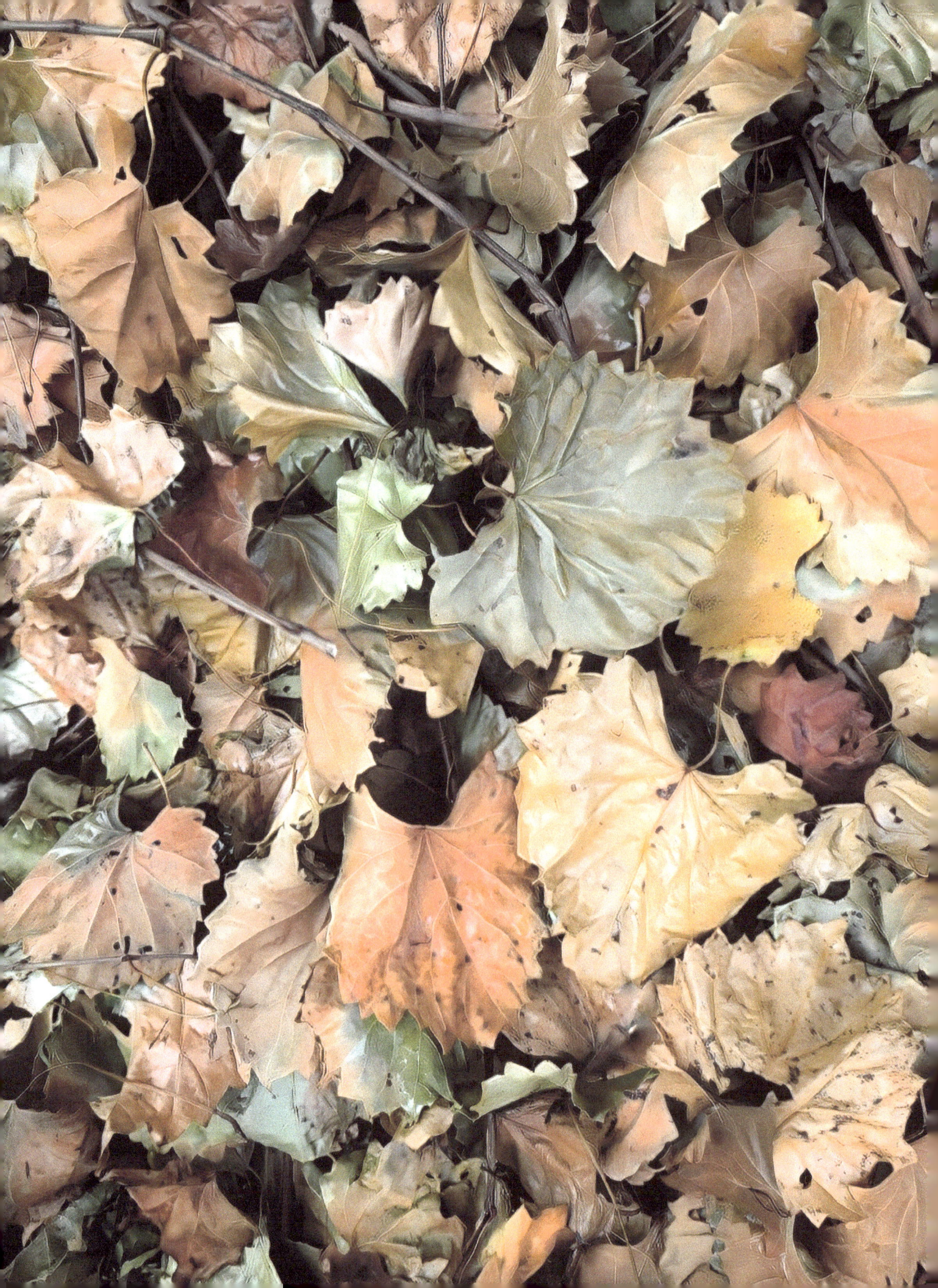

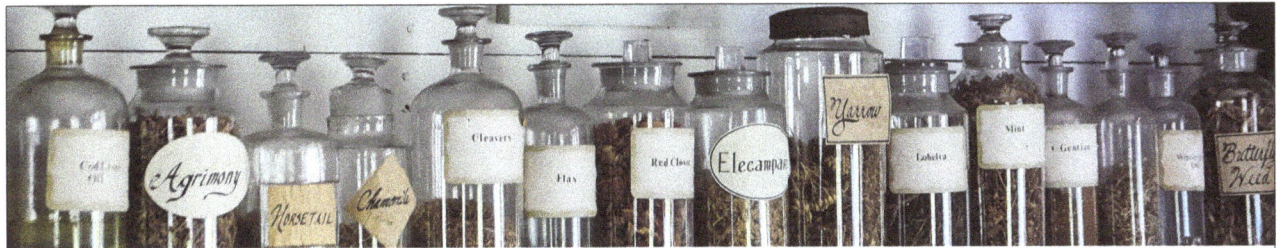

Therapeutic Index

The Therapeutic Index is a general guide to help you quickly find the right herb to treat a specific symptom or condition. Herbs shown in bold indicate a particular herb that is a known remedy for that symptom or condition.

To use the index, look up the symptom or condition and find one or more herbs that might be a good match for your symptoms. Then, review the monograph for each herb for current uses, actions and dosing recommendations.

Start with only one single herb. This simple approach helps you understand the herb's actions. If you're feeling more adventurous, you can create a simple formula by combining several herbs with complementary actions. For example, when treating a cold, you may need to address various symptoms, including fever, sore throat, and restlessness, with three individual herbs.

Sometimes, a single herb may offer all three actions, or you may need to combine two or more herbs to address all the symptoms. While the art of herb formulation is beyond the scope of this book, you could consider combining several herbs to create a simple formula. If you are just starting to learn about herbal actions, combine no more than three herbs and take them for a day or two (at the recommended dosage) before deciding whether they do or don't work for you. If you don't get symptom relief, try another herb. And, of course, be sure you are using high-quality herbal remedies!

Abscess (external)—Elder leaf, evening primrose, red root (internal)
Acne (external)—Sweetfern, jewelweed
Allergies (seasonal/hay fever)—Elder berry, elder flower, **goldenrod**, lobelia, **ragweed**
Amenorrhea—Partridgeberry
Anemia—**Ginseng**, rabbit tobacco, wild cherry
Appetite Loss—Boneset, **gentian**, ginseng, turtlehead, wild cherry
Anal Fistula—Goldenrod, red root (internal), sweetfern, **witch hazel**
Anxiety—Black cohosh, evening primrose, ginseng, **passionflower**, **skullcap**, wild cherry

Arthritis (see also Joint Pain/Stiffness)—**Black cohosh**, **black haw**, devil's walking stick (berries), wild yam, wood betony

Asthma (acute symptoms)—Black haw, bloodroot, blue cohosh, lobelia, rabbit tobacco

Bladder Infections—**Goldenrod**, Joe Pye weed, **pipsissewa**, wild cherry, wild hydrangea, wild yam

Bleeding (wounds)—Ragweed, sweetfern, sumac, **wild geranium**

Bleeding (internal)—Wild geranium, witch hazel

Blood Pressure (high)—Ginseng, **passionflower**

Boils (external)—Elder leaf, evening primrose

Breast Lumps/Cysts, Pain (Fibrocystic Breast Disease)—Poke root, red root

Bronchitis—Bee balm, black cohosh, bloodroot, blue cohosh, **boneset**, evening primrose, sarsaparilla, **wild cherry**

Burns (external)—Elder leaf, **goldenrod**, ragweed, red root, sumac, sweetfern, **witch hazel**

Breathing Difficulties and Wheezing—Goldenrod, **lobelia**

Bruises (external)—Elder leaf, fringetree, Solomon's seal, **witch hazel**

Bruises (internal)—Solomon's seal

Canker/Cold Sores—Red root, wild geranium, **yellowroot**

Congestion, Lung (see also Cold, Cough, Influenza, and Sinusitis)—Bee balm, bloodroot, **boneset**, **elder berry**, **elder flower**, goldenrod, pleurisy root, rabbit tobacco, ragweed, sassafras, spicebush, sweetgum, **wild cherry**

Circulation (stimulants)—Ginseng, red root, **wild ginger**

Colds (see also Bronchitis, Congestion)—Bee balm, boneset, **elder berry**, **elder flower**, goldenrod, Joe Pye weed, rabbit tobacco, sassafras, spicebush, sumac, sweetgum, wild cherry

Conjunctivitis (external)—Wild cherry, wild geranium, **yellowroot**

Constipation—Black walnut, **boneset**, elder berry, gentian, yellowroot

Cough (see also Bronchitis, Colds, Congestion)—Bee balm, **black cohosh**, bloodroot, blue cohosh, **elder berry**, elder flower, evening primrose, **pleurisy root**, rabbit tobacco, sarsaparilla, Solomon's seal, sumac, **wild cherry**, wild ginger

Cramps (see also Menstrual Cramps)—Black haw, lobelia, passionflower, skullcap, wild yam, wood betony

Cystitis—**Goldenrod**, Joe Pye weed,, wild hydrangea, wild yam

Debility/Weakness—Gentian, ginseng

Decongestant (See Congestion, Lung)

Diarrhea—Bee balm, goldenrod, ragweed, sumac, sweetfern, sweetgum, **wild geranium**, **witch hazel**

Diverticulitis—Black haw, Solomon's seal, wild yam

Drug/Alcohol Withdrawal—Skullcap

Earache (external)—Devil's walking stick

Eczema—Bloodroot, evening primrose, jewelweed, poke root, ragweed, red root (internal), sassafras (internal)

Endometriosis—Black cohosh, **blue cohosh**, partridgeberry, red root

Eye Irritation (external)—Evening primrose, ragweed, wild cherry, witch hazel

Fatigue—Gentian, **ginseng**, sarsaparilla, skullcap, Solomon's seal, wild cherry

Fever—Bee balm, **boneset**, elder berry, **elder flower**, mountain mint, sassafras, spicebush, sweetgum, sumac, wild cherry, wild ginger

Flatulence (gas)—Bee balm, mountain mint, sassafras, spicebush, sweetfern

Fibrocystic Breast Disease (see Breast Pain/Cysts)

Fibromyalgia—**Black cohosh**, partridgeberry, passionflower, skullcap

Fungal Infections—**Black walnut**, bloodroot, **yellowroot**

Gallbladder Inflammation/Stones—Fringetree, stoneroot, turtlehead

Gas (see Flatulence)

Gastritis—**Bee balm**, goldenrod, mountain mint, **Solomon's seal**, wild cherry, wild geranium, **wild yam**

Gingivitis—Bee balm, **bloodroot**, sumac, sweetfern, **yellowroot**

Glands (swollen)—Pleurisy root, **poke root, red root**

Gout—Sassafras, wild yam (acute)

Headache—Black cohosh, gentian, **passionflower, skullcap**

Hemorrhoids—Stoneroot, wild geranium, **witch hazel**

Heartburn—Bee balm, **gentian, goldenrod**, mountain mint, yellowroot

Hay Fever (see Allergies)

Hoarseness (see Laryngitis)

Immune Stimulant—**Boneset, elder berry**, elder flower, ginseng, sarsaparilla

Incontinence—Pipsissewa

Indigestion—**Bee balm**, bloodroot, boneset, **gentian**, ginseng, goldenrod, **mountain mint**, sassafras, **turtlehead**, wild cherry, yellowroot

Infections (See Bladder Infection, Respiratory Infection, Skin Infection, Viral Infection)

Infertility—Partridgeberry

Influenza—Bee balm, **boneset, elder berry**, elder flower, goldenrod, sassafras

Insect Bites (external)—Elder leaf, evening primrose, goldenrod, **jewelweed**, ragweed, wild geranium, **witch hazel**

Insomnia—Black cohosh, ginseng, **passionflower, skullcap**, wild cherry

Interstitial Cystitis—**Goldenrod**, Joe Pye weed, pipsissewa

Irritable Bowel Syndrome—Bee balm, black haw, passionflower, sassafras, sweetgum, wild cherry, **wild yam**

Itching/Skin Irritation (external)—Elder leaf, evening primrose, **jewelweed**, ragweed, sumac, sweetfern

Jaundice—Bloodroot, **fringetree**, red root, turtlehead

Joint Pain/Stiffness—Bee balm (external), black haw, devil's walking stick (berries), ginseng, Joe Pye weed, passionflower, **Solomon's seal**, **wood betony**

Kidney Stones—Goldenrod, **Joe Pye weed**, stoneroot, wild hydrangea

Kidney Tonic—Joe Pye weed, **pipsissewa**, wild hydrangea

Labor Tonics/Aids—**Black cohosh**, black haw, partridgeberry

Laryngitis (see also Sore Throat)—Elder flower, goldenrod, ragweed, **stoneroot**, wild cherry

Leucorrhea (see also Vaginitis)—Black walnut, partridgeberry, red root, sumac, sweetfern, wild geranium

Liver Tonics (Hepatic)—**Fringetree**, red root, turtlehead

Lung Congestion (see Congestion, Lung)

Menopause—**Black cohosh**, black haw, blue cohosh, partridgeberry, **skullcap**, wild yam

Menstruation (delayed)—Blue cohosh, partridgeberry, spicebush

Menstrual Cramps/Pain—**Black cohosh**, **black haw**, partridgeberry, passionflower, red root, **skullcap**, spicebush, wild yam

Menstruation (excessive bleeding)—**Black haw**, partridgeberry, sweetgum, wild geranium

Migraine headache—Lobelia, gentian, passionflower, **skullcap**

Miscarriage (threatened)—**Black haw**, partridgeberry

Morning Sickness—Bee balm, mountain mint, **wild ginger**, wild yam

Motion Sickness—Bee balm, mountain mint, **wild ginger**

Mouth ulcers (see also Canker/Cold Sores)—Bloodroot, red root, sumac, wild geranium, **yellowroot**

Muscle Stiffness/Sprains—**Black haw**, ginseng, passionflower, skullcap, **Solomon's seal**, wild yam, witch hazel, **wood betony**

Muscle Spasms—**Black haw**, lobelia, passionflower, skullcap, **wood betony**

Nausea—**Bee balm**, **mountain mint**, sassafras, sweetfern, sweetgum, **wild ginger**, wild yam

Nicotine (Cigarette) Withdrawal—Skullcap

Ovarian pain—Black haw, **blue cohosh**

Pain—Boneset, skullcap, wild ginger, wild hydrangea, wild yam, witch hazel, wood betony

Palpitations (Heart)—Black cohosh, black haw, **passionflower**, wild yam

Pertussis (see Whooping Cough)

Peptic Ulcers—Goldenrod, Solomon's seal, **yellowroot**

Poison Ivy Rash (external)—Elder leaf, **jewelweed**, ragweed, sassafras, sweetfern

Pre-Menstrual Syndrome (PMS)—**Black cohosh**, black haw, **blue cohosh**, **partridgeberry**, passionflower, skullcap, wild yam

Pregnancy (Fertility Tonics)—Blue cohosh, ginseng, **partridgeberry**

Pregnancy—Mountain mint, wild ginger, wild yam

Pregnancy (threatened miscarriage)—**Black haw**, blue cohosh, partridgeberry

Psoriasis—**Elder leaf**, evening primrose, goldenrod, jewelweed, red root (internal), sassafras (internal)

Prostatitis—Joe Pye weed, pipsissewa, stoneroot, wild hydrangea

Reproductive System Tonic (Female)—Partridgeberry

Respiratory Infections (see also Congestion, Lung, Cough, Decongestants, Viral Infections)—Bee balm, **boneset**, **elder berry**, **pleurisy root**, poke root, sarsaparilla, Solomon's seal, spicebush, stoneroot, **sweetgum**

Rheumatism—**Black cohosh**, black haw, boneset, devil's walking stick (berries), Joe Pye weed, poke root (berries), sassafras, wild yam, wood betony

Sciatica—Black haw, **skullcap**, wood betony

Skin Rash—**Elder leaf**, evening primrose, goldenrod, **jewelweed**, sumac, sweetfern, sweetgum, wild geranium

Skin Infection—Bloodroot, elder leaf, **sweetgum**, **yellowroot**

Sinusitis—Elder berry, elder flower, **goldenrod**, mountain mint, **ragweed**, yellowroot

Sore Throat—Evening primrose, goldenrod, **stoneroot**, sumac, sweetfern, **sweetgum**, wild cherry, wild ginger, witch hazel, yellowroot

Stress/Tension/Anxiety—**Evening primrose**, ginseng, **passionflower**, sarsaparilla, **skullcap**, wild cherry

Tinnitus—Black cohosh

Toothache (external)—Devil's walking stick (berries)

Uterine Fibroids—Blue cohosh, poke root

Uterine Pain—Black cohosh

Vaginitis (See Leucorrhea)

Varicose Veins—Stoneroot, witch hazel (external)

Vascular Tonic—Stoneroot

Viral Infections (see also Influenza)—**Boneset**, **elder berry**, poke root

Vomiting—Bee balm, mountain mint, sassafras, **wild ginger**

Warts—Bloodroot (external)

Whooping cough (see also Coughs, Decongestants)—**Black cohosh**, black haw, bloodroot, pleurisy root, wild cherry, wood betony

Worms/Parasites—Black walnut

Wounds (see also Bleeding)—Bloodroot, **elder leaf**, evening primrose, fringetree, goldenrod, **jewelweed**, sumac, sweet gum, yellowroot

Yeast Infections (Candidiasis)—Black walnut, yellowroot

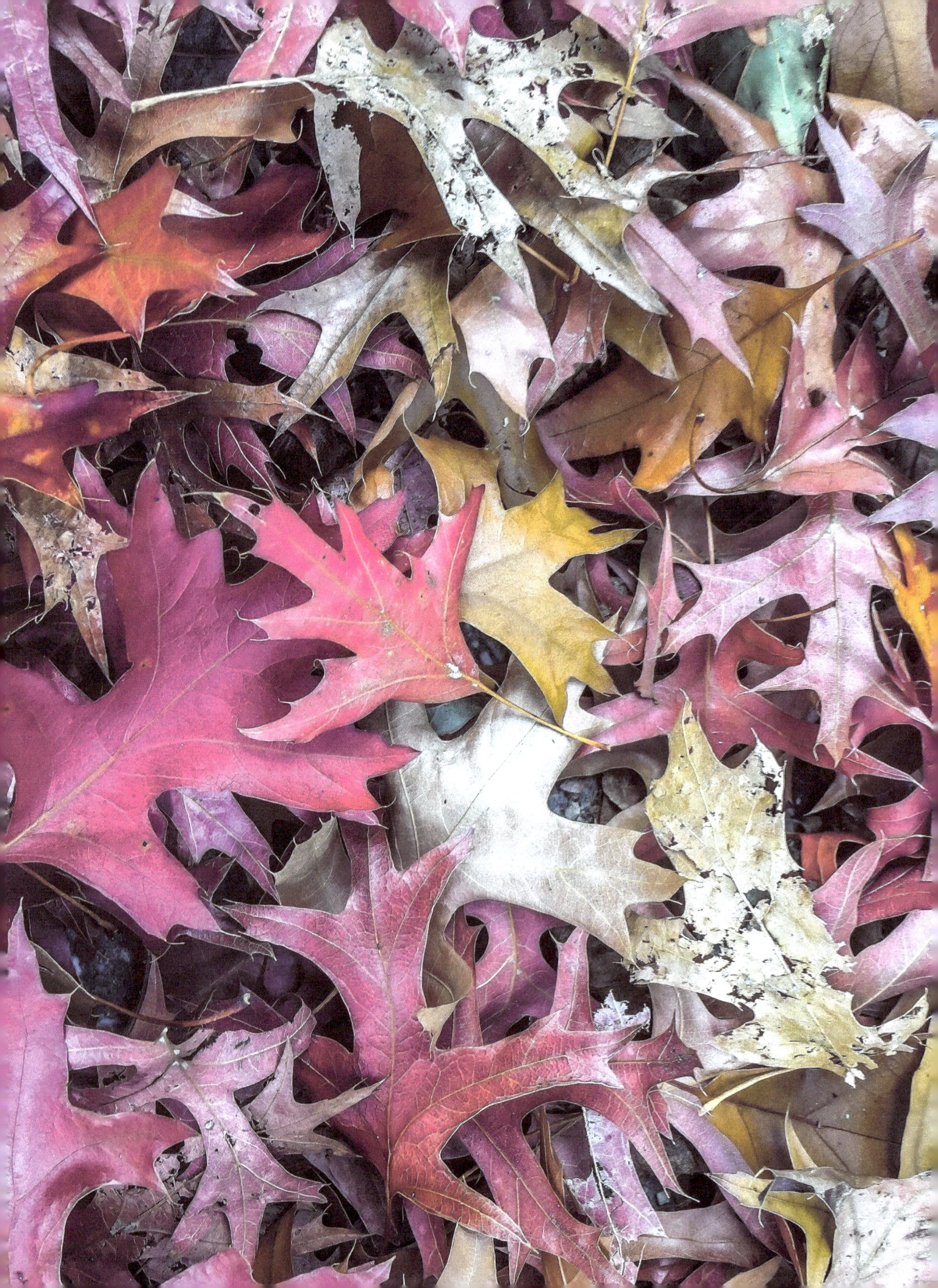

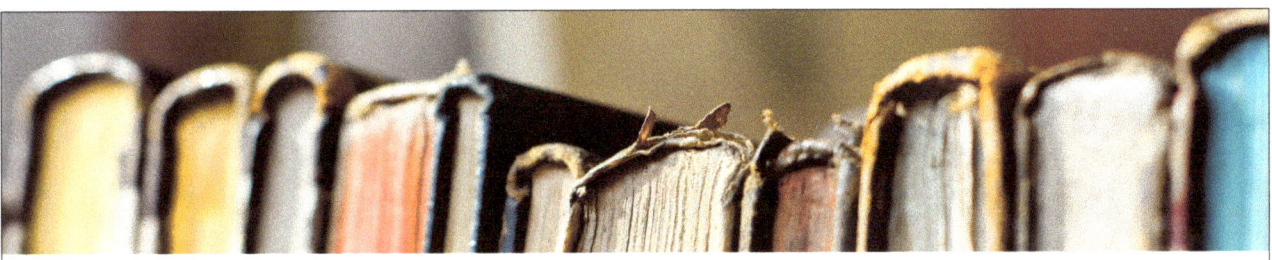

Bibliography

Bennett, Chris. *Southeast Foraging*. Timber Press. 2015.

Bergner, Paul. "Is Lobelia Toxic?" *Medical Herbalism,* Volume 10, No. 1 & 2. Spring and Summer, 1998.

Bergner, Paul and Jonathan Treasure. "The Lost Forms of Lobelia." *Medical Herbalism,* Volume 10, No. 1 & 2. Spring and Summer, 1998.

Brill, Steve "Wildman" with Evelyn Dean. *Identifying and Harvesting Edible and Medicinal Plants in Wild (and Not So Wild) Places.* Hearst Books/William Morrow and Co., Inc. 1994.

Brown, John Hull. *Early American Beverages*. C. E. Tuttle. 1966.

Brown, O. Phelps. *The Complete Herbalist, or The People Their Own Physicians*. Published by the author. 1897.

Carpenter, Jeff and Melanie Carpenter. *The Organic Medicinal Herb Farmer*. 2015.

Cavender, Anthony. *Folk Medicine of Southern Appalachia*. University of North Carolina Press. 2003.

Cech, Richo. *Making Plant Medicine*. Horizon Herbs Publications. 2000.

Cook, William H. *The Physio-Medical Dispensatory: A Treatise on Therapeutics, Materia Medica, and Pharmacy*. 1869. Reprint edition: Eclectic Medical Publications. 1985.

Covey, Herbert C. *African American Slave Medicine: Herbal and Non-Herbal*. Lexington Books, 2007.

Crellin, James A. and Jane Philpott. *A Reference Guide to Medicinal Plants: Herbal Medicine Past and Present*. 2 volumes. Duke University Press. 1990.

Dana, Mrs. William Starr. *How to Know the Wildflowers*. Dover Books. 1963.

Densmore, Frances. *How Indians Use Wild Plants for Food, Medicine and Crafts*. United States Government Printing Office.1928. Reprint edition: Dover Books. 1974.

Easley, Thomas and Steven Horne. *The Modern Herbal Dispensatory: A Medicine-Making Guide*. North Atlantic Books. 2016.

Elliott, Doug. *Wild Roots: A Foragers Guide to the Edible and Medicinal Roots, Tubers, Corms and Rhizomes of North America*. Healing Arts Press. 1995.

Elpel, Thomas. *Botany in a Day*. 4th edition. HOPS Press. 2001.

Erichsen-Brown, Charlotte. *Medicinal and Other Uses of North American Plants: A Historical Survey with Special Reference to Eastern Indian Tribes*. Dover Books. 1989.

Felter, Harvey, M.D. *The Eclectic Materia Medica, Pharmacology, and Therapeutics*. 1927. Reprint edition: Eclectic Medical Publications. 1989.

Felter, Harvey Wickes, and John Uri Lloyd. *King's American Dispensatory*. 18th edition. 1898. Reprint edition: Eclectic Medical Publications. 1983.

Foster, Steven and James A. Duke. *A Field Guide to Medicinal Plants and Herbs of Eastern and Central North America*. 2nd edition. Houghton Mifflin Company. 2000.

Gibbons, Euell. *Stalking The Wild Asparagus*. David McKay Company, Inc. 1962.

Gladstar, Rosemary and Pam Hirch, ed. *Planting the Future: Saving Our Medicinal Herbs*. Healing Arts Press. 2000.

Grieve, Mrs. M. *A Modern Herbal, Volumes I and II*. Dover Books. 1971.

Hamel, Paul B. and Mary U. Chiltoskey. *Cherokee Plants: Their Uses: A 400 Year History*. Cherokee Publications. 1975.

Harrington, H.D. and L.W. Durrell. *How to Identify Plants*. Swallow Press. 1957. 2nd edition. 1981.

Hemmerly, Thomas E. *Appalachian Wildflowers*. University of Georgia Press. 2000.

Hoffmann, David. *Medical Herbalism: The Science, Principles and Practice of Herbal Medicine*. Healing Arts Press. 2003.

Hutchins, Alma. *Indian Herbology of North America*. 9th edition. Merco. 1983.

Hutson, Robert W., William F. Hutson and Aaron J. Sharp. *Great Smoky Mountain Wildflowers*. 5th edition. Windy Pines Publishing. 1995.

Justice, William S. and C. Ritchie Bell. *Wildflowers of North Carolina*. University of North Carolina Press. 1968.

Kindscher, Kelly. *Medicinal Wild Plants of the Prairie*. University Press of Kansas. 1992.

Krochmal, Arnold, Russell Walters and Richard Doughty. *A Guide to Medicinal Plants of Appalachia*. Agricultural Handbook No. 400. Forest Service, US Department of Agriculture. 1971.

Kuhn, Merrily A. and David Winston. *Herbal Therapy and Supplements: A Scientific and Traditional Approach*. Lippincott Williams and Wilcox. 2000.

Lee, Michele E. *Working the Roots: Over 400 Years of Traditional African American Healing*. Wadastick. 2017.

Light, Phyllis D. *Southern Folk Medicine: Healing Traditions from the Appalachian Fields and Forests*. North Atlantic Books. 2018.

Lighthall, J. I. *The Indian Folk Medicine Guide*. Popular Library. 1973.

Matthews, Hugh A. *Leaves from the Notebook of an Appalachian Physician.* H. A. Matthews / Macon Graphics. 1980.

Moerman, Daniel E. *Native American Ethnobotany.* Timber Press. 1998.

Mooney, James. *"The Swimmer Manuscript: Cherokee Formulas and Medicinal Prescriptions."* Smithsonian Institution Bureau of American Ethnology, Bulletin 99. Revised and edited by Frans M. Olbrechts. United States Government Printing Office. 1932.

Moss, Kay K. *Southern Folk Medicine 1750 -1820.* University of South Carolina Press. 1999.

Newcomb, Lawrence, Gordon Morrison. *Newcomb's Wildflower Guide.* Little, Brown and Co. 1989.

Patton, Darryl. *Tommie Bass: Herb Doctor of Shinbone Ridge.* Back to Nature Publications. 1988.

Persons, W. Scott and Jeanine M. Davis. *Ginseng, Goldenseal & Other Woodland Medicinals.* 2nd edition. New Society Publishers. 2014.

Porcher, Frances P. *Resources of the Southern Fields and Forests.* Evans and Cogswell. 1863. Reprint edition: Arno Press. 1970.

Radford, Albert E., Harry E. Ahles and C. Ritchie Bell. *Manual of the Vascular Flora of the Carolinas.* University of North Carolina Press. 1968.

Romm, Aviva. *Botanical Medicine for Women's Health.* Churchill Livingston. 2010.

Shane, CoreyPine. *Southeast Medicinal Plants: Identify, Harvest, and Use 106 Wild Herbs for Health and Wellness.* Timber Press. 2021.

Shook, Edward. *Advanced Treatise in Herbology.* 1946. Reprint edition: Trinity Center Press. 1978.

Sinadinos, Christa. *The Essential Guide to Western Botanical Medicine.* Published by the author. 2020.

Skenderi, Gazmend. *Herbal Vade Mecum: 800 Herbs, Spices, Essential Oils, Etc. – Constituents, Properties, Uses, and Cautions.* Createspace. 2003.

Smith, Richard M. *Wildflowers of the Southern Mountains.* University of Tennessee Press. 1998.

Spira, Timothy P. *Wildflowers and Plant Communities of the Southern Appalachian Mountains and Piedmont.* University of North Carolina. 2011.

Sumner, Judith. *American Household Botany.* Timber Press. 2012.

Weakley, Alan S. *Plants of the Southern and Mid-Atlantic States.* 2010.

Winston, David. *"Nvwoti: Cherokee Medicine and Ethnobotany"* Journal of the American Herbalists Guild, Fall/Winter. 2001.

Wigginton, Elliot, ed. *Foxfire 3.* Anchor Press/Doubleday. 1975.

Wigginton, Elliot and Margie Bennett, ed. *Foxfire 9.* Anchor Press/Doubleday. 1986.

Wofford, B. Eugene. *Guide to the Vascular Plants of the Blue Ridge.* University of Georgia Press. 1989.

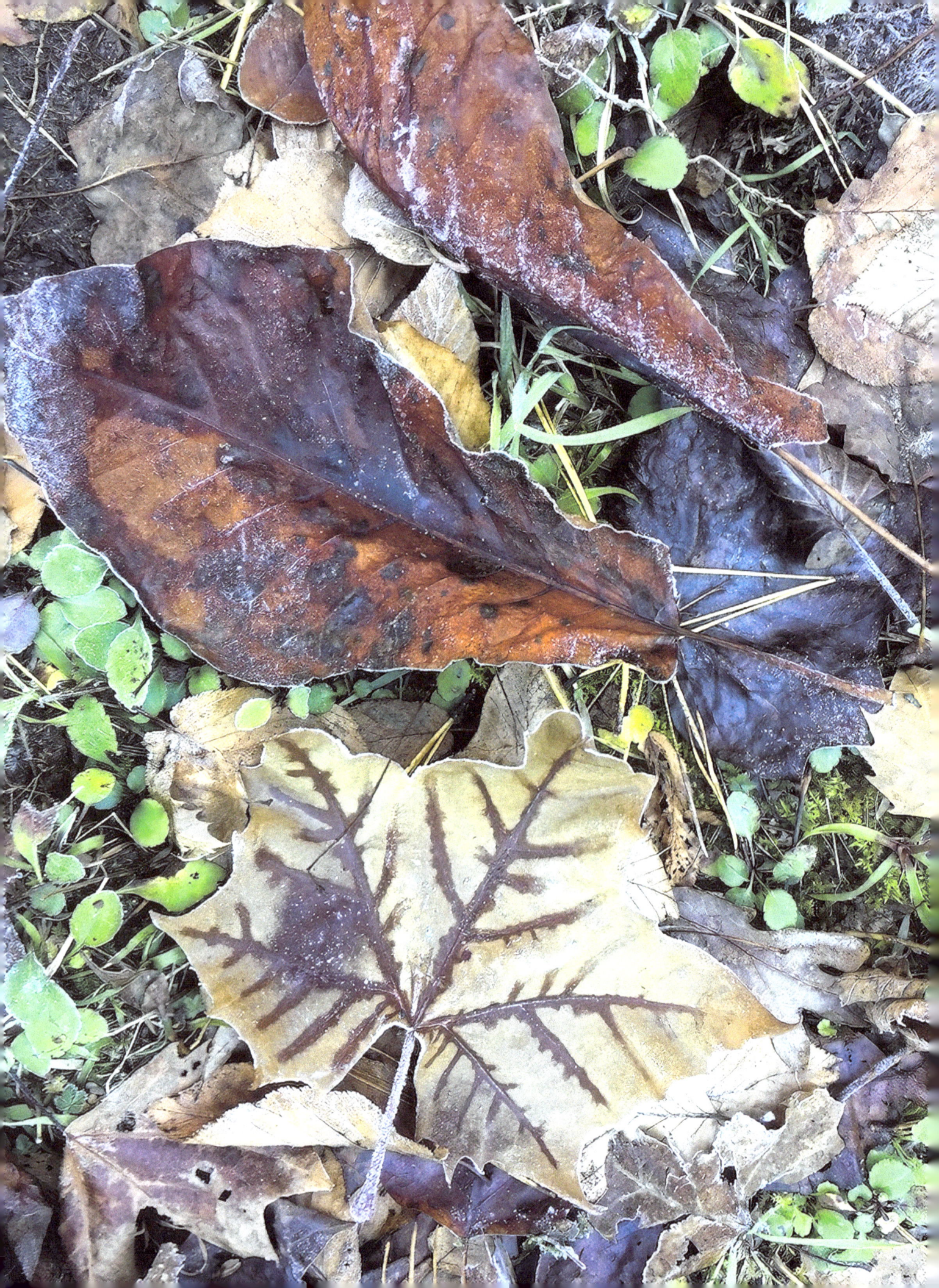

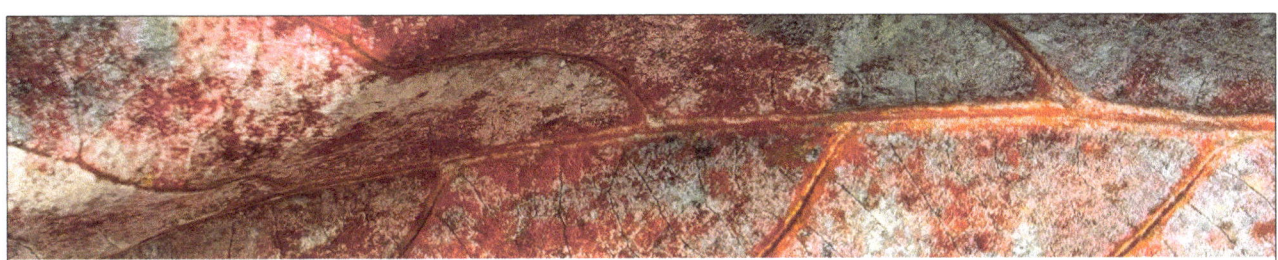

Index

A

Aaron's rod, 89
Abscess, see boils
Acne, 175, 237
Actaea pachypoda, 37
Actaea racemosa (Black cohosh), 35 – 37, 145, 160
Adaptogen
    Ginseng, 83
Ague tree, 149
Ague weed
    Boneset, 55
    Gentian, 79
Alcohol extracts, 18
Allergic reactions
    Blue cohosh, 35
    Lobelia, 101
Allergies, seasonal
    Elder, 65
    Goldenrod, 89
    Ragweed, 137
Alterative
    Pipsissewa, 119
    Poke root, 127
    Red root, 141
    Sarsaparilla, 145
    Sassafras, 149
    Sweetfern, 175
Alumroot, 195
Ambrosia spp. (Ragweed), 137 – 139
American ginseng *(Panax quinquefolius)*, 83 – 87, 146
American tormentil, 195
American walnut, 43
Anacardiaceae, 171
Anal fistula, 168 – 169

Analgesic
    Bee balm, 31
    Black cohosh, 35
    Boneset, 55
    Joe Pye weed, 97
    Wild hydrangea, 203
Angelica tree, 61
Anise-scented goldenrod, 89
Anodyne
    Blue cohosh, 51
Anti-catarrhal
    Boneset, 55
    Elder, 65
    Goldenrod, 90
    Pleurisy root, 123
Anti-depressant, 229
Anti-emetic, see nausea
Anti-fungal, 229
    Black walnut, 43
    Yellowroot, 219
Anti-helmintic
    Black walnut, 43
Antihistamine, 137
Anti-inflammatory
    Bee balm, 31
    Black cohosh, 35
    Black haw, 39
    Bloodroot, 47
    Devil's walking stick, 61
    Fringetree, 75
    Jewelweed, 93
    Joe Pye weed, 97
    Mountain mint, 107
    Pipsissewa, 119
    Pleurisy root, 123

Rabbit tobacco, 133
Stoneroot, 167
Turtlehead, 185
Wild cherry, 189
Wild geranium, 195
Wild yam, 207
Witch hazel, 211
Wood betony, 215

Anti-lithic, see kidney stones
Anti-rheumatic, see rheumatism
Antiseptic
Black walnut, 43
Pipsissewa, 119
Sweetgum, 179
Yellowroot, 219

Anti-spasmodic
Bee balm, 31
Black cohosh, 35
Black haw, 39
Bloodroot, 47
Blue cohosh, 51
Evening primrose, 71
Lobelia, 101
Mountain mint, 107
Rabbit tobacco, 133
Skullcap, 155
Wild cherry, 189
Wild yam, 207
Witch hazel, 211
Wood betony, 215

Anti-viral
Boneset, 55
Elder, 65
Sweetgum, 179

Anxiety
Black cohosh, 35
Passionflower, 115
Skullcap, 155
Sweetgum, 179

Appetite, lack of
Boneset, 55
Fringetree, 75
Gentian, 80
Pipsissewa, 119
Solomon's seal, 160
Turtlehead, 185

Aralia nudicaulis (Sarsparilla), 145 – 147
Aralia spinosa (Devil's walking stick), 61 – 63
Araliaceae, 61, 83, 145
Arrow-wood, 39
Arthritis (Osteoarthritis)
Black cohosh, 35
Black haw, 39
Blue cohosh, 51
Devil's walking stick, 61
Evening primrose (oil), 71
Poke root, 127
Wild yam, 207

Asarum canadense (Wild ginger), 48, 83, 199 – 201
Asclepiadaceae, 123
Asclepias tuberosa (Pleurisy root), 123 – 125
Asteraceae, 31, 55, 89, 97, 133, 137

Asthma
Black cohosh, 35
Black haw, 39
Blue cohosh, 51
Evening primrose, 71
Lobelia, 101
Rabbit tobacco, 133
Red root, 141

Asthma weed, 101

Astringent
Black haw, 39
Black walnut, 43
Elder, 65
Goldenrod, 89
Jewelweed, 93
Joe Pye weed, 97
Partridgeberry, 111
Rabbit tobacco, 133
Ragweed, 137
Red root, 141
Sumac, 171
Sweetfern, 175
Sweetgum, 179
Wild cherry, 189
Wild geranium, 195
Witch hazel, 211
Yellowroot, 219

Attention Deficit Disorder, 71, 230
Attention Deficit/Hyperactivity Disorder, 71, 230

B

Back pain, see anti-inflammatory, anti-spasmodic, analgesic, anodyne, nervine, sedative
    Black haw, 39
    Skullcap, 155
    Wild hydrangea, 203
    Wood Betony, 215
Balmony, 185
Balsaminaceae, 93
Bark, how to harvest sustainably, 183
Barberry family, 51
Basal cell carcinoma, 48
Bass, A.L. Tommie, 3, 31, 57, 61, 98, 220
Bath, herbal, 24
Bee balm *(Monarda spp.)*, 115 – 117
Beeswax, in salves, 27, 234
Belching, 32, 57, 80
Berberidaceae, 51
Bergamot oil, 44
Beverage teas
    Bee balm, 31
    Elder, 65
    Mountain mint, 107
    Red root, 141
    Sassafras, 149
    Spicebush, 163
    Sumac, 171
Bitters, about, 9, 91, 230
    Black walnut, 43
    Boneset, 55
    Fringetree, 75
    Gentian, 79
    Skullcap, 155
    Turtlehead, 185
    Yellowroot, 219
Black cherry, 189
Black cohosh *(Actaea racemosa)*, 3, 35 – 37, 51, 73, 83, 145, 160, 192
Black haw *(Viburnum prunifolium)*, 39 – 41, 76, 105
Black snakeroot, 35
Black walnut *(Juglans nigra)*, 43 – 45
Bladder disease, 98
Bladder infection, 92
Blakely, Tim, 13
Bleeding, see hemorrhage, menses (excessive), styptic

Bloating and gas
    Bee balm, 31
    Bloodroot, 47
    Boneset, 55
    Gentian, 79
    Red root, 141
    Spicebush, 163
    Sweetfern, 175
    Turtlehead, 185
Blood pressure, high (hypertension)
    Passionflower, 115
    Wild hydrangea, 203
Blood tonic, 145
Bloodroot *(Sanguinaria canadensis)*, 3, 47 – 49, 83, 160, 192
Bloom calendar, 224 – 225
Blue cohosh *(Caulophyllum thalictroides)*, 1, 2, 35, 51 – 53
Blue Mountain tea, 90
Boils, compresses for, 23
    Elder, 72
    Passionflower, 115
    Sweetgum, 179
    Turtlehead, 186
Boneset *(Eupatorium perfoliatum)*, 3, 22, 97, 192
Boneset Syrup recipe, 59
Botanical names, 13
Botany in a Day (book), 8
Bottle gentian, 79
Breast inflammation and pain
    Elder, 65
    Partridgeberry, 111
    Poke root, 127
    Red root, 133
    Solomon's seal, 159
    Stoneroot, 167
    Turtlehead, 185
    Wild ginger, 199
Breathing difficulties
    Black haw, 39
    Bloodroot, 47
    Ginseng, 83
    Lobelia, 101
    Passionflower, 115
    Pleurisy root, 123
    Solomon's seal, 159
Bronchial dilators, see bronchial spasm

Bronchial spasm, see bronchitis, congestion (respiratory), cough
    Bee balm, 31
    Bloodroot, 47
    Blue cohosh, 51
    Lobelia, 101
    Pleurisy root, 123

Bronchitis, see bronchial spasm, congestion (respiratory), cough
    Bee balm, 31
    Black cohosh, 35
    Blue cohosh, 51
    Bloodroot, 47
    Boneset, 55
    Ginseng, 83
    Pleurisy root, 123
    Red root, 141
    Sarsaparilla, 145
    Wild cherry, 189

Bruises
    Bee balm, 31
    Elder, 65
    Evening primrose, 71
    Fringetree, 75
    Solomon's seal, 159
    Stoneroot, 167
    Witch hazel, 211
    Buckthorn family, 141

Bugbane, 35
Bug bites, see insect bites
Bugwort, 35
Burns
    Elder, 65
    Goldenrod, 89
    Red root, 141
    Sumac, 171
    Sweetfern, 175
    Wild hydrangea, 203
    Witch hazel, 211
Butterfly weed, 123

C

Cabrera, Chanchal, 105
Campanulaceae, 101
Cancer salves, bloodroot in, 48
Candidiasis, 44

Canker sores, 195, 219
Caprifoliaceae, 39, 65
Cardamom, 81
Cardinal flower, 101
Cardio-stimulant
    Pleurisy root, 123
    Stoneroot, 167
Carminative
    Bee balm, 31
    Ginseng, 83
    Mountain mint, 107
    Sassafras, 149
    Sweetfern, 175
    Sweetgum, 179
    Wild ginger, 199
Carolina cranesbill, 195
Cashew family, 171
Cathartic
    Bloodroot, 47
    Poke root, 127
    Turtlehead, 185
Caulophyllum thalictroides (Blue cohosh), 2, 35, 51–53, 145, 160
Cavender, Anthony, 3
Ceanothus americanus (Red root), 141–143
Centers for Disease Control, 5
Ceremonial herbs
    Rabbit tobacco, 133
    Solomon's seal, 159
    Sumac, 171
    Sweetfern, 175
Checkerberry, 111
Chelone spp. (Turtlehead), 9, 185–187
Cherokee people, herbs used by, 2
    Bee balm, 31
    Black cohosh, 35
    Boodroot, 47
    Devil's walking stick, 61
    Jewelweed, 93
    Joe Pye weed, 97
    Lobelia, 101
    Mountain mint, 107
    Passionflower, 115
    Pipsissewa, 119
    Rabbit tobacco, 133
    Ragweed, 137

    Sarsaparilla, 145
    Skullcap, 155
    Solomon's Seal, 159
    Wild cherry, 189
    Wild ginger, 199
    Witch hazel, 211
    Yellowroot, 219
Chewing gum, 180
Chimaphila spp. (Pipsissewa), 119 – 121, 204
Chionanthus virginica (Fringetree), 75 – 77
Choke cherry, 189
Cholagogue
    Fringetree, 75
    Turtlehead, 185
Cimicifuga racemosa (Black cohosh), 35 – 37
Cinnamon wood, 149
Circulatory stimulant
    Devil's walking stick, 61
    Stoneroot, 167
Civil War, herbs used during
    Black walnut, 39
    Boneset, 55
    Pipsissewa, 119
    Poke root, 127
    Spicebush, 163
    Sumac, 171
    Sweetgum, 179
    Turtlehead, 185
Cleavers, 128
Closed gentian, 79
Cold sores, 196
Colds
    Bee balm, 31
    Black cohosh, 35
    Boneset, 55
    Elder, 65
    Goldenrod, 89
    Mountain mint, 107
    Pipsissewa, 119
    Pleurisy root, 123
    Rabbit tobacco, 133
    Sassafras, 149
    Sumac, 171
    Sweetgum, 179
    Wild cherry, 189

Colic
    Bee balm, 31
    Blue cohosh, 51
    Ginseng, 83
    Lobelia, 101
    Wild ginger, 199
    Wild yam, 207
Colic root
    Pleurisy root, 123
    Wild yam, 207
Collinsonia canadensis (Stoneroot), 167 – 169
Coltsfoot, 49, 192
Common names of plants, 7 – 8
Compresses, about, 23
Comptonia peregrina (Sweetfern), 175 – 177
Concentration, improved, 84
Congestion (respiratory)
    Bee balm, 31
    Bloodroot, 47
    Boneset, 55
    Elder, 65
    Goldenrod, 89
    Mountain mint, 107
    Pleurisy root, 123
    Rabbit tobacco, 133
    Sweetgum, 179
    Wild cherry, 189
    Wild ginger, 199
Conjunctivitis, 196
Constipation
    Boneset, 55
    Gentian, 79
    Ginseng, 83
    Red root, 141
    Solomon's seal, 159
    Turtlehead, 185
Contusions, see bruises
Convulsions, 102
Cough, see bronchial spasm, bronchitis, congestion (respiratory)
    Bee balm, 31
    Black cohosh, 35
    Bloodroot, 47
    Blue cohosh, 51
    Elder, 65
    Ginseng, 83

  Goldenrod, 89
  Lobelia, 101
  Pleurisy root, 123
  Rabbit tobacco, 133
  Red root, 141
  Sarsaparilla, 145
  Solomon's seal, 159
  Spicebush, 163
  Sumac, 171
  Sweetgum, 179
  Wild cherry, 189
  Wild ginger, 199
Cradle cap, 44
Crampbark, 39
Cramps, muscle, see menstrual cramps
  Bee balm, 31
  Black haw, 39
  Blue cohosh, 51
  Lobelia, 101
  Mountain mint, 107
  Partridgeberry, 111
  Passionflower, 115
  Skullcap, 155
  Wild yam, 207
  Wood betony, 215
Cranesbill, 195
Creole cooking, 149
Crohn's disease, 40
Croup, see colds, congestion (respiratory)
  Black cohosh, 36
  Lobelia, 101
Cystitis
  Goldenrod, 89
  Joe Pye weed, 97
  Pipsissewa, 119
  Wild hydrangea, 203

D

Decoctions, about, 16 – 17
Decongestant, see antihistamine, congestion (respiratory), anti-catarrhal
Delayed menses, see menses, delayed
Demulcent
  Evening primrose, 71
  Sassafras, 149
  Solomon's seal, 159

Deodorant, 167
Depression
  Black cohosh, 36
  Ginseng, 84
  Skullcap, 156
Devil's walking stick *(Aralia spinosa)*, 61 – 63
Diabetes (Type II)
  Fringetree, 75
  Joe Pye weed, 98
Diaphoretic
  Bee balm, 31
  Boneset, 55
  Elder, 65
  Goldenrod, 92
  Mountain mint, 107
  Sassafras, 149
  Spicebush, 163
  Stoneroot, 167
  Wild cherry, 189
  Wild ginger, 199
Diarrhea
  Goldenrod, 90
  Partridgeberry, 111
  Ragweed, 137
  Red root, 143
  Sassafras, 149
  Sumac, 172
  Sweetfern, 175
  Sweetgum, 179
  Wild cherry, 189
  Wild geranium, 195
  Witch hazel, 211
  Wood betony, 215
Digestive bitter
  Boneset, 55
  Gentian, 79
  Yellowroot, 219
Digestive Bitters recipe, 81
Dioscorea spp. (Wild yam), 207 – 209
Dioscoreaceae, 207
Diuretic
  Fringetree, 75
  Joe Pye weed, 97
  Pipsissewa, 119
  Wild hydrangea, 203
Diverticulitis, 207

Doll's eyes, 37
Dosage, about, 14
Douche, about, 33
Dove's foot, 177
Dowsing, 212
Dreams, 84
Drug and alcohol withdrawal, 156
Dry skin, 25, 27, 67, 160, 161
Dye plants
    Black walnut, 43
    Bloodroot, 47
    Sumac, 171
    Yellowroot, 219
Dysentery, see diarrhea

E

Earache
    Devil's walking stick, 61
    Passionflower, 115
Eclectic physicians, 44, 56, 76, 231
Eczema
    Black walnut, 43
    Bloodroot, 47
    Evening primrose, 71
    Fringetree, 75
    Poke root, 127
    Sassafras, 149
Edible plants, see wild foods
Elder (*Sambucus canadensis*), 10, 56, 58, 65 – 69, 97, 192
Elder Rob Syrup recipe, 69
Elecampane, 147, 197
Elpel, Thomas, 8
Emetic
    Bloodroot, 47
    Boneset, 55
    Devil's walking stick, 61
    Lobelia, 101
    Poke root, 127
Emmenagogue
    Bee Balm, 31
    Black cohosh, 35
    Bloodroot, 47
    Blue cohosh, 51
    Gentian, 79
    Skullcap, 155

Emollient
    Elder, 65
    Evening primrose, 71
    Jewelweed, 93
Endometriosis
    Black cohosh, 35
    Blue cohosh, 51
    Partridgeberry, 111
Enemas, about, 16, 24
Energy
    Ginseng, 83
    Pipsissewa, 119
    Sarsaparilla, 145
Engaging with Aromas (Tip), 176
Epilepsy (convulsions), 102
Escharotic, 47
Essential fatty acids, 72
Eupatorium perfoliatum (Boneset), 3, 22, 55 – 59, 97, 192
Eutrochium spp. (Joe Pye weed), 97 – 99, 204
Evening primrose (*Oenothera biennis*), 71 – 73
Exhaustion, see energy, fatigue
Expectorant
    Bloodroot, 47
    Boneset, 55
    Elder, 65
    Lobelia, 101
    Pleurisy root, 123
    Rabbit tobacco, 133
    Solomon's seal, 159
    Spicebush, 163
    Sumac, 171
    Sweetgum, 179
    Wild cherry, 189
Eye, irritation or inflammation, see conjunctivitis, sties
    Elder, 65
    Sassafras, 149
    Wild cherry, 189

F

Fairy torches, 35
False Solomon's seal, 159
Family names of plants, 7
Farewell-to-summer, 89
Fatigue
    Gentian, 79
    Ginseng, 83

  Goldenrod, 89
  Pipsissewa, 119
  Sarsaparilla, 145
  Skullcap, 155
Febrifuge, see fever
Fennel seed, 81
Fertility herbs for women, see infertility
Fever
  Bee balm, 31
  Boneset, 55
  Elder, 65
  Fringetree, 75
  Ginseng, 83
  Goldenrod, 89
  Joe Pye weed, 97
  Mountain mint, 107
  Pipsissewa, 119
  Sassafras, 149
  Spicebush, 163
  Sumac, 171
  Sweetgum, 179
  Wild cherry, 18
  Wild ginger, 199
  Witch hazel, 211
Fibrocystic breast disease
  Poke root, 127
  Red root, 141
Fibroid tumors, 58
Fibromyalgia, 36
Filé gumbo, 149
Fistula, anal, 168
Flameleaf sumac, 171
Fleas, 43
Folk method for tinctures, 20 – 21
Food and Drug Administration (FDA), 5, 150
Foot bath, 24
Foxfire books, 3
Fringetree *(Chionanthus virginica)*, 75 – 77
Fungal infections
  Black walnut, 43
  Bloodroot, 47
  Yellowroot, 219

G

Galium aparine, 128
Gallbladder inflammation
  Fringetree, 75
  Turtlehead, 185
  Wild hydrangea, 203
Gallstones
  Fringetree, 75
  Gentian, 79
  Stoneroot, 167
Gamma-linolenic acid, 72
Gas, see bloating
Gastric ulcers, 80
Gastritis, 160, see anti-inflammatory, demulcent, indigestion
Gentian *(Gentian spp.)*, 79 – 81
Gentian Digestive Bitters recipe, 81
Gentian family, 79
Gentianaceae, 79
Geraniaceae, 195
Geranium spp. (Wild geranium), 195
Geranium family, 195
Ginger, tropical, 200
Ginseng family, 61, 83
Ginseng, American *(Panax quinquefolius)*, 2, 3, 83 – 87
Ginseng, harvesting, 87
Gnaphalium obtusifolium (Rabbit tobacco), 48, 56, 59,
  133 – 135, 147, 192
Goldenrod *(Solidago spp.)*, 7, 8, 79, 89 – 91, 138, 139
Goldenseal, 3, 220
Gout, 203
Grain alcohol, about, 19
Granddad's beard, 75
Gravel root, 97
Greater Solomon's seal, 159
Gum disease or inflammation
  Bloodroot, 47
  Sumac, 171
  Sweetfern, 175
  Yellowroot, 219

H

Hairy Solomon's seal, 159
Hamamelidaceae, 179, 211
Hamamelis virginiana, 211 – 213
Hand bath, 24
Harvest calendar, 226 – 227
Harvesting plants, 11
Hayfever, see Allergies, seasonal

Hayfever weed, 137
Headache, 23
    Bee balm, 31
    Blue cohosh, 51
    Boneset, 55
    Gentian, 79
    Goldenrod, 89
    Mountain mint, 107
    Passionflower, 115
    Rabbit tobacco, 133
    Skullcap, 155
    Stoneroot, 167
    Sweetfern, 175
    Wild ginger, 199
Heart palpitations
    Black haw, 39
    Lobelia, 101
    Passionflower, 115
    Wild cherry, 189
Heartburn
    Goldenrod, 89
    Yellowroot, 219
Heartleaf, 199
Hemorrhage, 195
Hemorrhoids
    Evening primrose, 71
    Partridgeberry, 111
    Poke root, 127
    Stoneroot, 167
    Sumac, 171
    Turtlehead, 185
    Wild geranium, 195
    Witch hazel, 211
Hepatic
    Fringetree, 75
    Gentian, 72
    Turtlehead, 185
    Yellowroot, 194
Hepatitis, see hepatic
Herbal actions, about, 9
Herbal salves, about, 27
Herbal teas, about, 15 – 19
Hercules' club, 61
Herpes, 44
Hexastylis spp. (Wild ginger), 199
Hiccups, 51

High blood pressure, see blood pressure, high
High cholesterol, 72
Hives, see skin rash
Hoary mountain mint, 107
Honeysuckle family, 39, 65
Horehound, 192
Horsebalm, 167
Horsemint, 167
Horseweed, 167
Hot flashes, 36
How to Harvest Bark Sustainably (Tip), 183
Hydrangea arborescens (Wild hydrangea), 203 – 205
Hydrastis canadensis, 220
Hydrophobia, 155
Hypertension, see blood pressure, high

I

Ice cubes, jewelweed, 95
Immune stimulant
    Boneset, 55
    Ginseng, 83
Impatiens spp. (Jewelweed), 93 – 95, 97, 135, 185
Incontinence
    Joe Pye weed, 97
    Pipsissewa, 119
Indian paint, 47
Indian sage, 55
Indian tobacco, 101
Indigestion, 161
    Bee balm, 31
    Bloodroot, 47
    Boneset, 55
    Evening primrose, 71
    Fringetree, 75
    Gentian, 79
    Ginseng, 83
    Goldenrod, 89
    Mountain mint, 107
    Sassafras, 149
    Turtlehead, 185
    Wild ginger, 199
    Yellowroot, 219
Infants and children, herbs for
    Bee balm, 31
    Elder, 65
    Ginseng, 83

    Goldenrod, 89
    Jewelweed, 93
    Passionflower, 115
    Pipsissewa, 119
    Sarsaparilla, 145
    Stoneroot, 167
Infections, see bladder, fungal, skin, yeast
Infertility (women)
    Blue cohosh, 51
    Partridgeberry, 111
Influenza
    Bee balm, 31
    Boneset, 55
    Elder, 65
    Goldenrod, 89
Infused herbal oil, about, 25 – 27
Infusions, about, 15 – 17
Ink, 128
Insect bites
    Jewelweed, 93
    Ragweed, 133
    Witch hazel, 211
Insomnia, 24
    Black cohosh, 36
    Elder, 65
    Ginseng, 83
    Passionflower, 115
    Skullcap, 155
    Wild cherry, 189
Interstitial cystitis
    Goldenrod, 89
    Joe Pye weed, 97
    Wild hydrangea, 203
Intestinal cramps
    Bee balm, 31
    Black haw, 39
    Wild yam, 207
Intestinal worms and parasites, 40
Inula helenium (Elecampane), 147, 197
Irritable Bowel Syndrome (IBS), see intestinal cramps, demulcents
    Black haw, 39
    Sassafras, 149
    Wild yam, 207
Itching, see skin rash

J

Jaundice
    Bloodroot, 47
    Fringetree, 75
    Gentian, 79
    Turtlehead, 185
    Yellowroot, 219
Jewelweed (*Impatiens spp.*), 93 – 95
Joe Pye weed *(Eutrochium spp.)*, 97 – 99
Joint inflammation/pain
    Bee balm, 32
    Blue cohosh, 51
    Boneset, 55
    Devil's walking stick, 61
    Joe Pye weed, 97
    Lobelia, 105
    Pipsissewa, 119
    Sarsaparilla, 145
    Solomon's seal, 159
    Wood betony, 215
Jopi, 98
Juglandaceae, 43
Juglans nigra (Black walnut), 43

K

Kidney stones
    Fringetree, 75
    Goldenrod, 89
    Joe Pye weed, 97
    Pipsissewa, 119
    Stoneroot, 167
    Wild hydrangea, 203

L

Labor aid/tonics
    Black cohosh, 35
    Black haw, 39
    Partridgeberry, 111
    Skullcap, 155
    Wild cherry, 189
Lamiaceae, **31**, 107, 155, 167
Laryngitis
    Goldenrod, 89
    Stoneroot, 167
    Wood betony, 215

Lauraceae, 149
Laurel family, 149
Laxative
    Black walnut, 43
    Boneset, 55
    Elder, 65
    Gentian, 79
    Turtlehead, 185
Lemonade recipe, 173
Leucorrhea, see vaginitis
Life everlasting, 133
Liliaceae, 159
Lily family, 159
Lindera benzoin (Spicebush), 163 – 165
Linoleic acid, 72
Liquidambar styraciflua (Sweetgum), 179 – 181, 192
Lithotropic, see anti-lithic
Little brown jug, 199
Liver congestion, see hepatics
    Bloodroot, 47
    Fringetree, 75
    Red root, 141
    Turtlehead, 185
    Wild hydrangea, 203
Liver disease, see hepatics
Liver tonic, see hepatics
Lobelia (*Lobelia inflata*), 101 – 105
Lobelia spp., 101 – 105
Lobelia Liniment recipe, 105
Lobelia Traditional Tincture recipe, 104
Longevity tonic
    Ginseng, 83
    Solomon's seal, 159
Lousewort, 215
Love charm, 48
Lung congestion, see congestion (respiratory)
Lydia Pinkham's Vegetable Compound for Females, 39
Lymphatic, 142
    Pipsissewa, 119
    Pleurisy root, 123
    Poke root, 127
    Red root, 141
Lymphatic Herbs (Tip), 142

M

Mad dog skullcap, 155
Madder family, 111
Maianthemum racemosa, 159
Making Tea with Aromatic Herbs (Tip), 32
Mange (in dogs), 128
Marc, about, 18
Mastitis, 128
Maypop, 115
Meadow rue, 51
Measles
    Bee balm, 31
    Sassafras, 149
    Spicebush, 163
Menopause, general
    Black cohosh, 35
    Blue cohosh, 51
Menses, delayed
    Black cohosh, 35
    Blue cohosh, 51
    Mountain mint, 107
    Partridgeberry, 111
    Skullcap, 155
    Spicebush, 163
    Wild ginger, 199
Menses, excessive
    Black haw, 39
    Partridgeberry, 111
    Sweetgum, 179
    Wild geranium, 195
    Witch hazel, 211
Menses, irregular
    Partridgeberry, 111
Menstrual pain and cramps
    Bee balm, 31
    Black cohosh, 36
    Black haw, 39
    Blue cohosh, 51
    Skullcap, 155
Menstruums, about, 18
Menstruum charts, 21, 22
Mentha spp., 108
Middle Eastern cooking, sumac berries, 172
Migraines, see headache
Milk tea, 181, 197
Milkweed family, 123
Mint family, 31, 107, 155, 167
Miscarriage threatened

    Black haw, 39
    Blue cohosh, 51
    Partridgeberry, 112
    Wild yam, 207
Mitchella repens (Partridgeberry), 111 – 113
Monarch butterflies, 123
Monarda spp. (Bee balm), 31 – 33
Morning sickness, 207
Mountain mint (*Pycnanthemum incanum*), 32, 58, 59, 77, 107 – 109, 156
Mouth sores, see canker sores
Mullein, 4, 49, 56, 58, 59, 105, 120, 147, 191, 192
Muscle cramps, see cramps, antispasmodic
Myricaceae, 175

N

Nausea, see carminative
Nervine relaxants, see sedative
    Bee balm, 31
    Black cohosh, 35
    Elder, 65
    Evening primrose, 71
    Passionflower, 115
    Skullcap, 155
    Wild cherry, 189
Nervousness, see anxiety, nervine relaxants
New Jersey tea, 141

O

Oenothera spp. (Evening primrose), 71 – 73
Official part, definition, 10
Oils, see herbal oils infused
Old man's beard, 75
Oleaceae, 75
Olive family, 75
Omega-6 fatty acids, 72
Oxytocic, 51

P

Pale touch-me-not, 93
Panax spp. (Ginseng), 83
Papaveraceae, 47
Partridgeberry (*Mitchella repens*), 111 – 113
Partus preparator, 51, see labor aids
Passiflora incarnata (Passionflower), 115 – 117

Passiflora lutea, 120
Passionflower (*Passiflora incarnata*), 115 – 117
Passionflower, yellow, 115
Pedicularis canadensis (Wood betony), 215 – 217
Pelvic congestion, 76
Pemmican, 189
Penis wash, 107
Peppermint, 108
Pertussis (whooping cough), see cough, 37, 141
Phytolacca americana (Poke root), 127 – 131
Pipsissewa (*Chimaphila maculata*), 119 – 121, 185
Phytolaccaceae, 127
Plantago major, 49
Plantain, 49
Plaque, dental, 48
Pleurisy root (*Asclepias tuberosa*), 123 – 125
Pleurisy, 124
Pre-menstrual Syndrome (PMS)
    Black cohosh, 35
    Black haw, 39
    Blue cohosh, 51
    Partridgeberry, 111
    Passionflower, 115
    Skullcap, 155
    Wild yam, 207
Pneumonia, see cough, lung congestion
Poison ivy rash
    Jewelweed, 93
    Sarsaparilla, 145
    Sweetfern, 175
Poison sumac, 171
Poke root (*Phytolacca americana*), 127 – 131
Poke sallet, 131
Polycystic ovaries (PCOS), 52
Polygonatum biflorum (Solomon's seal), 159 – 161
Polygonatum multiflorum, 159
Polygonatum pubescens, 159
Poppy family, 47
Porcher, Dr. Frances P., 101, 127, 150, 164
Possum haw, 39
Postpartum bleeding, 40
Poultices, about, 31
    Evening primrose, 71
    Goldenrod, 89
    Jewelweed, 93
    Mountain mint, 107

Pregnancy, see labor tonics, miscarriage (threatened), morning sickness
Prickly ash, 62
The Problem with Common Names (Tip), 146
Prostatitis
    Joe Pye weed, 97
    Pipsissewa, 119
    Red root, 141
    Stoneroot, 167
    Wild hydrangea, 203
Prunus serotina (Wild cherry), 147, 183, 189 – 191
Prunus virginiana, 189
Psoriasis
    Evening primrose, 71
    Red root, 141
Puccoon, 47
Puke weed, 101
Pulmonary edema, 127
Purgative, 43
Purple boneset, 97
Pycnanthemum spp. (Mountain mint), 107 – 109

Q

Queen of the meadow, 97

R

Rabbit tobacco *(Gnaphalium obtusifolium)*, 48, 56, 59, 133 – 135, 147, 192
Ragweed *(Ambrosia artemesiifolia)*, 137 – 139
Ragweed, Greater, 137
Ragweed, Lanceleaf, 137
Ragweed Loves Goldenrod (Tip), 139
Ranunculaceae, 35, 219
Rash, see skin rash
Rat's bane/vein, 119
Rattlewort, 35
Red clover, 128
Red elder, 68
Red pucoon, 47
Red root *(Ceanothus americanus)*, 128, 141 – 143
Redneck goldenseal, 219
Redshank, 141
Respiratory infection, see bronchitis, congestion (respiratory), coughs, fever
Rhamnaceae, 141

Rheumatism, see analgesic, anti-inflammatory, anti-spasmodic
    Bee balm, 32
    Black cohosh, 35
    Black haw, 43
    Blue cohosh, 51
    Boneset, 55
    Devil's walking stick, 61
    Ginseng, 83
    Joe Pye weed, 97
    Partridgeberry, 111
    Pipsissewa, 119
    Poke root, 127
    Sassafras, 149
    Stoneroot, 167
    Wild hydrangea, 203
    Wild yam, 207
    Wood betony, 215
Rheumatism root, 207
Rhinitis (runny nose)
    Elder, 65
    Goldenrod, 89
    Ragweed, 137
Rhus spp. (Sumac), 59, 171 – 173, 192
Rich weed, 167
Ringworm, 44, 119
Root beer, herbs used in, 120, 146, 150
Rosaceae, 189
Rose family, 189
Rubiaceae, 111
Runny nose, see rhinitis

S

Safrole, 151
Sage *(Salvia officinalis)*, 192
Salve, about, 27
Sambucus spp. (Elder), 10, 56, 58, 65 – 69, 97, 192
Sang, 83
Sanguinaria canadensis (Bloodroot), 3, 47 – 49, 83, 160, 192
Sarsaparilla *(Aralia nudicaulis)*, 145 – 147
Sassafras *(Sassafras albidum)*, 138 – 141
Sassafras albidum, 138 – 141
Saxifragaceae, 203
Saxifrage family, 203
Scabies, 44

Sciatica
- Black haw, 39
- Skullcap, 155

Scutellaria spp. (Skullcap), 18, 73, 155 – 157

Sedative
- Bee balm, 31
- Black cohosh, 35
- Goldenrod, 89
- Passionflower, 115
- Rabbit tobacco, 133
- Skullcap, 155
- Solomon's seal, 159
- Sweetgum, 179
- Wild cherry, 189

Sevenbark, 203

Shoemac, 172

Sinusitis
- Elder, 65
- Goldenrod, 89
- Ragweed, 137

Skin infections, sores, wounds
- Black walnut, 43
- Elder, 65
- Evening primrose, 71
- Fringetree, 75
- Goldenrod, 89
- Partridgeberry, 111
- Passionflower, 115
- Sarsaparilla, 145
- Sumac, 171
- Sweetgum, 179
- Wild geranium, 195
- Witch hazel, 211
- Yellowroot, 219

Skin, rashes
- Evening primrose, 71
- Fringetree, 75
- Jewelweed, 93
- Rabbit tobacco, 133
- Ragweed, 137
- Sassafras, 149
- Sumac, 171
- Sweetfern, 175
- Sweetgum, 179
- Wild cherry, 189
- Wild hydrangea, 203

- Witch hazel, 211
- Yellowroot, 219

Skin, ulcers
- Bloodroot, 47
- Pipsissewa, 119

Skullcap *(Scutellaria spp.)*, 18, 73, 155 – 157

Smilacina racemosa, see *Maianthemum racemosa*

Smilax spp., 145

Smoking, Smoky Mountain Smokes recipe, 134
- Lobelia, 101
- Rabbit tobacco, 133
- Sumac, 171

Snakehead, 185

Snowball plant, 39

Snuff, 48, 200

Solidago spp. (Goldenrod), 7, 8, 79, 89 – 91, 138, 139

Solomon's plume, 159

Solomon's seal *(Polygonatum biflorum)*, 159 -161

Sore throat
- Bee balm, 32
- Elder, 65
- Evening primrose, 71
- Goldenrod, 89
- Poke root, 127
- Rabbit tobacco, 133
- Ragweed, 137
- Red root, 141
- toneroot, 167
- Sumac, 171
- Sweetfern, 175
- Sweetgum, 179
- Wild cherry, 189
- Wild geranium, 195
- Witch hazel, 211
- Wood betony, 215

Southern prickly ash, 61

Spasms and tics
- Bee balm, 31
- Black haw, 39
- Blue cohosh, 51
- Lobelia, 101
- Passionflower, 115
- Skullcap, 156
- Wild yam, 207
- Wood betony, 215

Spearmint, 108

Spicebush *(Lindera benzoin)*, 163 – 165, 192
Spicewood, 163
Spikenard, 145
Spotted Joe Pye weed, 97
Spotted pipsissewa, 119
Spotted touch-me-not, 93
Spp., definition of, 7
Squawvine, 111
Stachys officinalis, 215
Staghorn sumac, 171
Stansbury, Jill, 103
Staying Juicy (Tip), 161
Sties, 219
Stiff gentian, 79
Stomach ache, see carminatives, indigestion
Stoneroot *(Collinsonia canadensis)*, 167 – 169
Stork's bill, 195
Striped gentian, 79
Styptic, see hemorrhage
    Sumac, 171
    Wild Geranium, 195
Sumac *(Rhus glabra)*, 59, 171 – 173, 192
Sumac Berry Lemonade recipe, 173
Sumac, poison, 171
Sunburn, see burns
Sundrops, 71
Sweet everlasting, 133
Sweet goldenrod, 89
Sweet Joe Pye weed, 97
Sweetfern *(Comptonia peregrina)*, 175 – 177
Sweetgum *(Liquidambar styraciflua)*, 130, 174, 179 – 181
Swollen glands, 142, see lymphatics
    Elder, 65
    Red root, 141
Syrup, about, 22
    Boneset Syrup recipe, 59
    Elder (berry) Syrup recipe, 69
    Evening primrose, 71

T

Teething pain, 62, 145
Thalictrum spp., 51
Thomson, Samuel, 102
Thoreau, Henry David, 8
Throat irritation, see sore throat

Thrush
    Red root, 141
    Wild geranium, 195
    Yellowroot, 219
Thyme, 192
Tiarella cordifolia, 195
Tincture (alcohol extract) about, 18 – 19
    folk method, 20 – 21
    weight-to-volume method, 21 – 22
    weight-to-volume method chart, 21
Tips
    Engaging with Aromas, 176
    How to Harvest Bark Sustainably, 183
    Lymphatic Herbs, 142
    Making Tea with Aromatic Herbs, 32
    The Problem with Common Names, 146
    Ragweed Loves Goldenrod, 139
    Staying Juicy, 161
Tonic herbs, 10
    Blue cohosh, 51
    Boneset, 55
    Fringetree, 75
    Gentian, 79
    Ginseng, 83
    Joe Pye weed, 97
    Partridgeberry, 111
    Pipsissewa, 119
    Sarsaparilla, 145
    Sassafras, 149
    Skullcap, 155
    Solomon's seal, 159
    Spicebush, 163
    Stoneroot, 167
    Turtlehead, 185
    Wild cherry, 189
    Wild hydrangea, 203
    Yellowroot, 219
Toothache
    Devil's walking stick, 61
    Red root, 141
    Yellowroot, 219
Toothache tree, 61
Touch-me-not family, 93
Touch-me-not, 93
Trifolium pratense, 128
True Solomon's seal *(Polygonatum biflorum)*, 159 – 161

Tumors, 23
    Bloodroot, 47
    Poke root, 127
    Turtlehead, 185
Turtlebloom, 185
Turtlehead *(Chelone spp.)*, 185 – 187
Tussilago farfara, 192

U

United Plant Savers, about, 7
Urethritis, 124
Urinary tract infection
    Evening primrose, 71
    Goldenrod, 89
    Joe Pye weed, 97
    Pipsissewa, 119
    Wild hydrangea, 203
Uterine pain, 36
Uterine tonic
    Blue cohosh, 51
    Partridgeberry, 111

V

Vaginal discharge/infection, see vaginitis
Vaginal douche, about, 25
    Pipsissewa, 119
    Red root, 141
    Sumac, 171
    Sweetfern, 175
    Wild geranium, 195
    Yellowroot, 219
Vaginitis
    Black walnut, 39
    Partridgeberry, 111
    Pipsissewa, 119
    Red root, 141
    Sweetfern, 175
    Wild geranium, 195
    Yellowroot, 219
Varicose veins, 212
Vascular tonic, 167
Verbascum thapsus, 4, 49, 56, 58, 59, 105, 120, 147, 191, 192
Vermifuge, 43

Viburnum spp. (Black haw), 39 – 41, 105
Vomiting, see anti-emetic, nausea
Vulnerary
    Elder, 65
    Goldenrod, 90
    Pipsissewa, 119

W

Walnut family, 43
Walnut, American, 43
Warts, 54
Wax Myrtle family, 175
Weight-to-volume method
    Infusions and decoctions, 15 – 18
    Tinctures, 20 – 22
    Weight-to-volume chart, 21
White ash, 75
White baneberry, 35
Whooping cough (pertussis), see coughs
Wild allspice, 163
Wild basil, 107
Wild Cherry Brandy recipe, 193
Wild Cherry Cough Syrup recipe, 192
Wild cherry *(Prunus serotina)*, 48, 147, 183, 189 – 193
Wild foods
    Evening primrose, 71
    Passionflower, 115
    Poke root, 127
    Sassafras, 149
    Solomon's seal, 159
    Spicebush, 163
    Sumac, 171
Wild geranium *(Geranium maculatum)*, 195 – 197
Wild ginger *(Asarum canadense)*, 48, 199 – 201
Wild ginger *(Hexastylis spp.)*, 199 – 201
Wild hydrangea *(Hydrangea arborescens)*, 203 – 205
Wild sarsaparilla *(Aralia nudicaulis)*, 145 – 147
Wild Wormwood, 137
Wild yam *(Dioscorea spp.)*, 76, 207 – 209
Winged sumac, 171
Witch hazel *(Hamamelis virginiana)*, 211 – 213
Witch hazel family, 211
Wood betony *(Pedicularis canadensis)*, 215 – 217
Worms and parasites (intestinal), 44, 149
Woundwort, 89

X

Xanthorhiza simplicissima (Yellowroot), 219 – 221

Y

Yam family, 207
Yeast infection, see fungal infection, vaginitis
Yellow jewelweed, 93
Yellow passionflower, 115
Yellowroot *(Xanthorhiza simplicissima)*, 219 – 221

Z

Zanthoxylum clava-herculis, 61
Zingiber officinale, 200

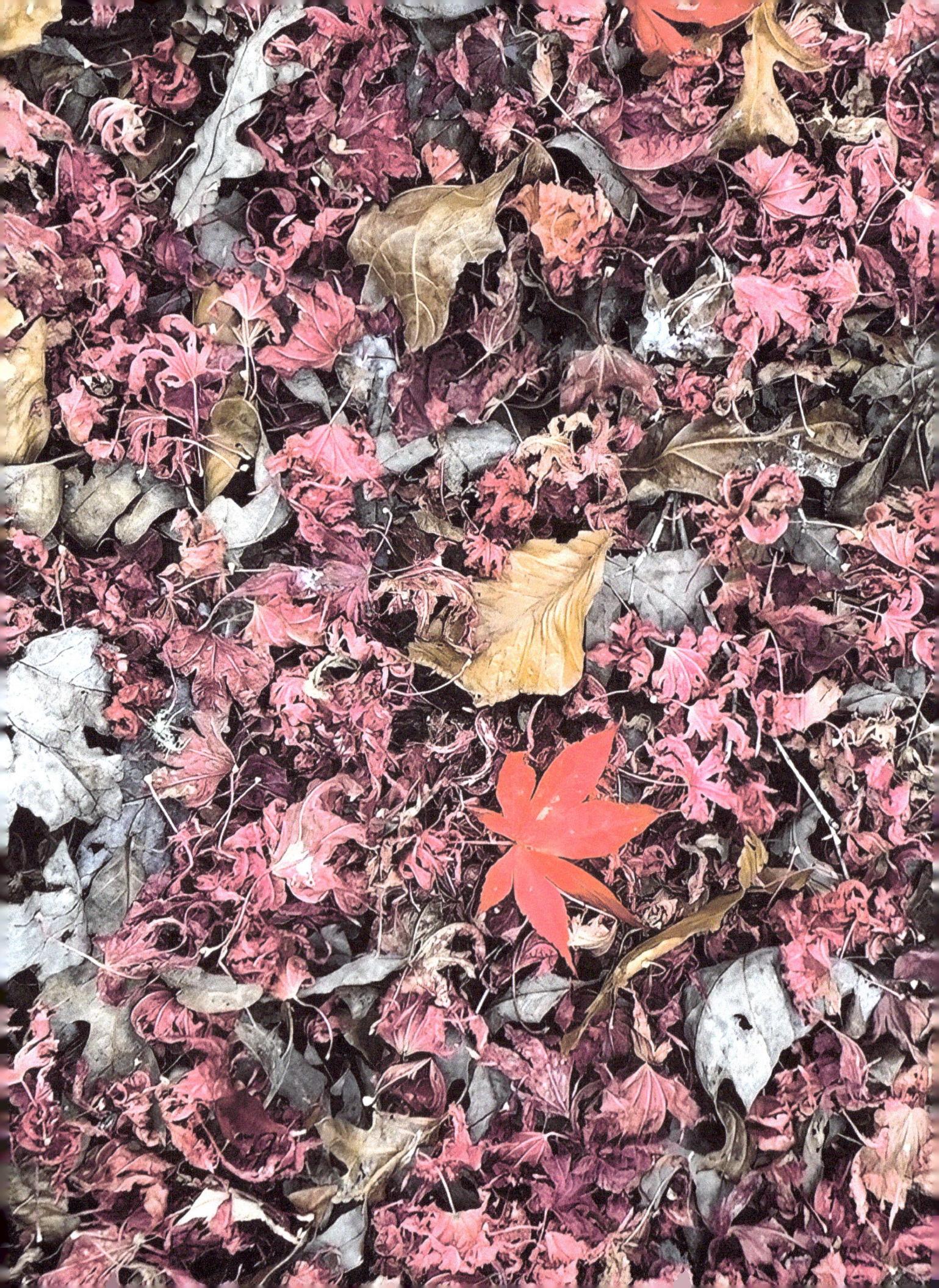

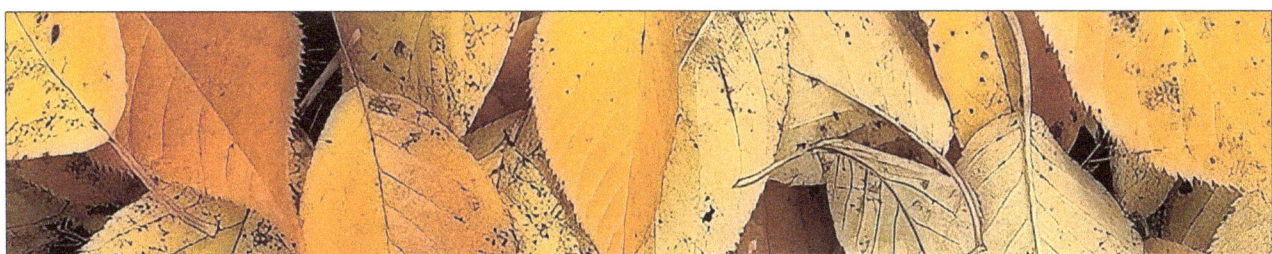

Acknowledgement

My friend Linda Anderson, an Appalachian folk artist, played a pivotal role in the birth of this book. Her unique blend of courage, artistic vision, and dedication to preserving family traditions through the rhythm of the seasons profoundly inspired me to write this book.

The information that graces these pages is a testament to the collective wisdom shared by my students at the BotanoLogos School of Herbal Studies and my clients over thirty years of clinical practice. Their contributions, along with the encouragement and inspiration from my herbal colleagues, family and friends, have been invaluable. I extend heartfelt thanks to Cassandra Alexander, Craig Burkhalter, Mary Ann Butler, Bob and Lydia Dalton, Jen Lynch Fitzgerald, Pam Gould, Jennafer Kummer, Rae Kyritsi, Cara-Lee Langston, Kat Maier, Helen Meadors, Althea Northage-Orr, Lorna Mauney-Brodek, Ronda Reynolds, Teresa Sena, Christa Sinadinos, Jen Stovall, and Leslie Williams. I am also profoundly grateful to Deb Goatcher, BotanoLogos' office manager, for her unwavering support and spectacular organizational skills.

The magic emanating from every page of this book is due to the incredible skill, creativity and endless patience of my book designer, Barbara Lande. Her artistic vision and attention to detail brought the text and images to life. It was a pleasure having her as my partner in creating this edition! Thanks to everyone who contributed their photos, especially Karen Lawrence.

My friend and colleague Leslie Williams graciously edited the manuscript using her considerable skills as an editor and herbalist. I am grateful for her support and encouragement over our many years of friendship. Any errors in the final version are solely mine.

Finally, I must acknowledge each of the plants in this book. They have been my companions in healing, my teachers in herbal medicine, and my inspiration, shaping my life and work; I am deeply grateful for their many blessings.

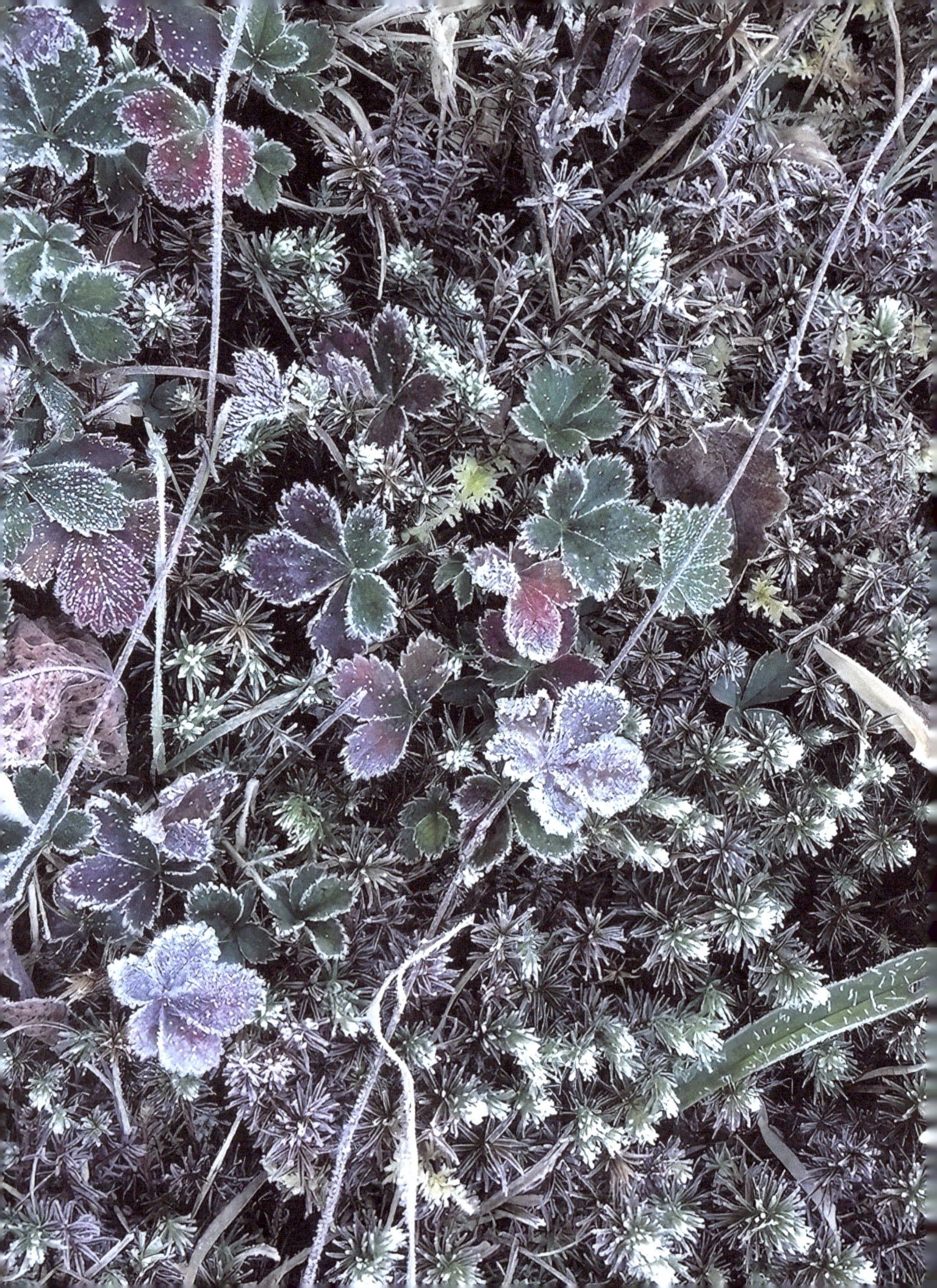

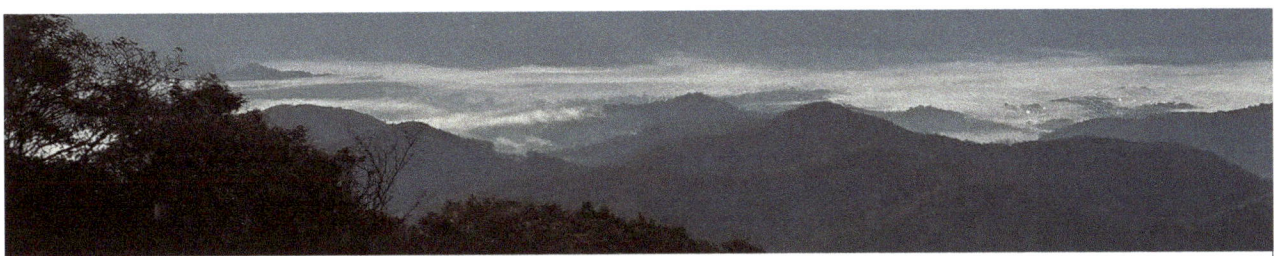

Photo Credits

Thank you to all my colleagues and friends who generously shared their fantastic photographs!

7Song—127, 143, 144, 145, 146, 182

Caleb Arnold—163, 165(2)

Steven J. Baskauf—(Wikimedia Commons) "*Lobelia inflata* fruit," 103

Rebecca Beyer—162, 164(2)

Craig Burkhalter—82, 83, 85

Roy Cohutta—(CC 2.0) "Monarch on *Asclepias tuberosa*," 124

Steven Foster—Cover, Title Page, 31(1), 33, 101(1), 102, 220(1)

Mary Clare Glabowicz—Author photo, 269

Michael Gras—(CC 2.0) "*Passiflora incarnata*," 117

Griffinsbray—(CC 1.0) "Butterfly Milkweed *(Asclepias tuberosa)*," 124

Patricia Kyritsi Howell—Table of Contents, 1, 3, 4, 6, 7, 10, 11, 14, 18, 23, 27, 28-29, 30, 31(2), 35(2), 41, 44, 45, 47, 51 (1, 2), 52, 53, 55(2), 56, 57, 60, 71, 73, 74, 74, 75(2), 77, 93,(1, 2, 3), 97(1), 101(2), 108, 111(1), 112, 118, 120, 134, 140, 142(2), 152, 156, 166, 167(2), 186, 201, 204, 206, 208, 211(1), 213, 216, 218, 219(1, 2), 220(2), 221, 222-223, 228, 229, 236, 246, 247, 264, 265, 266, 267, 268

Karen Lawrence—46, 55(1), 62, 64, 65, 70, 76, 79(2), 84, 88, 94, 95, 96, 98, 107(2), 115(1), 119(1), 123, 140, 141(1), 174, 187, 185, 194, 195, 197, 199(1, 2), 200, 202, 211

Andrea Koutros Lay—160

Peter McIntosh—"Devil's Branch," Preface to Second Edition, "Tennessee Rock Trail Overlook," 270

RockerBoo—(CC 2.0) "4123 Bumble Bees on Mountain Mint," 103

Martin Wall—49

Charlie Watts—17, 26

Eric Yarnell—147(2)

Vojtech Zavadil—(CC 3.0) "Viburnum berries and leaf," 40

H. Zell—(CC 3.0) "*Lobelia inflata* 0020," 103, "*Passiflora incarnata* 004," 116

All other photographs are from online stock sources.

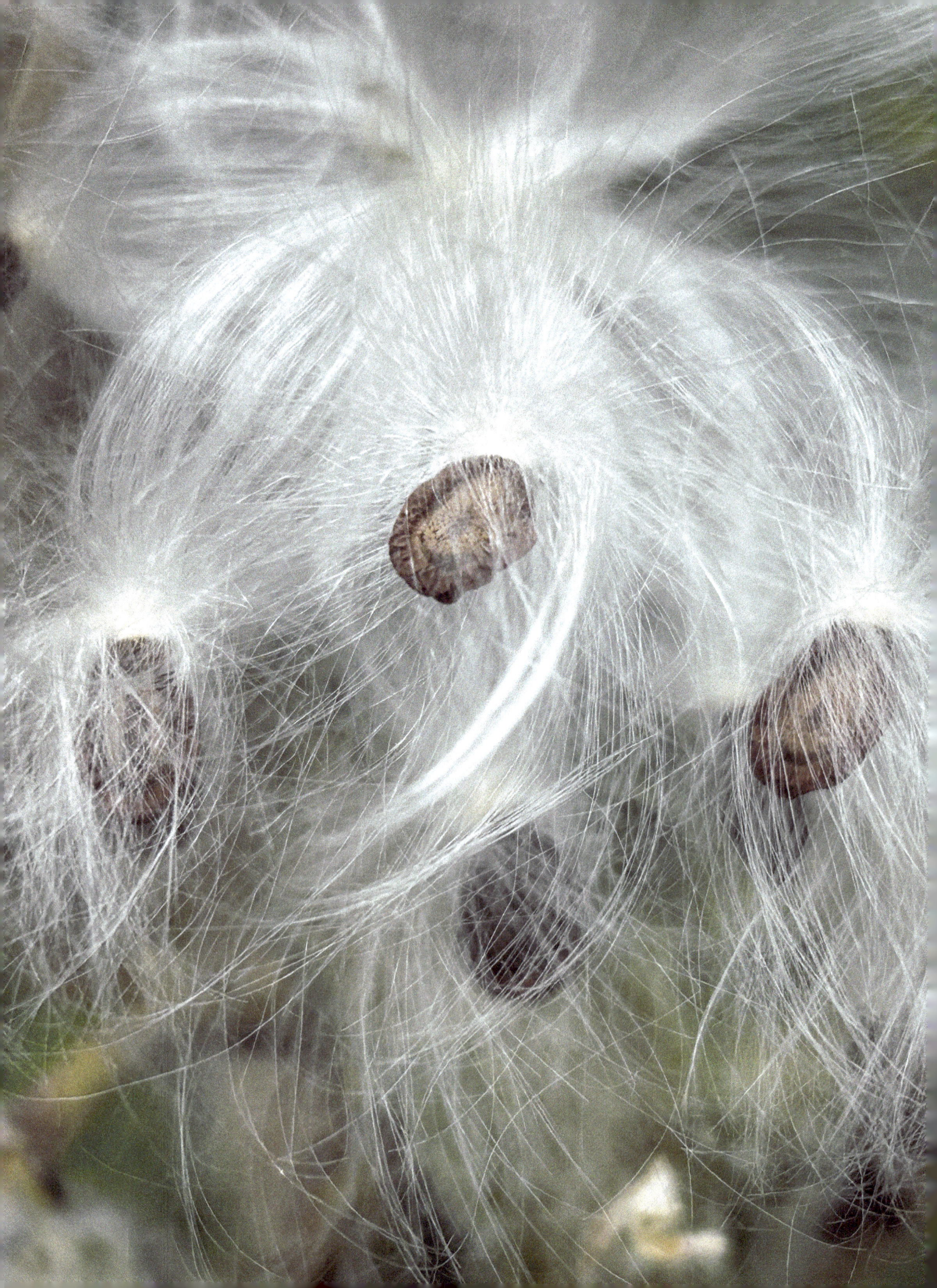

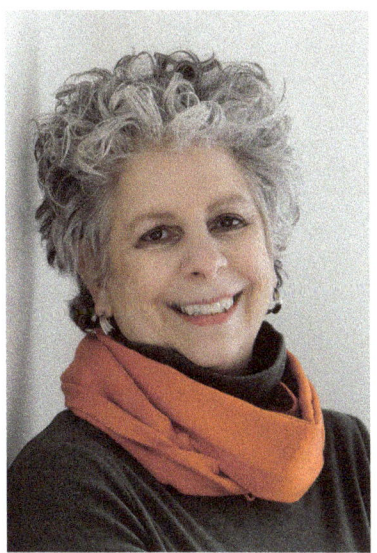

About the Author

Patricia Kyritsi Howell is a renowned herbalist, educator, and author with a deep connection to the medicinal plants of the Southern Appalachian Mountains. Early in her herbal career, Patricia moved her life and practice to North Georgia to surround herself with the centuries-old knowledge of Southern Appalachian plants. She has built her practice around her dedication to preserving and sharing Appalachia's rich herbal traditions. Patricia is known for blending traditional and modern practices while promoting the sustainable use of regional herbs.

Patricia is the founder and director of the BotanoLogos School of Herbal Studies. Over the past three decades, she has imparted her extensive knowledge of herbal medicine to many students, serving as a mentor and leader in the exploration of the medicinal plants of the Southern Appalachians.

Inspired by her Greek heritage, Patricia owns and operates Wild Crete Travel, a small travel company that offers trips to Greece to study Mediterranean herbs and enjoy traditional Cretan cuisine. Whether in the Appalachian Mountains or the rugged landscapes of Crete, Patricia aspires to empower others to embrace herbs as an essential part of healthcare.

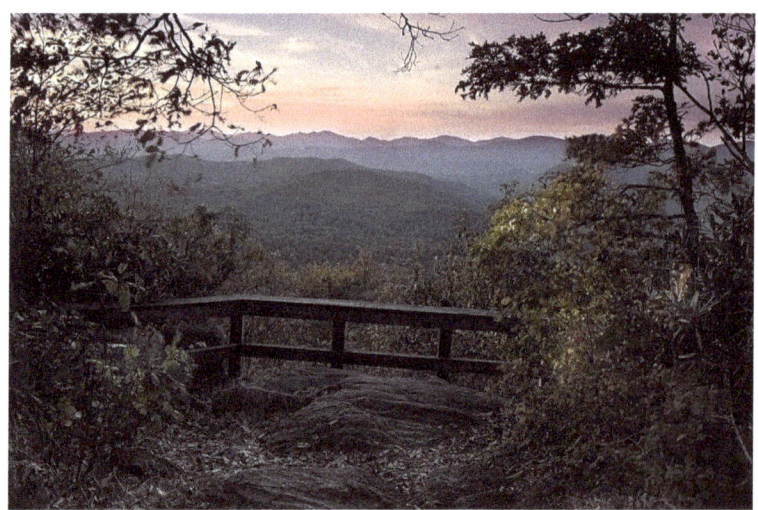

Thank You for Supporting a Self-Published Author!

As a self-published author, I pour my passion, effort, and resources into every step of the process — writing, editing, marketing, and distribution — without the backing of a big publishing house. It's a labor of love and a challenge, so reader support is essential.

I chose self-publishing for the sake of creative freedom. Traditional publishers frequently shy away from unconventional or controversial topics, particularly those related to herbal health care. Your support helps spread valuable knowledge to a broader audience.

When you buy a book from an indie author like me, more of your money directly supports my work. Each purchase, review, social media post and recommendation increases visibility, allowing independent voices to be heard.

And I, like many independent authors, rely on the unwavering backing of the many independent booksellers who stock our books. Please support your local bookstore!

To purchase additional copies, visit wildhealingherbs.com or scan the QR code below. For bulk orders, wholesale pricing or international orders, send an email to info@wildhealingherbs.com.

www.ingramcontent.com/pod-product-compliance
Lightning Source LLC
Chambersburg PA
CBHW040003040426
42337CB00033B/5212